Human Tumour Drug Sensitivity Testing *In Vitro*

Human Tumour Drug Sensitivity Testing *In Vitro*

Techniques and Clinical Applications

Edited by

PHILIP P. DENDY
Department of Medical Physics,
Addenbrooke's Hospital,
Cambridge, UK

BRIDGET T. HILL
Laboratory of
Cellular Chemotherapy,
Imperial Cancer Research Fund,
London, UK

1983

ACADEMIC PRESS

A Subsidiary of Harcourt Brace Jovanovich, Publishers
London   New York
Paris   San Diego   San Francisco   São Paulo
Sydney   Tokyo   Toronto

ACADEMIC PRESS INC. (LONDON) LTD.
24–28 Oval Road
London NW1 7DX

U.S. Edition published by
ACADEMIC PRESS INC.
111 Fifth Avenue
New York, New York 10003

British Library Cataloguing in Publication Data

Human tumour drug sensitivity testing in vitro.
1.Tumors
I. Dendy, P.P.   II. Hill, Bridget T.
616.99′2′061   RC254.5
ISBN 0-12-209860-9
LCCCN 83-71351

Printed in Great Britain at the Alden Press, Oxford

Contributors

G. M. Clark Department of Medicine, Division of Oncology, The University of Texas, Health Science Center at San Antonio, 7703 Floyd Curl Drive, San Antonio, Texas 78284, USA

D. Courtenay Institute for Cancer Research, Royal Marsden Hospital, South Downs Road, Sutton, Surrey SM2 5PX, UK

M. G. Daidone Oncologia Sperimentale C, Istituto Nazionale per lo Studio e la Cura dei Tumori, Via Venezian 1, 20133 Milan, Italy

J. L. Darling Gough-Cooper Department of Neurological Surgery, Institute of Neurology, The National Hospital, Queen Square, London WC1E 3BG, UK

P. P. Dendy Department of Medical Physics, The Radiotherapeutic Centre, Addenbrooke's Hospital, Hills Road, Cambridge CB2 2QQ, UK

W. J. Durkin Feigenbaum Smith Ruben & Durkin MDPA, 570 Memorial Circle, Ormond Beach, Florida 32074, USA

M. J. Embleton Cancer Research Campaign Laboratories, University of Nottingham, University Park, Nottingham NG7 2RD, UK

L. M. Franks Cellular Pathology Laboratory, Imperial Cancer Research Fund, P.O. Box 123, Lincoln's Inn Fields, London WC2A 3PX, UK

R. I. Freshney Department of Oncology, University of Glasgow, 1 Horselethill Road, Glasgow G12 9LY, UK

V. K. Ghanta Department of Microbiology, University of Alabama School of Medicine, University Station, Birmingham, Alabama 35294, USA

A. W. Hamburger Department of Cell Culture, American Type Culture Collection, 12301 Parklawn Drive, Rockville, Maryland 20852, USA

Bridget T. Hill Laboratory of Cellular Chemotherapy, Imperial Cancer Research Fund Laboratories, P.O. Box 123, Lincoln's Inn Fields, London WC2A 3PX, UK

R. N. Hiramoto Department of Microbiology, University of Alabama School of Medicine, University Station, Birmingham, Alabama 35294, USA

J. A. Houghton Division of Biochemical and Clinical Pharmacology, St. Jude Children's Research Hospital, 332 North Lauderdale Street, P.O. Box 318, Memphis, Tennessee 38101, USA

P. J. Houghton Division of Biochemical and Clinical Pharmacology, St. Jude Children's Research Hospital, 332 North Lauderdale Street, P.O. Box 318, Memphis, Tennessee 38101, USA

M. Kaufmann Institut für Experimentelle Pathologie, Deutsches Krebsforschungs-zentrum, Im Neuenheimer Feld 280, D-6900 Heidelberg 1, West Germany

C. L. Laboisse Laboratoire de Biologie et Physiologie des Cellules Digestives de Médicine Faculté Xavier Bichat, 16 rue H. Huchard, 75018 Paris, France

J. R. W. Masters Department of Pathology, St. Paul's Hospital, 24 Endell Street, London WC2H 9AE, UK

J. Mattern Institut für Experimentelle Pathologie, Deutsches Krebsforschungszen-trum, Im Neuenheimer Feld 280, D-6900 Heidelberg 1, West Germany

S. A. Metcalfe Department of Pathology, St. Paul's Hospital, 24 Endell Street, London WC2H 9AE, UK

T. Nederman Department of Physical Biology, Gustav Werners Institute, University of Uppsala, Box 531, S-751 21 Uppsala, Sweden

S. E. Salmon Department of Internal Medicine, Section of Hematology and Oncology, University of Arizona Health Services Center, Tucson, Arizona 85724, USA

O. Sanfilippo Oncologia Sperimentale C, Istituto Nazionale per lo Studio e la Cura dei Tumori, Via Venezian 1, 20133 Milan, Italy

R. Silvestrini Oncologia Sperimentale C, Istituto Nazionale per lo Studio e la Cura dei Tumori, Via Venezian 1, 20133 Milan, Italy

L. A. Smets Department of Experimental Cytology, Netherlands Cancer Institute, 121 Plesmanlaan, 1066 CX Amsterdam, The Netherlands

D. G. T. Thomas Gough-Cooper Department of Neurological Surgery, Institute of Neurology, The National Hospital, Queen Square, London WC1E 3BG, UK

K. M. Tveit Department of Biochemistry, Norsk Hydro Institute for Cancer Research, The Norwegian Radium Hospital, Montebello, Oslo 3, Norway

M. Volm Institut für Experimentelle Pathologie, Deutsches Krebsforschungszen-trum, Im Neuenheimer Feld 280, D-6900 Heidelberg 1, West Germany

D. D. Von Hoff Department of Medicine, Division of Oncology, The University of Texas, Health Science Center at San Antonio, 7703 Floyd Curl Drive, San Antonio, Texas 78284, USA

Foreword

Having had experience of culture studies with human tumours since early days, it is a pleasure for me to be asked to write a preface to this book. I can remember the time when tissue culture resembled somewhat the activities of a club in which white-coated operators carried out mysterious activities behind the closed doors of the sterile room. This was before antibiotics came into general use to hide our mistakes. In those days it was a major achievement to devise a culture medium in which cells could be grown successfully, particularly as cell lines maintained by sub-culture for many years. Those outside the field could not see the relevance of this work either to general biology or to the cancer problem.

However, without this painstaking work by pioneers in tissue culture, the important developments in culture work, which have a direct bearing on the treatment of cancer patients, as described in this book, could not have taken place. It has become evident, both from culture work and from experience in the clinic, that cancers which, according to histological characteristics, are identical, nevertheless are highly individualistic in their sensitivity to drugs; the biochemical or structural factors responsible for these differences are at present largely unknown. In practice, this means that a rapid predictive test on which the clinician could rely would be of immense value for cancer chemotherapy. Culture methods are the only techniques that can provide information within the time that a clinician is prepared to wait before starting treatment.

It is most encouraging to read in this book how a number of clinicians are now working closely with the tissue culture experts. For short-term information and treatment the soft agar method has given strikingly good correlations with clinical results. But the method selects out a small fraction of the tumour population, possibly the fastest growing fraction. It may be necessary, eventually, to develop two types of test, a rapid test and a more detailed examination of the whole spectrum of response of the mixed cell population, possibly using labelling methods and xenografts so that further treatment can be given to avoid reoccurrence of tumour growth.

There is every reason to believe that, as the result of the dedicated work of biologists, predictive tests will become a standard hospital facility. I think that Dr Hill and Dr Dendy have made a timely presentation of work in this field.

May 1983   E. J. AMBROSE
                                                                               East Sussex

Contents

Part III
Laboratory Predictions and Clinical Correlations

1. Introduction

P. P. DENDY and B. T. HILL

It has been recognized for many years that the experimental systems most extensively used to study carcinogenesis, notably continuous cell lines and tumours propagated in animals, have severe limitations as models for human cancers. In particular they fail to take into consideration the marked differences both in the appearance, in terms of histology, vascularity, and stromal involvement, and in the behaviour of tumours in individual patients.

With the advent of cancer chemotherapy it soon became clear that another source of variation was in the response of tumours to anticancer drugs. Furthermore it was apparent that the drug sensitivity of a tumour could not be predicted entirely either from clinical symptoms or from histological examination. Thus a number of groups began to investigate the possibility of using the patient's own tumour material for *in vitro* experiments to predict drug sensitivity (Wright *et al.*, 1957; Di Paolo and Dowd, 1961).

In 1964 Limburg and Krahe reported substantial improvement in the median survival time of patients with advanced ovarian carcinomas if treatment was based on the results of an *in vitro* predictive test. Since median survival time is very susceptible to the presence of one or two very long surviving patients in the group, the improvement achieved with the methods available at that time was probably rather less than the authors suggested. Nevertheless this work gave considerable impetus to the subject and over the next decade a number of short-term culture systems were developed. Disaggregated biopsies containing either single cells or small clumps of cells, tissue explants, or tumour slices were used to establish suspension, monolayer or organ cultures.

Most groups reported evidence of variations in chemosensitivity, and in 1970 Tanneberger and Bacigalupo introduced the term onkobiogramm to describe the characteristic and unique response of tumour cells from one patient to a spectrum of cytotoxic drugs.

In late 1974 a meeting was held in Cambridge (Dendy, 1976) to review this

1

rapidly developing subject of human tumours in short-term culture. The purpose of the meeting was threefold: to report what was already known; to identify technical difficulties limiting progress at that time; to discuss some of the clinical problems that these model systems might help to solve.

It was already clear that a major potential application was the development of predictive assays to characterize the drug sensitivity spectrum of individual tumours. However, a number of outstanding problems were recognized, including:

(i) Can adequate numbers of representative cultures be prepared?
(ii) How should the malignant origin of the cultured cells be confirmed?
(iii) Are the properties of cells in culture a true reflection of their properties *in vivo*?
(iv) Is there sufficient knowledge of the biochemical actions of these drugs for *in vitro* observations to be correctly interpreted?
(v) Is the response spectrum to a given series of drugs always different for cells from specific tumour types?
(vi) Can suitable quantitative assay techniques be developed for the *in vitro* work?
(vii) Is it feasible to make a correct evaluation of the predictive approach in terms of clinically assessed patients' responses, and is the level of collaboration between clinicians and scientists adequate?

Many early publications made little reference to the identity of the cells established in culture, but since 1974 there has been a much greater awareness that such studies must be carried out in parallel with the main experiments. In the first section of this book the various morphological, physical, biochemical, and immunological methods currently available for identification of human tumour cells are presented, and their suitability for recognizing such cells quickly and easily in short-term culture is considered.

A major limitation in 1974 was the lack of a clonogenic assay for freshly cultured human tumour cells. Attempts to extend the pioneering work of Puck and Marcus who cloned HeLa cells as early as 1955 had been unsuccessful. A break-through came in the 1970s with the development of a method that permitted mouse myeloma cells to be cloned *in vitro* (Park *et al.*, 1971) and the subsequent publication by Courtenay (1976) of details of a soft agar assay for solid tumours taken directly from the mouse. The first reported extension of these methods to human tumours was by Hamburger and Salmon (1977) who successfully grew tumour colonies from various human neoplasms including multiple myeloma, non-Hodgkin's lymphoma, ovarian adenocarcinoma, melanoma, and neuroblastoma. Subsequent progress has been extremely rapid and successful colony formation has been reported for many different human carcinomas and sarcomas. The cloning efficiency is, however, invariably low with sometimes as few as 10 tumour colonies per 500 000 cells plated. For this and other reasons many groups have continued to work with alternative assay methods.

Culture *in vitro* is still unsuccessful with many specimens. Furthermore some researchers consider that growth *in vitro* is too far removed from reality. Therefore other systems have been developed, for example growth in diffusion chambers (Heckmann, 1967; Smith *et al.*, 1976) or as xenografts in immune-deprived mice (Houghton *et al.*, 1977; Bateman *et al.*, 1979). These approaches are most likely to remain research investigations because if a predictive test is to be widely accepted as a routine procedure it must be quick, technically simple, and inexpensive, criteria met realistically only by *in vitro* methods. Nevertheless the major methodological approaches that have been attempted are all considered in the second section of this book, with critical comment on their strengths and weaknesses.

In recent years our understanding of the relevance of certain aspects of cell cycle kinetics to cancer chemotherapy has been greatly extended (see e.g. Hill, 1978) and, as discussed in Chapter 17, we are now much more aware of the need to study the pharmacological behaviour of commonly employed antitumour drugs. Since it is unreasonable to suppose that the *in vitro* drug concentration, expressed as a function of time, will imitate *in vivo* behaviour, deductions must be based on differences in relative sensitivity between different tumour specimens treated with the same drug under standard conditions. Nevertheless it is reasonable to select a range of doses for testing *in vitro* on the basis of the dosage that can be achieved pharmacologically.

Clinical investigators will have a particular interest in the final section of this book which concentrates on correlations of laboratory predictions with clinical response to treatment. It is encouraging to report clear evidence of increasing cooperation between clinicians and scientists, and an increasing tendency, within the requirements imposed by the needs of individual patients, to adopt a more uniform approach to testing and evaluating chemotherapy regimens. This greater degree of standardization is essential if valid deductions are to be made from the data. However, the breadth of contributions in this section reflects once again the current broad spectrum of opinion over the best approach to this problem of predictive drug sensitivity testing.

Throughout this book contributors have adopted a critical approach and, as a result, the reader may find conflicting views expressed. We make no apology for this. Indeed we hope it will help to emphasize that the present position is fluid and many problems remain to be resolved.

References

Bateman, A. E., Peckham, M. J. and Steel, G. G. (1979). Assays of drug sensitivity for cells from human tumours: *in vitro* and *in vivo* tests on a xenografted tumour. *Br. J. Cancer* **40**, 81–88.

Courtenay, V. D. (1976). A soft agar colony assay for Lewis lung tumour and B16 melanoma taken directly from the mouse. *Br. J. Cancer* **34**, 39–45.

Dendy, P. P. (ed.) (1976). *Human Tumours in Short Term Culture: Techniques and Clinical Applications.* Academic Press, London and New York.

Di Paolo, J. A. and Dowd, J. E. (1961). Evaluation of inhibition of human tumour tissue by cancer chemotherapeutic drugs with an *in vitro* test. *J. Nat. Cancer Inst.* **27**, 807–815.

Hamburger, A. W. and Salmon, S. E. (1977). Primary bioassay of human tumour stem cells. *Science* **197**, 461–463.

Heckmann, U. (1967). Neue Möglichkeiten einer Resistenzprüfung menschlicher Karzinomgewebe gegen Zytostatika im *in vivo* test. *Deutsch. Med. Wochenschr.* **92**, 932.

Hill, B. T. (1978). Cancer chemotherapy: the relevance of certain concepts of cell cycle kinetics. *Biochem. Biophys. Acta* **516**, 389–417.

Houghton, P. J., Houghton, J. A. and Taylor, D. M. (1977). Effects of cytotoxic agents on TdR incorporation and growth delay in human colonic tumour xenografts. *Br. J. Cancer* **36**, 206.

Limburg, H. and Krahe, M. (1964). Die Züchtung von menschlichem Krebsgewebe in der Gewebekultur und seine Sensibilitätstestung gegen neuere Zytostatika. *Deutsch. Med. Wochenschr.* **89**, 1938–1946.

Park, C. H., Bergasgel, D. E. and McCulloch, E. A. (1971). Mouse myeloma tumour stem cells: a primary cell culture assay. *J. Nat. Cancer Inst.* **46**, 411–422.

Puck, T. T. and Marcus, P. I. (1955). A rapid method of viable cell titration and clone production with HeLa cells in tissue culture: the use of X-irradiated cells to supply conditioning factors. *Proc. Nat. Acad. Sci.* **41**, 432–437.

Smith, I. E., Courtenay, V. D. and Gordon, M. Y. (1976). A colony-forming assay for human tumour xenografts using agar in diffusion chambers. *Br. J. Cancer* **34**, 476–483.

Tanneberger, S. and Bacigalupo G. (1970). Einige Erfahrungen mit der individuellen zytostatischen Behandlung maligner Tumoren nach prätherapeutischer Zytostatika Sensibilitätsprüfung *in vitro* (Onkobiogramm). *Arch. Geschwulstforsch.* **35**, 44–53.

Wright, J. C., Cobb, J. P., Gumport, S. L., Golomb, F. M. and Safodi, D. (1957). Investigation of the relation between clinical and tissue culture response to chemotherapeutic agents of human cancer. *New Engl. J. Med.* **257**, 1207–1211.

Part I
Tumour Cell Identification in Biopsy Specimens, in Mixed Culture and in Isolated Colonies

2. Morphological Criteria for Tumour Cell Identification

L. M. FRANKS

I. Introduction

There are no features that absolutely identify every tumour cell, and a few moments thought about the nature of the neoplastic process makes it plain that this objective is not likely to be achieved. Alterations in structure and in behaviour appear at a relatively late stage in this process. In an experimental situation, with a known carcinogen, the initiating event which follows the application of a carcinogen usually produces no change that can be identified as neoplastic, nor do such changes appear during the greater part of the long subsequent latent period, yet the treated cells have been altered and can be induced to form tumours by the application of promoting agents. Even after morphologically altered cells appear, there may be no direct relationship between the degree of structural alteration and the "malignancy" of the cells. Although well differentiated tumours usually are less "malignant" than more anaplastic tumours, this is not invariably the case. Some well differentiated "grade 1" tumours may metastasize while other apparently more "malignant" tumours may not. Over the years a pattern of tumour structure and behaviour has been established. To take a simple example, confident predictions can be made if a lump in the breast of a woman is found to have a specific microscopic structure, e.g. grade 1 adenocarcinoma. Experience has shown that 80% of women with this particular pattern will be alive 5 years later although 20% will be dead. The pattern and structure will not allow a distinction to be made between individuals in the two subgroups, i.e. morphology alone is not enough. Even this behaviour pattern is only identifiable in a group in which there is clinical evidence of tumour growth, i.e. a lump. In circumstances in which the morphological change is found by chance no prediction can be made. A classic example of this situation is found in the latent carcinomas that occur so frequently in the prostate (Franks, 1956). These lesions, although they have the morphological structure of tumours, are considered by some not to be true tumours since they do not appear to be growing. Hence there is the need for methods to measure growth (or growth potential). Logically tumours that are growing most actively in the host would be expected to grow most rapidly in tissue culture. Unfortunately this too is not the case, and again there seems to be no direct relationship between structure *in vivo* and growth rate *in vitro* or even the ability of tumour cells to grow at all *in vitro*. On the relatively small proportion of cells that will grow *in vitro* a number of behavioural tests can be applied. Results of some of these can be assessed by alterations in structure, and some may be correlated with "malignancy". Morphology alone can identify altered cells. Can functional morphology identify cells with increased or decreased growth potential or other characters associated with "malignancy"? There are many reviews on markers of neoplastic transformation (e.g. Cameron and Pool, 1981; Busch and Yeoman, 1982; Franks, 1979, 1982) but most of these markers have been established using mesenchymal cells transformed *in vitro*, whereas the common tumours are epithelial in origin. In most experiments changes in cells grown from normal tissues have been recorded after the application of a transforming agent. The well known appearance of "transformed foci" of irregular fusiform cells in a random criss-cross pattern was first described in experiments of this sort and is regarded as a reliable indicator of transformation. Unfortunately a careful study (Sanford *et al.*, 1974) showed that, although some treated cultures contained fusiform cells growing in a random criss-cross pattern, these cultures did not form tumours in untreated hosts. Most of the cell lines that developed from carcinogen-treated cultures and were tumour-producing showed neither a fusiform shape nor a criss-cross pattern. Others (e.g. Tomei and Bertram, 1978) have shown that this kind of transformed phenotype can be returned to normal (as can contact inhibition of growth) by growing the "transformed" cells in chemically defined medium, so that appearances in culture seem to reflect environmental conditions. Reversion to the transformed pattern could be obtained by adding 2% serum or 0.1% albumin to the medium in the log phase of growth or by exposure to trypsin for 30–60 s. Other markers for transformation, e.g. growth in agar, fibronectin production, cytoskeletal changes, etc., also show a dissociation between the presence or absence of the markers and malignancy, especially in epithelial systems (see, for example, Marshall *et al.*, 1977; Franks, 1982, for review). Some of these problems have also been discussed in detail (Franks, 1979). Here they will be considered in the specific context of identification of tumour cells. Most of the commonly used markers require mass populations of cells, so methods that can be applied to single cells would be invaluable.

II. Tumour cells *in vivo*

The morphology of tumour cells has been described and illustrated many times, and a more or less generally accepted description and nomenclature is given in standard text books of pathology and in particular the World Health Organization series on the Histological Typing of Tumours. Diagnosis of neoplasia is based on the degree of departure from the normal in either histology or cytology. Histological differentiation is concerned with alterations in tissue structure, i.e. the relationship of cells to each other and to their supporting stroma. Cytological changes are concerned with alterations in structure in individual cells. In brief, malignant tumours differ from benign tumours in that the degree of tissue disorganization is greater and there is no well defined tumour capsule. The cells are cytologically abnormal although in some well differentiated tumours abnormalities may not be easily detectable. Standard criteria are an increase in cell number, loss of normal regular arrangement of cells, variation in cell shape and size, increase in nuclear size and density of staining (both of which reflect an increase in total DNA), and increase in mitotic activity and the presence of abnormal mitoses. When all these features are present, diagnosis is easy. Diagnosis of carcinomas *in situ* depends on recognition of these changes in an area of epithelium, usually on a surface, the cervix of the uterus or skin, but it may occur in the bladder or other organs. Changes only involve the epithelium and there is no invasion of underlying tissues, i.e. the neoplastic cells remain where they began—*in situ*. The only definite evidence of malignancy is invasion of underlying tissues. The electron microscope is of little help in identification of tumour cells except in a few well defined areas (see Ghadially, 1980, for ultrastructure of tumours). Transmission electron microscopy (TEM) may be of value in establishing the cellular origins of tumours, e.g. by morphological identification of specific cell products or by identifying tumours as epithelial by the presence of specific epithelial cell contacts, particularly desmosomes. Unfortunately these tend to be preserved mainly in well differentiated tumours which are easily diagnosable using light microscopy. Recognition of invasion by electron microscopy is also unreliable since it has recently been shown that some tumour cells actually make basement membrane material (Leivo *et al.*, 1982; Franks, unpublished). The only cytological feature of value in diagnosis is the presence of abnormal mitochondria in tumour cells, although alterations in structure or distribution of most cell organelles, including cell surface, cell contacts, microtubules and microfilaments, nuclear and nucleolar pattern, have been described. Cell surface changes in particular have been studied with the scanning electron microscope (SEM). Kenemans *et al.* (1981), Koss and Domagala (1980), Domagala and Koss (1980), and others have described alterations in pattern and distribution of microvilli in precancerous and tumour cells from different organs. Freeze fracture techniques have also been used to study surface features, especially of cell contacts (Weinstein *et al.*, 1980). As with every other technique used, SEM, TEM, and replica methods show that there is a progressive disorder or loss of specialized cell structure, i.e. there is a loss of differentiation, so the value of these techniques is that they may show differences on a scale not visible with the light microscope; however, as Kenemans *et al.* (1981) conclude, they have "no early diagnostic, prognostic or therapeutic significance".

If the whole tumour is available for study, diagnosis is usually easy, but in biopsy material there are complications. An obvious one is concerned with sampling, particularly if only small fragments, which may not be representative of the whole tumour, are removed. These small fragments are also much more liable to damage either during removal, by direct trauma, by torsion in punch biopsies, or by heat coagulation if removed by diathermy. Even after removal, small fragments are much more easily damaged by handling, fixation, etc. The importance of damage before or after removal is that it may cause distortion of normal tissue arrangements and of cell structure which may lead to an erroneous diagnosis of neoplasia.

III. Tumour cells *in vitro*

The problems involved in identification of tumour cells *in vivo* are also present in tissue cultures but are made even more difficult as a consequence of the culture conditions. An essential preliminary to culture is preparation of cell suspensions by trypsinization or of small tissue fragments by chopping. Both produce cell damage and disruption of normal tissue and tumour architecture. Both give rise to mixed cell populations containing tumour cells and normal cells in unknown proportions. Although many cells may survive for a short time, only a small number will go on to divide and populate the culture vessel, and these are not necessarily tumour cells. Many normal mesenchymal cells seem to have a greater proliferation capacity in the early stages of culture than do some tumour cells. Buehring and Williams (1976), using human biopsy material from breast cancers, breast atypias and normal breast, as well as breast fluid and four established human breast tumour cell lines, found that: (a) malignant cells divided at a slower mean rate than normal cells; (b) population doubling time values of malignant cells were more heterogeneous than those of normal cells; (c) cultures from non-malignant atypias showed population doubling time means and standard deviations between those of normal and malignant cells; and (d) long-term mammary tumour cell lines divided more slowly than normal cells. These findings have been confirmed by others (cited by Buehring and Williams, 1976) and are further confirmed by the difficulties of establishing cell lines from any human tumours. Even if the cells that do survive in early cultures can be identified as tumour cells, they may not be representative of the tumour as a whole and may well differ metabolically from similar cells *in vivo*. The only cells that will survive *in vitro* are those that can adapt to the standardized conditions of culture, so they inevitably have many features in common with each other. Ideally it should be possible to establish the proportion of tumour cells in a mixed population, particularly if the assay to be used involves biochemical or other methods that require the tissue to be homogenized. There are as yet no biochemical or biophysical markers that allow this to be done. Can it be done cytologically?

IV. Morphology of tumour cells *in vitro*

Using the standard light microscope and morphological criteria outlined in the preceding section on *in vivo* diagnosis, organized groups of surviving tumour cells can be recognized easily, but a firm diagnosis is impossible with single cells or groups of cells without an organized pattern. Many cells derived from normal tissues show nuclear, chromosomal, and cytoplasmic abnormalities in culture, particularly as they reach a terminal growth phase, and these changes are exaggerated by the effects of cytotoxic agents. The most convincing indicator of malignancy—invasion—cannot of course be applied to cells *in vitro*.

The ultrastructural features of neoplastic transformation in cells in culture have been described in detail elsewhere (Franks and Wilson, 1977; Franks, 1982), and Seman and Dmochowski (1975) have described the ultrastructure of human tumour cell lines. Most of the changes in general and cell surface morphology, glycocalyx, plasma membrane, cytoskeleton and enzyme patterns are a reflection of alteration or loss of differentiated characters rather than specific indicators of neoplastic changes, but may be a guide, particularly if a comparison can be made with cells of the same origin known to be non-neoplastic. Original papers should be consulted for details. Sanford and her colleagues (Handleman *et al.*, 1977) made a detailed study of the cytology of spontaneous transformation *in vitro*. Cultures were examined for 19 cytological abnormalities and 5 of these were found to correlate with the ability of the cells to form tumours: cytoplasmic basophilia, high nuclear/cytoplasmic ratio, reduced cytoplasmic spreading on substrate, clumping, and cording (end-to-end alignment of cells). Many of these are of course interrelated and reflect the cytological criteria for malignancy already referred to. It is suggested that each of the properties can be measured directly or by computerized image analysis, and some preliminary results have been reported (e.g. Fox *et al.*, 1977). None of the features correlated absolutely with tumorigenicity.

In epithelial systems there is a similar lack of correlation between morphology and malignancy (see Franks and Wigley, 1979, for full review and references). In skin Fusenig *et al.* (1979) could find no "reliable criteria for discriminating the typical transformed phenotype". In rat liver Williams *et al.* (1973) found no uniform, characteristic alterations in carcinogen-treated cells, as did Schaeffer and Heintz (1978) who found no correlation with "cytopathological morphology, formation of cell foci, growth in soft agar or irregular fibroblast-like growth patterns". In mouse mammary gland Voyles and McGrath (1976) found that normal and premalignant epithelial cells were morphologically indistinguishable from malignant mouse mammary epithelial cells in primary monolayer culture. Growth rates and saturation densities were also indistinguishable. In mouse salivary gland and bladder systems (see Wigley, 1979; Summerhayes, 1979, for reviews) altered foci developed but many of these, although morphologically abnormal, were not tumour-producing on transplantation into syngeneic mice and many regressed. Only a small number of foci developed into fully transformed tumour-producing cells and none showed any predictable markers.

In human cell lines Smith *et al.* (1979), using semiquantitative assessment, compared cells derived from a variety of human tumours with others derived from normal tissues, and described ultrastructural nuclear differences. Nuclear bodies and perichromatin granules were found only in tumour-derived lines. Margination of chromatin, irregularity of nuclear outline, and redistribution of nucleolar components were much more marked in tumour cells, and dilatation of the nuclear envelope was not seen in cells derived from normal organs. Unfortunately, as the authors point out, all these markers have been found in normal and diseased cells, as well as in tumours, so none can be considered absolute markers, although there appeared to be quantitative differences. Zimmer *et al.* (1981) also used an electron microscopic counting method to compare the amount of polymerized tubulin in virus transformed and non-transformed 3T3 cells and found a reduced amount in transformed cells, confirming earlier observations, using immunofluorescence, on disturbances in distribution and amount in the microtubules and the cytoskeleton but no obvious changes in kind (see Zimmer *et al.*, 1981, for references) on transformed cells.

Particular features that may be of help in identifying tumour cells are mitochondrial changes, changes in cell surface pattern and function, and DNA changes.

A. Mitochondrial changes in tumour cells

The presence of morphologically abnormal mitochondria in tumour cells has already been referred to (see Franks and Wilson, 1977; Pedersen, 1978, for reviews), and differences in glycolysis between normal and tumour cells are well known. But most tumour cells contain all normal respiratory enzymes, and isolated tumour mitochondria are similar in behaviour to those from normal cells (Weinhouse, 1974) in spite of abnormalities in structure, so differences in behaviour must depend on quantitative differences or on differences in control systems in the cell. A method for detection of mitochondrial changes in cells *in situ* may therefore be very valuable. Johnson *et al.* (1982) have shown that uptake and retention of a mitochondria-specific membrane potential probe, Rhodamine 123, was reduced in virus transformed mink cells. The probe can be detected and measured by quantitative fluorescence microscopy of living cells.

B. Changes in cell surface pattern

Changes in cell surface pattern as shown by SEM have been described in normal and tumour cells in culture. Heatfield *et al.* (1980) described SEM changes in human bladder epithelium in culture. These illustrate the general pattern. Within 2–3 days differentiated cells were lost and replaced by cells having short microvilli with strands of fine filamentous material attached. These completely covered the culture by 1–2 weeks. By 4 weeks microvilli were more variable, and by 10 weeks the surface epithelium was flattened (squamous-like) or cuboidal, with irregular microvilli. They considered that these changes reflect failure of normal cell maturation *in vitro*, and state that similar features have been described *in vivo* by others in ageing, benign hyperplastic and preneoplastic epithelium. Surface changes have been described in other cells in culture. Haugen and Laerum (1978), for example, described a high degree of surface activity in culture as shown by microvilli, filopodia, ruffling membranes, and zeiotic blebs in glioma-like tumour-producing cells derived from rat embryo brain treated *in vivo* with a carcinogen. Cells producing neurinoma-like tumours had a low surface activity.

Perhaps the most instructive findings are those of Koss and Domagala. They selected clumps of tumour cells and mesothelial cells present in pleural and peritoneal effusions, identified by their light microscopic appearance (Koss and Domagala, 1980), and compared the appearance with those found in human tumour tissue obtained by needle biopsy (Domagala and Koss, 1980). They described the surface configuration in normal urothelial cells, macrophages, and polymorphs, and showed that these changed when the cells altered their attachment or functional activity. For example, *in situ*, urothelial cells had many microvilli, but when free the surface was covered by irregular blebs. Macrophages were usually covered by veil-like ridges. Tumour cells in effusions had many irregular microvilli, but in tumour cells from needle biopsies a varied pattern was found, ranging from numerous microvilli, especially in breast tumours and melanoma, to blebs, ridges, or almost entirely smooth surfaces. They concluded that there were no specific surface features for any of the tumour cells studied except for small cell carcinoma of lung. Their final comment could be considered unenthusiastic: "The possibility that SEM may prove to be of diagnostic value in selected special clinical or diagnostic situations cannot be ruled out".

Although these observations are not based on cells in culture, they clearly indicate the changes that may be induced by a change of environment, and particularly the surface changes induced by transfer into a fluid environment, a similar situation to that in tissue culture, and clearly illustrate the difficulties of specifically identifying individual cells morphologically.

C. Functional changes in the cell surface

Changes in cell surface enzymes and other proteins, e.g. fibronectin, have been described in tumour cells, and other functional markers, such as the ability to grow in agar or differences in substrate attachment or lectin binding, are almost certainly due to alterations in surface proteins. Many of these changes can be studied cytologically, and although none is an absolute indicator for transformed cells (see Franks, 1982, for review) they may be of value in some circumstances. Alkaline phosphatase, for example, has been used as a cell surface marker for transformation in some mouse and hamster cell systems, and a derepressed placental isoenzyme phenotype has been described in some human tumour cells (e.g. Fishman *et al.*, 1968), but a more extensive study on several mouse, rat, and human mesenchymal, lymphoblastoid and bladder tumours has shown that changes in the enzyme or its isozymes are not invariable markers for transformation (Wilson *et al.*, 1977).

Concanavalin A (Con A) binding can also be demonstrated cytologically. Voyles and McGrath (1976) compared normal, premalignant, and malignant cells from mouse mammary carcinoma; although they could detect no differences in morphology, growth rate, or saturation densities, Con A binding demonstrated by haemadsorption, using Con A coated red cells, was present only in malignant and premalignant cells, in primary and secondary cultures and in cell lines.

Changes in other cell surface proteins, e.g. fibronectins, discussed in more detail in Chapter 4, can also be studied, using immunocytochemical methods, but again there are no absolute differences.

D. Changes in chromosomes and DNA

One of the few consistent changes in tumour cells is the presence of abnormal chromosomes (see e.g. Cowell, 1979), and this often occurs in the preneoplastic stages (e.g. Barrett, 1980), but in primary and mixed cultures chromosome studies are difficult since it is usually not possible to obtain a sufficient number of mitotic cells, or to be sure that the cells obtained are tumour cells. An alternative method, which is particularly useful for studying small groups of cells, is quantitative microfluorimetry of total DNA. Both of these approaches are considered in more detail in Chapter 3.

E. Immunocytological methods for tumour cell detection

Immunocytological methods (discussed in more detail in Chapter 5) are potentially of great value. They may be used to identify cell types if they produce a specific cell product, e.g. a cytokeratin, or specific enzymes or hormones, or an ectopic tumour-associated product such as chorioembryonic antigen. They are also useful in comparing the pattern and distribution of normal cell structures, e.g. cytoskeleton or cell surface proteins, as indicators of transformation. Detection of true tumour-specific proteins in cells in culture would provide absolute markers. For example, Boone *et al.* (1979) have described such proteins in transformed mesenchymal cells, and Duhl *et al.* (1982) have described tumour-associated chromatin antigens in human carcinoma cell lines. Recently Harris and his colleagues (Ashall *et al.*, 1982) described a glycoprotein, the Ca antigen, recognizable by a monoclonal antibody, which was present in many malignant tumours (McGee *et al.*, 1982) and in tumour-producing hybrid cells. This should be of value in diagnosis. Developments in this field are of obvious importance. Unfortunately these early reports have not been confirmed (Krausz *et al.*, 1983).

V. Conclusions

There are no absolute markers for transformed cells in any systems. Many of the markers reflect quantitative differences rather than differences in kind, although these may be of value if a normal cell is available for comparison. Comparisons may be complicated by the fact that many markers that can be cytologically characterized, e.g. cytoskeletal and cell surface changes, are influenced by culture conditions and stages in the cell cycle. Given the conditions in primary cultures of tumours, where both tumour and normal cells are present, the most reliable method of identification is tumour cell morphology, although this may be strengthened by applying quantitative methods, particularly single-cell DNA measurements. Again this is most reliable in assessing the distribution of aneuploid cells in a group rather than in assigning a single cell into a normal or malignant compartment.

Immunocytochemical methods can be developed for the identification of cell types by the presence of cell-specific products and ultimately by detection of tumour-specific proteins. Another promising approach is selective killing of normal or tumour cells by immunological methods.

References

Ashall, F., Bramwell, M. E. and Harris, H. (1982). A new marker for human cancer cells. 1. The Ca antigen and the Cal antibody. *Lancet* **ii,** 1–6.

Barrett, J. C. (1980). A preneoplastic stage in the spontaneous neoplastic transformation of Syrian hamster embryo cells in culture. *Cancer Res.* **40,** 91–94.

Boone, C. W., Vembu, D., White, B. J., Takeichi, N. and Paranjpe, M. (1979). Karyotypic, antigenic, and kidney-invasive properties of cell lines from fibrosarcomas arising in C3H/10T$\frac{1}{2}$ cells implanted subcutaneously attached to plastic plates. *Cancer Res.* **39,** 2172–2178.

Buehring, G. C. and Williams, R. R. (1976). Growth rates of normal and abnormal human mammary epithelia in cell culture. *Cancer Res.* **36,** 3742–3747.

Busch, H. and Yeoman, L. C. (eds) (1982). *Methods in Cancer Research*. Vol. 19. *Tumour Markers*. Academic Press, New York and London.

Cameron, I. L. and Pool, T. B. (eds) (1981). *The Transformed Cell*. Academic Press, London.

Cowell, J. K. (1979). Chromosome changes associated with epithelial cell transformation with special reference to *in vitro* systems. In *Neoplastic Transformation in Differentiated Epithelial Cell Systems in Vitro* (ed. L. M. Franks and C. B. Wigley), pp. 159–286. Academic Press, London.

Domagala, W. and Koss, L. G. (1980). Surface configuration of human tumor cells obtained by fine needle aspiration biopsy. In *Scanning Electron Microscopy* (ed. A. M. F. O'Hare), pp. 101–108. SEM Inc., U.S.A.

Duhl, D. M., Banjar, Z., Briggs, R. C., Page, D. L. and Hnilica, L. S. (1982). Tumor-associated chromatin antigens of human colon adenocarcinoma cell lines HT-29 and LoVo. *Cancer Res.* **42,** 594–600.

Fishman, W. H., Inglis, N. R., Stolbach, L. L. and Krant, H. J. A. (1968). Serum alkaline phosphatase isoenzyme of human neoplastic cell origin. *Cancer Res.* **28,** 150–154.

Fox, C. H., Caspersson, T., Kudynowski, J., Sanford, K. K. and Tarone, R. E. (1977). Morphometric analysis of neoplastic transformation in rodent fibroblast cell lines. *Cancer Res.* **37,** 892–897.

Franks, L. M. (1956). Latency and progression in human tumours. *Lancet* **2,** 1037–1039.

Franks, L. M. (1979). What is a cancer cell? Phenotypic markers in *in vitro* carcinogenesis in epithelial systems. In *Neoplastic Transformation in Differentiated Epithelial Cell Systems in Vitro* (ed. L. M. Franks and C. B. Wigley), pp. 287–300. Academic Press, London.

Franks, L. M. (1982). The neoplastic cell and its analysis by cell hybridization. 1. The nature of the transformation process and its markers. 2. Analysis of transformation by cell hybridization. In *Gene Expression in Normal and Transformed Cells* (ed. J. E. Celis). Plenum Publishing Company (in press).

Franks, L. M. and Wigley, C. B. (1979). *In vitro* transformation in the respiratory tract. In *Neoplastic Transformation in Differentiated Epithelial Cell Systems in Vitro* (ed. L. M. Franks and C. B. Wigley), pp. 163–170. Academic Press, London.

Franks, L. M. and Wilson, P. D. (1977). Origin and ultrastructure of cells *in vitro*. *Int. Rev. Cytol.* **48**, 55–139.

Fusenig, N. E., Breitkreutz, D., Boukamp, P., Lueder, M., Irmscher, G. and Worst, P. K. M. (1979). Chemical carcinogenesis in mouse epidermal cell cultures. Altered expression of tissue specific functions accompanying cell transformation. In *Neoplastic Transformation in Differentiated Epithelial Cell Systems in Vitro* (ed. L. M. Franks and C. B. Wigley), pp. 37–98. Academic Press, London.

Ghadially, F. N. (1980). *Diagnostic Electron Microscopy of Tumours*. Butterworth, London.

Handleman, S. L., Sanford, K. K., Tarone, R. E. and Parshad, R. (1977). The cytology of spontaneous neoplastic transformation in culture. *In Vitro* **13**, 526–536.

Haugen, A. and Laerum, O. D. (1978). Scanning electron microscopy of neoplastic neurogenic rat cell lines in culture. *Acta Path. Microbiol. Scand. (A)* **86**, 101–110.

Heatfield, B. M., Sanefuji, H., El-Gerzawi, S., Urso, B. and Trump, B. F. (1980). Surface alterations in urothelium of normal human bladder during long-term explant culture. In *Scanning Electron Microscopy* (ed. A. M. F. O'Hare), p. 61. SEM Inc., U.S.A.

Johnson, L. V., Summerhayes, I. C. and Chen, Lan Bo (1982). Decreased uptake and retention of Rhodamine 123 by mitochondria in feline sarcoma virus-transformed mink cells. *Cell* **28**, 7–14.

Kenemans, P., Davina, J. H. M., de Haan, R. W., van der Zanden, P., Vooys, G. P., Stolk, J. G. and Stadhouders, A. M. (1981). Cell surface morphology in epithelial malignancy and its precursor lesions. In *Scanning Electron Microscopy* (ed. A. M. F. O'Hare), pp. 23–36. SEM Inc., U.S.A.

Koss, L. G. and Domagala, W. (1980). Configuration of surfaces of human cancer cells in effusions: a review. In *Scanning Electron Microscopy* (ed. A. M. F. O'Hare), pp. 89–100. SEM Inc., U.S.A.

Krausz, T. J., Van Noorden, S. and Evans, D. J. (1983). *Lancet* **i**, 1097 (letter).

Leivo, I., Alitalo, K., Risteli, L., Vaheri, A., Timpl, R. and Wartiovaara, J. (1982). Basal lamina glycoproteins laminin and type IV collagen are assembled into a fine-fibered matrix in cultures of a teratocarcinoma-derived endodermal cell line. *Exp. Cell Res.* **137**, 15–23.

Marshall, C. J., Franks, L. M. and Carbonell, A. W. (1977). Markers of neoplastic transformation in epithelial cell lines derived from human carcinoma. *J. Nat. Cancer Inst.* **58**, 1743–1751.

McGee, J. O'D., Woods, J. C., Ashall, F., Bramwell, M. E. and Harris, H. (1982). A new marker for human cancer cells. 2. Immunohistochemical detection of the Ca antigen in human tissues with the Cal antibody. *Lancet* **ii**, 7–10.

Pedersen, P. L. (1978). Tumor mitochondria and the bioenergetics of cancer cells. *Progr. Exp. Tumor Res.* **22**, 190–274.

Sanford, K. K., Handleman, S. L., Fox, C. H., Burris, J. F., Hursey, M. L., Mitchell, J. T., Jackson, J. L. and Parshad, R. (1974). Effects of chemical carcinogens on neoplastic transformation and morphology of cells in culture. *J. Nat. Cancer Inst.* **53**, 1647–1659.

Schaeffer, W. I. and Heintz, N. H. (1978). A diploid rat liver cell culture. IV. Malignant transformation by aflatoxin B_1. *In Vitro* **14**, 418–427.

Seman, G. and Dmochowski, L. (1975). Ultrastructural characteristics of human tumor cells in vitro. In *Human Tumor Cells in Vitro* (ed. J. Fogh), pp. 395–486. Plenum Press, New York and London.

Smith, H. S., Springer, E. L. and Hackett, A. J. (1979). Nuclear ultrastructure of epithelial cell lines derived from human carcinomas and nonmalignant tissues. *Cancer Res.* **39,** 332–344.

Summerhayes, I. C. (1979). Influence of donor age on *in vitro* transformation of bladder epithelium. In *Neoplastic Transformation in Differentiated Epithelial Cell Systems in Vitro* (ed. L. M. Franks and C. B. Wigley), pp. 137–160. Academic Press, London.

Tomei, L. D. and Bertram, J. S. (1978). Restoration of growth control in malignantly transformed mouse fibroblasts grown in a chemically defined medium. *Cancer Res.* **38,** 444–451.

Voyles, B. A. and McGrath, C. M. (1976). Markers to distinguish normal and neoplastic mammary epithelial cells *in vitro*: comparison of saturation density, morphology and concanavalin A reactivity. *Int. J. Cancer* **18,** 498–509.

Weinhouse, S. (1974). Isozyme alterations and metabolism of experimental liver neoplasms. In *Control Processes in Neoplasia* (ed. A. M. Mehlman and R. W. Hanson), pp. 1–30. Academic Press, New York.

Weinstein, I. B., Mufson, R. A., Lee, L.-S., Fisher, P. B., Laskin, J., Horowitz, A. D. and Ivanovic, V. (1980). Membrane and other biochemical effects of the phorbol esters and their relevance to tumor promotion. In *13th Jerusalem Symposium Carcinogenesis: Fundamental Mechanisms and Environmental Effects* (ed. B. Pullman, P. O. P. Ts'o and H. Gelboin), pp. 543–563. Reidel Publishing Co., Amsterdam.

Wigley, C. B. (1979). Transformation *in vitro* of adult mouse salivary gland epithelium: a system for studies on mechanisms of initiation and promotion. In *Neoplastic Transformation in Differentiated Epithelial Cell Systems in Vitro* (ed. L. M. Franks and C. B. Wigley), pp. 3–34. Academic Press, London.

Williams, G. M., Elliott, J. M. and Weisburger, J. H. (1973). Carcinoma after malignant conversion *in vitro* of epithelial-like cells from rat liver following exposure to chemical carcinogens. *Cancer Res.* **33,** 606–612.

Wilson, P. D., Benham, F. and Franks, L. M. (1977). Alkaline phosphatase phenotypes in tumour and non-tumour cell lines: not an invariable marker for neoplastic transformation. *Cell Biol. Int. Rep.* **1,** 229–238.

Zimmer, D. B., Turner, D. S., Goldstein, M. A. and Brinkley, B. R. (1981). A quantitative ultrastructural study of microtubules in transformed and nontransformed cells *in vitro*. *Cell Biol. Int. Rep.* **5,** 1115–1125.

3. Physical Methods of Tumour Cell Identification

P. P. DENDY

I. Introduction

Positive identification of tumour cells is of paramount importance to experiments designed to investigate drug sensitivity using *in vitro* techniques. It is of course a problem that has concerned diagnostic cytologists for many years, and the considerable corpus of knowledge that they have accumulated must be examined (see Chapter 2). However, there is a major change of emphasis when the question is considered in the context of *in vitro* drug sensitivity testing. Now we are no longer trying to find a small number of tumour cells in a largely normal population to provide early detection of a malignant or premalignant condition, but require a rapid and reliable determination of the proportions of tumour and normal stromal cells in a mixed population. In this context, properties chosen for identification must satisfy three criteria: specificity, stability, and simplicity.

Several properties are considered to be specific to chemically or virally transformed cells but few critical attempts have been made to check that these are also specific properties for human tumour cells. Recent work suggests that some properties, for example colony formation in Methocell, and on density-inhibited monolayers, as well as tumour induction in immuno-suppressed mice, are *related* to malignancy but are non-essential markers and cannot therefore be used for unequivocal identification (Smith, 1979).

Regarding stability, it has been shown that growth properties change after extensive subculturing *in vitro*. Some traditional morphological criteria of malignancy, notably cell size and shape, may change simply because the metabolic activity of the cells is different *in vitro*. In other cases the change may be more fundamental and may reflect the acquisition of properties thought to represent the malignant phenotype. For example Faulk and Galbraith (1979) showed that transferrin receptors found on human breast tumour cells were

19

absent from normal cells at biopsy but, if the latter were maintained in culture, transferrin receptors appeared. Clearly this property could not be used for tumour cell identification *in vitro*.

The final criterion is simplicity. Since tumour cell identification is subsidiary to the main purpose, it must be simple, straightforward, and quick.

These criteria are of greater importance than high precision; an estimate of the proportion of tumour cells to 10% accuracy would be perfectly adequate for most purposes. Hence physical techniques that permit rapid data analysis may provide the best prospects for solving the problem, and this section places emphasis on physical methods of measurement that may be readily automated.

II. Morphological criteria

A major difficulty in using morphological criteria is the subjective nature of the assessment, so the introduction of quantitative techniques based on predefined features represents a major step forward. For an excellent general review of the frontiers of quantitative cytochemistry the reader is referred to Bahr (1979).

Since no single morphological feature is diagnostic for malignancy, tumour cell identification relies on a multiparameter approach. Hence automated techniques coupled with the data storage capability and speed in performing routine processes of a computer based system are invaluable. It is important not only to select features that are relevant to the distinction between normal and tumour cells but also to appreciate that some features are more relevant than others. Statistical approaches have been discussed by Bartels (1979) but virtually no attempts have been made to identify the most relevant discriminatory features for normal and tumour cells maintained in short-term culture.

Preston (1980) reviewed automated analysis of cell images but concluded that significant commercial hardware for cytologic pattern recognition was only available in the area of haematology. Systems capable of analysing human epithelial tumour cells still seem to be at a developmental stage but some specific examples can be given.

Rheinhard *et al.* (1979) classified cervical cells using a television scanned image. Each nucleus was first digitized and several hundred features were then derived. When 1000 cell images in each Papanicolou-stained specimen were examined for the 10 most important morphological features, correct classification as either normal or suspicious was better than 91%. Using special hardware processors, classification of 1000 cells with up to 200 coefficients can be performed in about 1 min.

Stenkvist *et al.* (1978) used a slightly different technique linking a microscope to a diode array scanner and computer. Cells in which DNA and RNA had been stained with gallocyanin chrome alum were described by various indices concerned with density, shape, and texture. The indices were given numerical gradings and the total numerical score for each nucleus correlated well with the degree of nuclear atypia. Results also showed good reproducibility.

Although most efforts to identify cells by computer assisted pattern recognition have been orientated primarily towards automated diagnosis, some of the methods may be applicable to cells in culture. For example MacKillop *et al.* (1982) carried out a density/volume analysis of cellular heterogeneity in human ovarian carcinoma. Using an ovarian carcinoma cell line and ascites cells from two human ovarian carcinomas, they made a computer analysis of the cell volume spectra of density gradient fractions. MacKillop *et al.* concentrated on analysis of cellular heterogeneity within the tumour cell population, mapping both the proliferative state (labelling index) and growth potential (clonogenicity) in terms of density/volume measurements. However, the work could be extended to identify normal and tumour cells and is clearly applicable to several problems related to *in vitro* drug sensitivity prediction.

III. Chromosome karyotype

Tumour cells frequently show abnormalities both in their number and shape of chromosomes. Karyotyping or chromosome mapping has long been used to assist in differentiating between tumour and normal cells. A review of chromosome changes associated with epithelial transformation, with special reference to *in vitro* systems, is provided by Cowell (1979).

Introduction of chromosome banding techniques has greatly improved the specificity of this method of tumour cell identification and has allowed all previously studied neoplasms to be re-examined. Many neoplasms carry a marker chromosome, which not only demonstrates the clonogenic nature of the disease but also provides the most definitive single piece of information that can be used to relate an isolated cell to its origin when comparing primary tumour material with cultured cells.

When attempting identification by chromosome karyotyping as an adjunct to predictive drug sensitivity testing, the third requirement, that of simplicity, creates most problems. First, the cells must divide before the karyotype can be measured. Thus the method may be readily applied to cells that are actively cycling, but its use is limited with primary tumour material. Sonta and Sandberg (1978) pointed out that, because (a) primary solid tumours have a low mitotic index, (b) banding is difficult owing to the chromosomes being rather contracted, and (c) cancerous chromosomes are often resistant to banding, results for solid tumours are much less numerous than for haematological disorders. Trent and Salmon (1981) have reported detailed chromosome banding analyses of six cases of ovarian adenocarcinoma cultured in agar for up to 4 days to promote cell division. Results of G & C banding revealed a variety of changes with most frequent involvement of chromosomes #1 and #6. The use of short-term agar culture may greatly facilitate chromosome karyotyping of certain solid tumours that have so far proved refractory.

Similar problems occur *in vitro* if the mitotic index is very low. Although chromosome numbers together with cytological and electron microscope appearances were used by Guner *et al.* (1977) to identify tumour cells in lines derived from astrocytoma, we found the method somewhat unsatisfactory for identification of tumour cells from ovarian biopsies in short-term culture (Wright and Dendy, 1976). On one occasion we harvested only two countable spreads from a population of 10^6 ovarian tumour cells. This means the method is highly selective, giving information about only a tiny fraction of the population and no information about cells that may be temporarily out of the cell cycle.

Secondly, there are several reasons why this method cannot be used to estimate the proportion of tumour cells in a mixed population. Normal chromosomes may spread more easily than tumour chromosomes, so normal cells are more likely to be selected for analysis. In addition, both the proportion of cells in cycle and the duration of the cell cycle will determine the number of cells trapped in mitosis and available for examination.

Finally, chromosome analysis is time-consuming.

IV. DNA content

Closely related to chromosome karyotyping is identification of malignant cells by measurement of nuclear DNA content. In the strictest sense this method is non-specific since there is little doubt that a small percentage of malignant tumours contain cells in which the DNA content is indistinguishable from normal. However, there is evidence to suggest that abnormal DNA values are more common in de-differentiated tumours (Tribukait and Esposti, 1976) and in later stages of the disease (Bohm and Sandritter, 1975). Biopsy specimens cultured for predictive sensitivity testing will generally come from these categories. Note also that reported normal DNA values for tumour cells may be spurious unless the malignant origin of the cells has been convincingly verified by other methods.

Traditionally, DNA values are obtained by quantitative microdensitometry. Cells are stained with a dye that is stoichiometric for DNA (usually
Feulgen's reagent), and the attenuation of a beam of monochromatic light as
it passes through the cell nucleus is measured. The machine may be calibrated
using a standard cell type, for example bull sperm or diploid, tetraploid, and
octaploid nuclei from adult liver.

For normal cells in culture, a range of DNA values is observed because
many cells are in S phase and have DNA values intermediate between G_1 and
G_2. These cells might erroneously be identified as tumour cells in an unknown
population, so to avoid this problem the cells are exposed to ^{3}H-thymidine, a
specific precursor of DNA, immediately prior to fixation. After DNA
measurements have been made, autoradiographs are prepared and S-phase
cells are separately identified.

Dendy and Algüneş (1979) evaluated this technique for identification of
tumour and normal cells *in vitro*, and Ling *et al.* (1981) used it to examine
cultured abdominal tumours. Fig. 1 shows results obtained for a vascular
infiltrating anaplastic carcinoma, probably of the ovary, with little evidence of
stroma. In the smear and primary culture normal and tumour cells were
present, but after passage the normal cells had disappeared. Unfortunately
this was not always the outcome; sometimes only normal cells survived in
culture. Table 1 summarizes the results of this study.

Fig. 1 highlights other problems with this type of work. As the culture
progresses, we see not only a change in the proportion of normal and tumour
cells but also a marked change in the DNA distribution of supposed abnormal
cells (mainly due to cell cycle effects) and variations in the proportion of cells
labelled with ^{3}H-thymidine.

Fluorescent stains may be used instead of Feulgen's reagent. Cowell and
Franks (1980) described a rapid method for accurate measurement of single
cells *in situ* using Hoechst 33258 as a quantitative fluorochrome and
ultraviolet illumination through a Zeiss photomicroscope. To permit examination of cells growing on plastic surfaces, which are unsuitable for use with
transmitted light, epillumination was used. A shutter system minimized the
duration of exposure to ultraviolet light, thereby almost eliminating errors
due to fluorochrome fading, and standard deviations of less than 5% were
obtained.

V. Flow methods for tumour cell identification

When only a small number of cells is available, static cytophotometry may be
the only feasible method. However, developments in automated techniques of
impulse cytophotometry are providing very rapid analysis in cases where

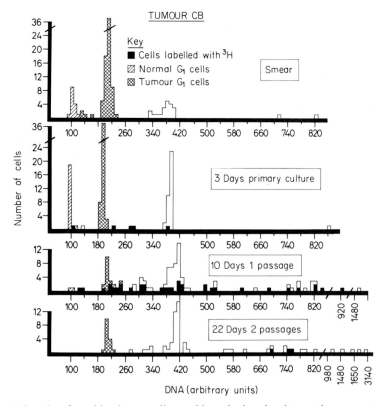

Fig. 1 Results of combined autoradiographic and microdensitometric measurements on cells from an anaplastic carcinoma, probably ovarian in origin.

Table 1 Summary of results on cultures derived from human abdominal surgical specimens (Ling *et al.*, 1981)

	Number of specimens examined	Number cultured successfully	Cells with abnormal DNA values for:		
			smear	primary culture	after first passage
Normal specimens	3	3/3	0/3	0/2	0/2
Borderline malignancy	3	1/3	1/3	—	—
Abdominal malignancies	9	8/9	9/9	4/7	2/5

sufficient single cells can be obtained. A fluorescent dye is used for staining, and each cell flowing through a measuring chamber is illuminated with an intense beam of light. Since the transit time for each cell is only 10–20 μs, a very high light intensity, for example from a laser, is required to obtain an adequate signal from suitably stained material. Use of a laser also ensures good focussing and a very constant light output at fixed wavelength so there is good reproducibility for constant stain intensity.

Mørk and Laerum (1980a) used this method to study the modal DNA content of human intracranial neoplasms and found a much larger proportion of poorly differentiated gliomas with a near-diploid DNA mode than had been reported previously. Mørk and Laerum (1980b) also reported that, when gliomas were maintained *in vitro* for periods up to 180 days, changes in ploidy characteristics were sometimes observed. From 10 poorly differentiated gliomas, two that were heteroploid changed to near-diploid in culture, and two initially near-diploid cultures developed heteroploidy (Fig. 2).

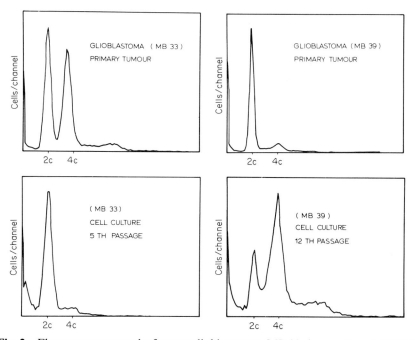

Fig. 2 Flow cytometry results for two glioblastomas. MB 33 shows a bimodal DNA content in the primary tumour but only the near-diploid population survived in culture. MB 39 is an example where the primary tumour was near-diploid but cells with a near-tetraploid DNA culture gradually appeared after passage in culture (Mørk and Laerum, 1980b).

There are many possibilities for fluorochrome staining, with DNA, double- and single-stranded RNA, and proteins among the most popular. Watson (1980) used fluorogenic substrates to determine the cellular activity in mouse tumour cells *in vitro*, and also the reaction kinetics of phosphatases located in the plasma membrane. Since identification of tumour cells by nucleic acid or protein content has been rather disappointing, this new capability to analyse enzyme patterns is of considerable interest.

There are numerous advantages to flow cytometry (Mendelsohn, 1980). The first is precision of measurement. Coefficients of variation of fluorescence or scatter are about 1–2%, much lower than for any other form of cytometry. The second is speed. A suspension of cells can be fixed in ethanol, washed, treated with ribonuclease, and stained with, say, propidium iodide in less than 20 min. A histogram for 10 000 cells from each sample can be recorded in about 4 min, and thus results for a whole series of replicate cultures treated in different ways can be obtained in about half a day.

Third, there are several ways in which measurement of two properties can be made on the same cell:

(a) Acridine orange intercalates with double-stranded helical DNA and gives a green fluorescence when excited with blue light, but stacks on single-stranded nucleic acid and fluoresces red. Thus, if all the RNA is denatured to the single-stranded form, RNA and DNA may be measured simultaneously. An excellent account of this method to stain unfixed cells is given by Traganos *et al.* (1977).

(b) Two different fluorescent stains may be used. Bentley *et al.* (1979) used, simultaneously, propidium iodide which fluoresces with DNA and RNA, and fluorescein isothiocyanate which fluoresces with protein, to examine cervical material.

(c) Two laser beams, focussed either to the same point or to two different points in a vertical plane may be used. If an argon laser, which gives a blue line, and a krypton laser, which gives lines in the ultraviolet, are used together, the flexibility of the system is greatly increased.

As a further elaboration of the basic system, not only the fluorescent beam but also light scattered in the forward direction by the cells may be measured using solid-state photodetectors. Several detectors may be arranged at different angles, and by collecting information on the pulse height, pulse width, and the area under the pulse, a large amount of data relating to the size and shape of the cells, and also to their surface properties and internal structure, may be obtained. This approach has the additional advantage for chemosensitivity testing that cells do not need to be stained, so cell killing by the stain or synergistic interactions between stain and drug are not a problem.

VI. Cell sorting and related problems

The other major advantage of pulse cytophotometry is that it is capable of cell sorting. If a fine jet of fluid issues from a nozzle oscillating at very high frequency, the stream will break up into a highly regular pattern of droplets. The flow rate, cell concentration, and oscillating frequency are adjusted so that approximately 1 in 50 droplets contains a cell and the jet is examined with a laser beam before it breaks up. If the required properties are detected, a few droplets are charged so that, when they pass between permanently charged electrodes, the droplet containing the required cell is deflected out of the main stream. The method used by Stovel and Sweet (1979) to produce a fluorescence micrograph of a 10×10 array of droplets could readily be adapted to fill a microtiter tray with tumour cells.

There are three other problems closely related to tumour cell identification where flow cytophotometry and cell sorting may assist. (i) Is it possible to distinguish living cells from dead cells at this stage? (ii) Can cycling cells be distinguished from non-cycling cells? (iii) Could one distinguish clonogenic from non-clonogenic cells, because it can be argued that only the drug sensitivity of clonogenic cells is really important?

Some progress has been made on all these questions. For example, a viability test may be carried out using fluorescein diacetate, and Stohr and Vogt Schaden (1980) have extended this method to a dual staining technique able to give information on drug induced cell killing that is cell cycle phase specific. Swartzendruber (1977) has shown that one way to monitor for cycling cells is to grow them in bromodeoxyuridine (BUdR) which is only incorporated during the DNA synthetic phase. The amount of fluorescence on subsequent staining with mithramycin is proportional to the BUdR incorporated, so one may identify cells that have cycled once, twice, or not at all. Watson (1980) has discussed the third question and presented evidence to suggest that simultaneous estimation of RNA content and non-specific esterase activity might distinguish between clonogenic and non-clonogenic cells.

It must be emphasized that there are still a number of problems with flow cytophotometry for the identification of tumour cells from biopsies. The first is the preparation of single cell suspensions. Neither mechanical nor enzymatic methods, using various combinations of trypsin, collagenase, pronase, and hyaluronidase, give good results with all specimens. Cells may easily be damaged during disaggregation, and care is also required to ensure that they are not mechanically damaged in the flow apparatus.

Secondly, no one parameter is specific for human tumour cell identification, and most commercially available cytophotometers operate at low dimensionality. That is to say only one or two measurements are made on each object. Also measurements are generally made at zero resolution, thus representing the whole object, so any morphological features that might help with identification are lost. One system has been reported that can measure three different parameters, for example, cell volume, nuclear DNA content, and cell membrane density of carcinoembryonic antigen, on 100 000 cells min^{-1}. However, as progressively more stringent criteria of tumour cell identification are applied, although the purity of the tumour cell suspension may improve, the yield decreases rapidly.

Thirdly, if cells are to be identified and sorted prior to culture, they must remain viable. Most fluorescent stains are either used on fixed cells or will themselves kill the cells. Some of the benzimidazole stains (Hoechst) appear to be non-toxic, and measurement of scattered light at multiple small angles in the forward direction does not require prior staining.

Finally, most flow cytometers on the market are versatile but very expensive. An instrument of more limited capability designed and built specifically for the purpose of sorting cell suspensions from biopsies is required at a realistic price.

VII. Conclusions

1. The cell population in a disaggregated human tumour biopsy is very heterogeneous and methods of tumour cell identification and purification are required to improve the reliability of data from drug sensitivity tests.

2. The philosophy behind this work is somewhat different from that of the diagnostic cytologist. The problem is not to find the occasional tumour cell within a largely normal population, but to assign cells quickly and accurately to the normal or abnormal category.

3. No single property is diagnostic for individual tumour cells. Discrimination can be improved by a multiparameter approach but this increases the complexity of the measuring equipment and reduces the yield of positively identified cells.

4. Both static and flow methods have been used with some success to identify tumour cells, generally on the basis of abnormal DNA values. They have confirmed that the primary culture usually contains both normal and abnormal cells and in subsequent growth either may dominate.

5. The next logical step is purification of the initial population. Since upwards of 10^6 cells may be required for meaningful analysis of chemosensitivity to a range of drugs, rapid flow methods combined with cell sorting would appear to provide the most feasible prospects, perhaps using dedicated equipment.

Acknowledgement

This work has been supported by the Cancer Research Campaign.

References

Bahr, G. F. (1979). Frontiers of quantitative cytochemistry: development and potential. *Anal. Quant. Cytol.* **1**, 1–19.

Bartels, P. H. (1979). Numerical evaluation of cytologic data. 3. Selection of features for discrimination. *Anal. Quant. Cytol.* **1**, 153–159.

Bentley, S., Smith, E., Halbersett, M. and Herman, C. (1979). A pattern classification system for automated cervical cytologic screening based on flow microfluorometric analysis. *Anal. Quant. Cytol.* **1**, 61–66.

Bohm, N. and Sandritter, W. (1975). DNA in human tumours: a cytophotometric study. *Curr. Top. Pathol.* **60**, 151–219.

Cowell, J. K. (1979). Chromosome changes associated with epithelial cell transformation with special reference to *in vitro* systems. In *Neoplastic Transformation in Differentiated Epithelial Cell Systems in Vitro* (ed. L. M. Franks and C. B. Wigley), pp. 159–286. Academic Press, London.

Cowell, J. K. and Franks, L. M. (1980). A rapid method for accurate DNA measurements *in situ* using a simple microfluorimeter and Hoechst 33258 as a quantitative fluorochrome. *J. Histochem. Cytochem.* **28**, 206–210.

Dendy, P. P. and Algüneş, C. (1979). Human tumour cell identification in short term culture by combined microdensitometry and autoradiography. *Anal. Quant. Cytol.* **1**, 217–227.

Faulk, W. P. and Galbraith, G. M. P. (1979). Trophoblast transferrin and transferrin receptors in the host–parasite relationship of human pregnancy. *Proc. Roy. Soc.* **B204**, 83–98.

Guner, M., Freshney, R. I., Morgan, D., Freshney, M. G., Thomas, D. G. T. and Graham, D. I. (1977). Effects of dexamethasone and betamethasone on *in vitro* cultures from human astrocytoma. *Br. J. Cancer* **35**, 439–447.

Ling, C. R., Dendy, P. P. and Abramovich, D. R. (1981). The use of quantitative cytochemistry to monitor human tumour cells in culture. *Arch. Geschwulstforsch.* **51**, 80–86.

MacKillop, W. J., Stewart, S. S. and Buick, R. N. (1982). Density/volume analysis in the study of cellular heterogeneity in human ovarian carcinoma. *Br. J. Cancer* **45**, 812–820.

Mendelsohn, M. L. (1980). The attributes and applications of flow cytophotometry. In *Flow Cytometry*. IV (ed. O. D. Laerum, T. Lindmo and E. Thorud), pp. 15–27. Bergen Nor Universitets Floraget.

Mørk, S. J. and Laerum, O. R. (1980a). Modal DNA content of human intracranial neoplasms studied by flow cytophotometry. *J. Neurosurg.* **53**, 198–204.

Mørk, S. J. and Laerum, O. R. (1980b). DNA distribution in human glioma *in vivo* and *in vitro*. In *Flow Cytometry*. IV (ed. O. D. Laerum, T. Lindmo and E. Thorud), pp. 403–406. Bergen Nor Universitets Floraget.

Preston, K. (1980). Automation of the analysis of cell images. *Anal. Quant. Cytol.* **2**, 1–14.

Rheinhard, E., Erhardt, R., Schwarzmann, P., Bloss, W. and Ott, R. (1979). Structure, analysis and classification of cervical cells using a processing system based on TV. *Anal. Quant. Cytol.* **1**, 143–150.

Smith, H. S. (1979). *In vitro* properties of epithelial cell lines established from human carcinomas and non-malignant tissue. *J. Nat. Cancer Inst.* **62**, 225–230.

Sonta, S. J. and Sandberg, A. A. (1978). Chromosomes and causation of human cancer and leukaemia. XXX. Banding studies of primary intestinal tumours. *Cancer* **41**, 163–173.

Stenkvist, B., Westmann-Naeser, S., Holmquist, J., Nordin, B., Bengtsson, E., Vegelius, J., Eriksson, O. and Fox, C. (1978). Computerised nuclear morphometry as an objective method for characterizing a human cancer cell population. *Cancer Res.* **38**, 4688–4695.

Stohr, M. and Vogt Schaden, M. (1980). A new dual scanning technique for simultaneous flow cytophotometric DNA analysis of living and dead cells. In *Flow Cytometry.* IV (ed. O. D. Laerum, T. Lindmo and E. Thorud), pp. 96–99. Bergen Nor Universitets Floraget.

Stovel, R. T. and Sweet, R. G. (1979). Individual cell sorting. *J. Histochem. Cytochem.* **27**, 284–288.

Swartzendruber, D. E. (1977). A bromodeoxyuridine–mithramycin technique for detecting cycling and non-cycling cells by flow microfluorimetry. *Exp. Cell Res.* **109**, 439–443.

Traganos, F., Darzynkiewicz, Z., Sharples, T. and Melamed, M. R. (1977). Simultaneous staining of ribonucleic and deoxyribonucleic acids in unfixed cells using acridine orange in a flow cytofluorometric system. *J. Histochem. Cytochem.* **25**, 45–56.

Trent, J. M. and Salmon, S. E. (1981). Karyotype analysis of human ovarian carcinoma cells cloned in short-term agar culture. *Cancer Genet. Cytogenet.* **3**, 279–291.

Tribukait, B. and Esposti, P. (1976). Comparative cytofluorometric and cytomorphologic studies in non-neoplastic and neoplastic human urothelium. In *Pulse Cytophotometry* (Applications in cancer research and haematology with special reference to cell kinetics), 2nd Int. Symp., Nijmegen, The Netherlands (ed. W. Gohde, J. Schumann and T. L. Buchner), pp. 176–187. European Press, Ghent, Belgium.

Watson, J. V. (1980). Identification of different cell types and their separation using flow cytophotometric systems. In *Cancer Assessment and Monitoring* (ed. T. Symington, A. E. Williams and J. C. McVie), pp. 77–95. Churchill Livingstone, Edinburgh.

Wright, J. E. M. and Dendy, P. P. (1976). Identification of abnormal cells in short term monolayer cultures of human tumour specimens. *Acta Cytologica* **20**, 328–334.

4. Biochemical Methods of Tumour Cell Identification

L. A. SMETS

I. Introduction

In the past decade the concept has been established that tumour cells have accumulated a number of qualitatively different, mutation-like events (e.g. gene transpositions) affecting editing of genetic information. Tumour cells therefore do not produce new chemical entities but rather normal substances in wrong amounts or combinations, and they may even synthesize compounds normally found in cells of different developmental lineages. Biochemical identification of tumour cells should therefore not aim at unique properties since there are probably no parameters universally discriminating any tumour cell from all normal cells. However, the phenotypic schizophrenia associated with most tumour cells will possibly allow discrimination of explanted tumour cells of known pathology and clinical history from their most likely normal contaminants.

Within the scope of this book, tumour cell identification means recognition of malignant cells in short-term cultures of explanted tumours. Specific problems in this particular situation are well known: low cell numbers, loss of morphological features and of three-dimensional texture, and contamination with cells of (sometimes) unknown origin. The ideal test therefore should be accomplished in a non-destructive way at the single-cell level with high discriminative power. Methods satisfying one or more of these criteria include radioautography, radioimmune assays, fluorescence microscopy, and micro-spectrophotometry. In contrast, several detection procedures successfully applied by clinical biochemistry are not suited for the present purpose since their detection threshold is too high or the products that they measure are not permanently associated with the cell.

This chapter is meant to stimulate investigators to find solutions for tumour cell identification problems using biochemical methods. As will become apparent, there are no methods generally applicable, and consequently no easy solutions. Instead of enumerating exhaustively the many biochemical differences described between malignant and normal cells, or the parameters serving as clinical markers, a selection will be presented of biochemical properties that might serve as tools in (tumour) cell recognition at the tissue culture level.

II. Nuclear properties

A. Alterations in structure and amount of nucleic acids

According to the somatic mutation theory, alterations at the base-pair level of DNA must have occurred in all tumours. In virally transformed cells, specific DNA sequences (oncogenes) and their translation products are detectable at the single-cell level by molecular hybridization while similar observations in spontaneous tumours are now being reported (Cooper *et al.*, 1980). Thus, molecular hybridization with radioactive or fluorescent DNA probes could possibly be used as a marker of tumour cells. Until recently these methods were still too insensitive for routine application and only multiple copies of amplified genes were directly detectable by radioautography. However, improved methods can now detect single gene copies (Kirsch *et al.*, 1982). Yet, the possibility that different tumours contain different, lineage-specific oncogenes still leaves one with considerable logistical problems. Since progress in this area of molecular tumour biology is extremely fast, it is a reasonable assumption that a number of its sophisticated techniques will soon feature as routine methods.

Other candidates for tumour cell identification at the nucleic acid level could be the RNA transcripts of oncogene sequences. The technical and logistical problems in their detection are basically similar to those described for DNA sequences.

Many tumours develop chromosomal aberrations, either *ab initio* or during progressive development in the host. Chromosomal abnormalities are usually accompanied by alterations in total DNA content. Measurement of DNA content per cell can serve as a convenient and reliable parameter for the malignant origin in a rather broad range of applications as has been outlined in Chapter 3.

B. Chromatin changes

Malignant transformation involves reprogramming of chromosomal activity and hence changes in interaction between DNA and the associated proteins that regulate chromatin structure and transcriptional control. Of these, changes in the non-histone nuclear protein have been described and antisera against them have been raised (e.g. Yeoman *et al.*, 1978). Such antisera display tissue specificity and even cell specificity and are often directed against the complex of DNA and non-histones. While such antisera can probe cells at the single-cell level, they certainly are not general tumour markers. On the other hand, tissue identification by such antisera might appear sufficient for practical purposes in specialized areas.

III. Cytoplasmic changes

A. Cytoskeletal elements

The cytoskeleton is composed of microfilaments, microtubules, and intermediate-sized fragments. Gross changes in organization of the cytoskeleton are a ubiquitous accompaniment of cell transformation and could be helpful in tumour cell identification. However, the structural appearance of the cytoskeleton is highly modulated by growth conditions, degree of cell stretching, and culture history, which may compromise the validity of such assays. Apart from the structure of the cytoskeleton as a whole, the intermediate-sized fragments are composed of several specific proteins, e.g. keratin, desmin, and vimentin, which are highly tissue-specific in their distribution. Specific antisera raised against these proteins can differentiate epithelial, mesenchymal, myogenic, neural, and glial cells, and they have been successfully applied in the diagnosis of metastases from tumours with unknown primary site (Ramaekers *et al.*, 1981) as illustrated in Fig. 1. A similar application in tissue culture systems could be an elegant way of distinguishing tumour cells from the most likely contaminants.

B. Isoenzymes and hormones

Several specific changes in enzymes and hormones have been detected in body fluids of cancer patients and are clinically used as indices for tumour progression or therapeutic response. Also at the cellular level, tumour cells by virtue of their deprogramming can differ in the activity profiles of various (iso)enzymes to the extent that each individual tumour has a characteristic "enzyme signature". Modern technology allows detection of enzyme activities in samples containing as few as 50–100 cells. With a reference enzyme activity profile of the original tumour, its explanted progeny in tissue culture could be monitored by a similar set of parameters.

Of particular interest are the X-linked isoenzymes. In women, functional

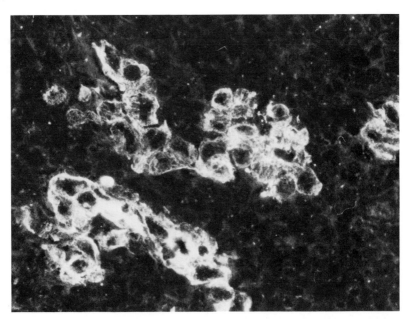

Fig. 1 Lymph node metastasis of a poorly differentiated adenocarcinoma of unknown primary site. The tumour cells have been visualized with a rabbit anti-keratin antiserum by indirect immunofluorescence. Magnification × 600 (Ramaekers *et al.*, 1981).

hemizygotism of one of the X-chromosomes is established by random inactivation of one of these chromosomes (the Barr body). Since tumours are of monoclonal origin, all cells from tumours in women who are heterozygote for a given enzyme are of either type whereas normal tissues are 50:50 mixtures of both allelic phenotypes. The best-documented example at the moment is the X-linked glucose-6-phosphate dehydrogenase isoenzymes observed in heterozygotic form in about 25% of non-caucasian women (Fialkow, 1976). The isoenzymes can be detected by gel electrophoresis, and this assay recognizes tumours as being of monoclonal origin. However, other enzyme systems may become of similar importance upon further exploration of this system.

In addition, several tumours contain increased levels of cell-bound and tissue-specific enzymes or hormones which may serve as useful markers. The terminal deoxynucleotidyl transferase in leukaemia and lymphoma, the amylase enzyme of serous ovarian carcinoma, the prolactin associated with trophoblastic tumour cells, and the S-100 protein described by Gaynor *et al.* (1981) in tissues of neural origin (e.g. melanoma), all detectable by immuno-histochemical methods, are of potential interest for small-scale application.

C. Other proteins

Apart from specific isoenzymes and altered hormone production, tumours may accumulate new proteins detectable by antisera and characterized by their apparent molecular weight on separation on gels. Such proteins may be translation products of oncogenes or derepressed foetal genes. In most cases these proteins are not functionally characterized and many of them will probably appear to be growth-associated rather than tumour-associated products.

IV. Plasma membrane and cell surface

A. Membrane fluidity

The rotation of a fluorescent probe inserted into the plasma membrane lipid bilayer causes depolarization of the emitted light. The degree of depolarization is proportional to the fluidity of the lipids into which the probe is embedded and can be measured at the single-cell level with laser-equipped detectors. Increased membrane fluidity has been forwarded as a specific accompaniment of malignant transformation. However, earlier claims on tumour specificity and on exclusive localization of the probes in the plasma membrane cannot be upheld (Collard and De Wildt, 1978). Increased fluidity probably monitors some functional property of the cellular lipids associated with growth or activated state. Since membrane fluidity is largely determined by the amount of cholesterol, a compound that equilibrates with the concentration in the serum, cells initially different in membrane fluidity tend to reach similar values upon prolonged incubation in tissue culture (Inbar *et al.*, 1977). For these reasons it is doubtful whether fluidity measurements can discriminate cells with sufficient reliability for the purposes under discussion.

B. Glycolipids

Glycolipids are integral components of the plasma membrane, extending their antigenic carbohydrate determinants into the outer phase of the cell. The relative composition as well as the expression of membrane glycolipids may change as a consequence of cell transformation (Hakamori, 1975), resulting for instance in alterations in the relative amounts of blood-group specificities or even in the appearance of new species. As with many potential markers, such changes are not always undirectional and require calibration against the original tumour for useful application in explanted tumour cells. In addition, there are technical difficulties in analysing glycolipids isolated from small numbers of cells. In view of their antigenic properties, immunological detection methods are to be preferred in this area.

C. Glycoproteins

Surface labelling of integral membrane glycoproteins and subsequent separation by gel electrophoresis can serve for the recognition of subsets of tissue types but not for safe recognition of their tumour origin. On the other hand, tumour-specific changes in the fucose-containing carbohydrate units of these membrane molecules have been described for a wide variety of tumours (Warren *et al.*, 1978). These changes are brought about by increased branching and augmented levels of terminal sialic acids, and are detected by shifts in overall size-distribution on gel filtration columns. Such shifts are largely independent of differentiation state and proliferative activity, and their presence in human cells is of demonstrated clinical relevance (Van Beek *et al.*, 1978). Accordingly, alterations in surface carbohydrates seem to fulfil many conditions for being an ideal tumour marker. Unfortunately assessment of these changes requires a few million cells and comparison with matching normal control cells. Unlike the situation with glycolipids (see above), the use of sensitive monoclonal antibodies might not be the magic formula in this situation. If the changes involve only relative amounts of certain carbohydrate classes, considerable cross-reactivity with normal cells can be expected, added to which the highly sialylated species may be non-immunogenic by nature. Accordingly, any conclusion regarding the usefulness of this intriguing change as a tumour marker awaits isolation and identification of the chemical determinants.

D. Lectins

Lectins are saccharide binding (glyco)proteins isolated from a wide variety of plants and animals. They probe the cell surface in two ways: by recognition of specific complementary sugar binding sites, and by mediating agglutination of cells in a process involving lateral movement and clustering of binding sites. Cells with similar binding properties may yet differ in agglutinability, and most transformed cells agglutinate better than corresponding untransformed counterparts. In spite of this, the agglutination response is not a good marker for tumour cells since many stimulating and inhibiting factors determine the final response (Nicolson *et al.*, 1975). Many differences may be indirectly related to tumorigenicity via differences in growth, cell density, and cell cycle distribution. A special application is the differential haemagglutination of concanavalin A coated erythrocytes to normal, preneoplastic or neoplastic mammary tumour cells (Voyles and McGrath, 1976). This method may have broader applications using erythrocytes coated with tissue-specific antibodies or lectins. The latter possibility is of increasing potential interest. Most commercial lectin preparations contain fractions that, after purification, can recognize subsets of cells, e.g. a fraction from pokeweed mitogen can distinguish monocytes from other nucleated blood cells. Visualization can be achieved at the single-cell level in a non-destructive way by haemagglutination with red blood cells coated with specific antibodies or lectin preparations.

E. Other cell surface markers

Tumour cells differ from corresponding normal cells in various other surface determinants such as receptors for hormones or growth factors and differentiation antigens (Embleton, 1983, see Chapter 5). Overlap between determinants detected by immunological methods and those revealed by functional tests or chemical analyses is to be expected, and for many determinants tumour specificity remains to be confirmed. In general, such properties are dynamic and sensitive to modulation by receptor-mediated endocytosis, growth rate, and state of differentiation. Therefore positive as well as negative findings in explanted cells should be interpreted with caution. Another trivial yet relevant notion regarding the situation in tissue culture might be that many surface properties may pass undetected as a consequence of specific binding to components already present in tissue culture medium or by mere physical covering with serum components.

V. Extracellular compounds

A. Fibronectin

Fibronectin is a high molecular weight glycoprotein, derived from the cell surface or from blood plasma, which forms part of the extracellular matrix. Many but not all transformed cells are unable to retain the fibronectin on their surface. Studies to investigate whether this deficiency also holds for tumours *in vivo*—notably metastatic tumours—have revealed that fibronectin retention is far from being a simple yes-or-no phenomenon, let alone a simple tumour marker (Yamada and Olden, 1978).

B. Plasminogen activators

Plasminogen activators (PA) are proteolytic enzymes which can convert plasminogen into its active form, plasmin. The enzyme urokinase is the activator best studied in human tissues. There are multiple forms with different molecular weights and/or immunogenic specificities (Christman, 1978). Elevated levels of PA are found in some normal tissues and in many tumours. The diversity in PA species and the existence of sensitive methods for their detection, viz. degradation of radiolabelled fibrin, plaque lysis of fibrin overlays, immunohistology, would make these molecules interesting candidates for tissue typing at the cellular or colony level. There are reports that tumours produce PA at elevated levels but in relative amounts similar to the parent normal tissue, thus offering another possibility for tissue typing.

C. Other released products

Apart from fibronectin and plasminogen activators, tumours may release several other products into the circulation with narrower specificity: acid and alkaline phosphatases, α-foetoprotein, carcinoembryonic antigens, and many others (for reviews see Ruddon, 1978; Sell, 1980; Bush and Yeoman, 1982). The production of such compounds is often a recapitulation of foetal characteristics and therefore frequently associated with tumours from the major sites of production in foetal stages. α-Foetoprotein for that reason is most frequently associated with hepatocarcinoma and with teratocarcinoma of ovary and testes. These and other products are of extreme importance in the clinical management of specific tumours. However, routine application for tissue typing in cultures has not been achieved yet, a major problem being the weak association of the product with the producer cell.

VI. Conclusions

Characterization of tumour cells in explants serves two goals. First to establish that the cells under investigation are indeed derivatives of the original tumour, but potentially also to assess effects of antitumour drugs in special cases.

For the time being, there are no (practical) biochemical procedures that, in a simple assay, can recognize the neoplastic cell in tissue culture. However, several suggestions may be found in the literature on how to recognize the histiogenetic origin of cells in mixed populations, some of them being mentioned in this chapter. As most investigators are engaged in the study of diagnostic subcategories of tumours, discrimination of, for instance, carcinoma cells from fibroblastic or endothelial contaminants is achievable by tissue typing alone. The approach that will best fit the demands of the investigator is largely dependent on the particular tumour under investigation. However, immunohistochemical characterization of cytoskeleton proteins may seem the best candidate among the methods already available.

Literature services such as the Oncology Information Service, section Tumour Markers (Medical and Dental Library, University of Leeds, U.K.), or the International Cancer Research Data Bank (U. S. Department of Health and Human Services, Philadelphia, PA, U.S.A.) can be very helpful.

Perhaps many of the answers to identification problems that have been suggested here may eventually fail for lack of specificity or for practical reasons. However, most of them are fascinating tools in tumour cell biology. As such, they may ultimately contribute, albeit along completely different routes, to the management of neoplastic diseases.

References

Bush, H. and Yeoman, L. C. (1982). *Methods in Cancer Research*, Vol. XIX. Academic Press.

Christman, J. K. (1978). Multiple forms of plasminogen activator. In *Biological Markers of Neoplasia: Basic and Applied Aspects* (ed. R. W. Ruddon), pp. 433–449. Elsevier, Amsterdam.

Collard, J. G. and De Wildt, A. (1978). Localization of the lipid probe 1,6-diphenyl-1,3,5-hexatriene (DPH) in intact cells by fluorescence microscopy. *Exp. Cell Res.* **116**, 446–450.

Cooper, G. M., Okenquist, S. and Silberman, L. (1980). Transforming activity of DNA of chemically transformed and normal cells. *Nature* **284**, 418–421.

Fialkow, P. J. (1976). Clonal origin of human tumors. *Biochim. Biophys. Acta* **458**, 283–321.

Gaynor, R., Irie, R., Herschman, H. R., Jones, P. and Cochran, A. (1981). S100 protein: a marker for human malignant melanomas? *Lancet* **1**, 869–871.

Hakamori, S. (1975). Structures and organization of cell surface glycolipids: dependency on cell growth and malignant transformation. *Biochim. Biophys. Acta* **417**, 55–89.

Inbar, M., Goldman, R., Inbar, L., Bursuker, I., Goldman, B., Akstein, E., Segal, P., Ipp, E. and Ben-Bassat, I. (1977). Fluidity differences of membrane lipids in human normal and leukemic lymphocytes as controlled by serum components. *Cancer Res.* **37**, 3037–3041.

Kirsch, I. R., Morton, C. R., Nakahara, K. and Leder, P. (1982). Human immunoglobulin heavy chain genes map to a region of translocations in malignant B lymphocytes. *Science* **216**, 303.

Nicolson, G. L., Lacorbiere, M. and Eckhart, W. (1975). Qualitative and quantitative interactions of lectins with untreated and neuraminidase-treated normal, wild-type and temperature-sensitive Polyoma-transformed fibroblasts. *Biochemistry* **13**, 196–204.

Ramaekers, F., Puts, J., Kant, A., Moesker, O., Jap, P. and Vooys, G. P. (1981). Use of antibodies to intermediate filaments in the characterization of human tumors. *Cold Spring Harbor Symp. Quant. Biol.* **46**, 331–339.

Ruddon, R. W. (ed.) (1978). *Biological Markers of Neoplasia: Basic and Applied Aspects*. Elsevier, New York.

Sell, S. (1980). *Cancer Markers: Diagnostic and Developmental Significance*. Humana Press, Clifton, New Jersey.

Van Beek, W. P., Smets, L. A., Emmelot, P., Roozendaal, K. J. and Behrendt, H. (1978). Early recognition of human leukemia by cell surface glycoprotein changes. *Leukemia Res.* **2,** 163–171.

Voyles, B. A. and McGrath, C. M. (1976). Markers to distinguish normal and neoplastic mammary epithelial cells *in vitro*: comparison of saturation density, morphology and concanavalin A reactivity. *Int. J. Cancer* **18,** 498–509.

Warren, L., Buck, C. A. and Tuszynski, G. P. (1978). Glycopeptide changes and malignant transformation: a possible role for carbohydrate in malignant behavior. *Biochim. Biophys. Acta* **516,** 97–127.

Yamada, K. M. and Olden, K. (1978). Fibronectins: adhesive glycoproteins of cell surface and blood. *Nature* **275,** 197–184.

Yeoman, L. C., Woolf, L. M., Taylor, C. W. and Busch, H. (1978). Nuclear antigens of tumor cell chromatin. In *Biological Markers of Neoplasia: Basic and Applied Aspects* (ed. R. W. Ruddon), pp. 409–416. Elsevier, New York.

5. Immunological Methods of Tumour Cell Identification (with special reference to monoclonal antibodies)

M. J. EMBLETON

I. Introduction

The concept of identifying human tumour cells by means of surface antigenic markers stems originally from the observation that artificially induced animal tumours tend to be characterized by tumour-specific antigens. These antigens are often capable of inducing tumour rejection responses in immunized syngeneic hosts, and cell surface antigens with similar specificities are demonstrable using *in vitro* assays to detect cell-mediated or humoural immune reactions to isolated tumour cells or tumour extracts. The same *in vitro* techniques applied to cultured human tumours gave results that, for a time, led to simplistic and misleading analogies. As in many other fields, there are numerous pitfalls in the transition of immunology from animal to human tumours, and it is only recently that immunological means of identifying human tumour cells have begun to be practicable.

Techniques for detecting cell-mediated immunity using effector cells from cancer patients or lymphocytes stimulated *in vitro* can be dismissed, on several counts, as wholly inappropriate for identifying tumour cells. For example, none of the various assays available allows discrimination between subpopulations of target cells, routine provision of effector cells presents logistic problems, and the principal cytotoxic cells detectable *in vitro* are natural killer (NK) cells which display no specificity with regard to tumour type. For these and other reasons immunological identification of tumour cells must rely upon the use of antibodies. The antibody sources available are sera from cancer patients, absorbed xenogeneic antisera, and monoclonal antibodies.

II. Antibody reagents

A. Cancer patient sera

Sera from cancer patients have often been reported to contain antibodies reacting preferentially with certain tumour types, this being particularly so for malignant melanoma and for sarcomas of various types. In early studies serum reactivity was apparently directed primarily towards tumours of the type borne by the serum donor, with only minimal reactivity reported towards tumours of other types and normal cells. However, more recent reports have shown that sera from cancer patients have a high frequency of reactivity for normal cells as well as tumours, and this has been variously ascribed to the presence of antibodies to blood group antigens, culture medium components, foetal antigens, and normal tissue autoantigens. To some extent these problems might be overcome by appropriate absorption (Thorpe *et al.*, 1977), but in order to obtain sera with any degree of specificity it is necessary to screen a large number against a range of known target cells and to select the small minority that show the desired pattern of reactivity (Old, 1981). This is not always practicable and in any case the available stock of useful reagent will ultimately be small. In view of these limitations and the paucity of reports of serum antibodies to tumour types other than melanoma and sarcomas, sera from cancer patients cannot be regarded as a practical source of antibodies for tumour cell typing.

B. Xenogeneic sera

Xenogeneic sera are raised, usually in rabbits but also in other foreign species, by immunizing the animal with tumour tissue or fractions. The immunized animals may be pre-tolerized to normal human tissues, or alternatively the antiserum is extensively absorbed with normal tissues to remove antibodies against antigens common to all human cells. It should be pointed out that antigens detected by such antisera are almost certainly irrelevant from the point of view of tumour immunity in humans, but they can provide important markers for tumour cells. It is difficult to prepare xenogeneic antibodies specifically against cell surface antigens associated with a particular tumour type, and absorption extensive enough to remove all unwanted antibodies can leave little or no remaining reactivity against the tumour. Conversely, it is difficult to be sure that antibodies reacting with tumour cells are completely devoid of reactivity towards any normal component. The most useful and reproducible xenogeneic antibodies have been raised against components that are common to a variety of tumour tissues and are expressed, usually at a reduced level, also on some normal tissues. Examples are antibodies to so-called oncofoetal antigens such as carcinoembryonic antigen (Gold and Freedman, 1965), and α-foetoprotein (Abelev *et al.*, 1963), and common membrane-associated antigens such as that of the milk fat globule membrane (Ceriani *et al.*, 1977). These reagents, although not necessarily tumour-specific, can be used to identify tumour cells (particularly metastases) within a mixed population of cells (De Lellis *et al.*, 1979). It is necessary with this type of reagent to be aware of the extent of reactivity of the antibody, and to design its experimental application in such a way as to avoid confusing cross-reactions (e.g. to avoid its use in tissues where it is known to react with normal cells).

C. Monoclonal antibodies

The monoclonal antibody technique was originally devised by Kohler and Milstein (1975) and has been described in detail elsewhere (Goding, 1980). Basically, mature B lymphocytes are fused with cells of a cultured myeloma using polyethylene glycol to promote fusion. This results in megakaryons, a large number of which are hybrids of both cell types. These inherit the growth potential of the myeloma and the antibody specificity of the B lymphocytes. The myelomas used are biochemically deficient mutants and B lymphocytes do not survive and grow in culture, so the use of selective media ensures growth only of hybrid cells (termed hybridomas). Some of the hybridomas have the ability to secrete immunoglobulins of the parental B cells, thus immortalizing the production of certain antibodies. These are identified by screening against appropriate target antigens, and a chosen hybridoma is cloned, either in soft agar or by limiting dilution, to derive cell lines producing monoclonal antibodies.

The myelomas currently available are derived from mouse, rat, and man, and the relevant sources of B lymphocytes are spleen cells from mice or rats immunized against human tumours, or lymphocytes from human cancer patients, respectively. It is possible to produce interspecies hybridomas, but these tend to be less stable chromosomally than hybridomas produced within a single species and are prone to die out or to lose the ability to secrete antibody. For the study of human tumours the two principal avenues of choice are to use human hybridomas which presumably react against antigens recognized as foreign by the cancer host (which could either be tumour-associated antigens or autoantigens), or murine hybridomas which react against a wide range of human cell components. By screening against a panel of normal and tumour targets it is possible to eliminate hybridomas of unwanted specificity, and by this means many murine monoclonal antibodies with exquisitely defined specificity have been derived. One point to bear in mind is that monoclonal antibodies are specific only for epitopes, not for whole molecules or given cell types, so the sole fact that an antibody is monoclonal does not mean that it will not be cross-reactive when tested against cells from different tissues. The limits of specificity are readily determined, however, and murine monoclonal antibodies offer the best possible means of immunologically identifying human tumour cells.

III. Reactions of monoclonal antibodies against human cell surface antigens

A. Tumour-associated antigens

Malignant melanoma has received the most attention, and a number of groups have reported production of monoclonal antibodies to cultured melanoma cell lines (Koprowski et al., 1978; Yeh et al., 1979; Carrel et al., 1980; Old, 1981). In these reports, some monoclonal antibodies reacted only with the melanoma line used to immunize the murine spleen donor, but others reacted with antigens common to a number of melanomas. Reactivity with normal cells and other tumours was variable for different hybridomas, but all groups identified several antibodies that were apparently specific for cultured melanoma cells and did not cross-react with other cultured cell lines. Later investigations have extended these observations to show that some antibodies also recognize antigens on melanoma cells freshly obtained from surgical specimens thereby excluding culture artefacts (Steplewski et al., 1979). In some cases, however, it has been shown that monoclonal antibody-defined antigens that were hitherto believed to be melanoma-specific are also shared (albeit often at a low level) by some normal cells (Brown et al., 1980; Imai et al., 1982). Of particular interest is the finding that some melanoma antigens are shared by neural tumours such as neuroblastoma and glioma, since melanocytes are of neural crest origin (Old, 1981). This indicates that antitumour monoclonal antibodies can be useful in delineating differentiation antigens that are of significance in ontogeny.

Another tumour against which apparently specific monoclonal antibodies have been produced is colorectal carcinoma. Thus Herlyn et al. (1979) made murine monoclonal antibodies against colorectal carcinoma cell lines which reacted with both cultured and freshly prepared colorectal carcinoma cells, but not with normal colonic mucosa, leucocytes, or embryonic cells, or cultured tumour cells of various types. Some antibodies reacted with carcinoembryonic antigen (CEA), but in most cases the colorectal carcinoma antigens detected were distinct from CEA (Steplewski, 1980).

Monoclonal antibodies have been prepared against a variety of other human tumours, but with generally less evidence of specificity towards the particular tumour type. Antibodies to breast carcinomas, for example, showed preferential binding to breast carcinomas compared with normal breast and other normal tissues, but reacted also with benign breast tumours and adenocarcinomas of other organs (Colcher et al., 1981; Nuti et al., 1982). One of these antibodies was referred to as a "pan-carcinoma" reagent (Colcher et al., 1981). Similarly, a monoclonal antibody raised against a cell line derived from small cell carcinoma of the lung reacted against various types of lung carcinoma in preference to normal lung and other tissues, but bound also to neuroblastoma and breast carcinoma cell lines (Cuttitta et al., 1981). It was negative, however, for a range of other human tumour lines. An anti-neuroblastoma monoclonal antibody originally reported to be specific for neural tumours (neuroblastomas, retinoblastoma, and glioma) and foetal brain (Kennet and Gilbert, 1979) was subsequently found to bind to acute lymphoblastic leukaemia and normal B lineage cells (Greaves et al., 1980).

A number of murine anti-sarcoma monoclonal antibodies have been reported, sometimes showing specificity restricted to the immunizing tumour type. For example, Deng et al. (1981) produced a monoclonal antibody to freshly isolated leiomyosarcoma cells, which did not react with a variety of fresh normal cells or cultured tumours. Anti-osteogenic sarcoma antibodies, again raised against fresh tumour, also showed preferential reactivity for sarcoma tissue (osteogenic sarcoma and chondrosarcoma) although they also bound weakly to apparently normal chondrocytes (Hosoi et al., 1982). However, two monoclonal antibodies raised against a cultured osteogenic sarcoma cell line (791T) were less restricted in their activities (Embleton et al., 1981a,b). One of these antibodies (791T/36) reacted with 7 of 13 osteogenic sarcoma lines but was negative for 10 fibroblast lines, including 3 derived from the donor of sarcoma line 791T. This antibody was not specific for osteogenic sarcoma, however, since it reacted also with 5 of 25 unrelated tumour cell lines (carcinomas of lung, prostate, cervix, and colon).

Monoclonal antibodies that are apparently specific for tumours of a single type are particularly useful for positive identification of that tumour type. However, for the purposes of general discrimination between tumour and normal cells it might be better to use one of the less restricted "pan-tumour" reagents described above. Perhaps the most impressive monoclonal antibody of this type is one recently reported by Ashall et al. (1982). This antibody, designated Ca1, was raised by fusing mouse myeloma cells with spleen cells from a mouse immunized against the cultured laryngeal carcinoma cell line

H.Ep.2. It was screened against a series of hybrids prepared from a human cervical carcinoma and diploid fibroblasts, some of which were malignant in character and some of which were not. The Ca1 antibody bound only to the malignant hybrids, and it was also found to bind to a high proportion of human tumour cell lines, but not to normal cells. In a companion paper, McGee *et al.* (1982) showed by immunohistochemistry that the antibody reacted with sections of most malignant tumours, but not benign tumours or normal tissues. Since this technique avoided possible artefacts of culture, the authors have suggested that the antibody may be useful in diagnosis of cancer in biopsies or cytological smears.

B. Normal differentiation antigens

Antibodies to normal differentiation antigens may be useful in the identification of tumour cells on several counts. First, some tumours may express antigens that are abnormal within the context of their tissue of origin although they may be normal antigens with respect to differentiated tissue elsewhere in the body; second, some tumours may lose expression of a normal differentiation antigen characteristic of the normal tissue from which they arose; third, antibodies to differentiation antigens marking different stages of ontogeny may be capable of identifying tumour cells that have undergone some degree of de-differentiation or for some other reason express antigens normally expressed on immature cells of the same lineage.

Probably the best-studied differentiation antigens are those of lymphoid and related cells, particularly T and B lymphocytes. One of the most widely used series of monoclonal antibodies to T cell markers is the OKT series developed by Schlossman's group (Kung *et al.*, 1979; Reinherz *et al.*, 1980). This group have also developed a monoclonal antibody designated OM1, which is specific for monocytes (Breard *et al.*, 1980), and others have prepared monoclonal antibodies that detect B cells (Trucco *et al.*, 1978). Markers such as these are particularly valuable in determining functions of lymphocyte subsets, and in the analysis of stem cells and leukaemias, which has already provided valuable information on the origin and classification of leukaemias (Greaves and Janossy, 1978; Greaves *et al.*, 1980). In some cases, lymphocyte markers may be of use in distinguishing cells other than lymphocytes or leukaemias. This is particularly the case with DR (Ia-like) antigens which are markers of normal B cells and monocytes. DR antigens are often expressed on malignant melanoma cells and could perhaps be used in the identification of this tumour in biopsies or cultures. At one time it was believed that other human solid tumours might express abnormal amounts of DR antigen, but it now seems that this is a property particularly characteristic of melanomas (Old, 1981; Howe *et al.*, 1981).

Inappropriately expressed blood group antigens may also be diagnostic of tumour cells. For example, many colorectal and stomach carcinomas express blood group antigens, and several monoclonal antibodies to colorectal carcinomas have been identified as reacting towards these antigens. Koprowski's group have described two anti-colon carcinoma antibodies reacting with Lewis[a] and Lewis[b] structures (Brockhaus et al., 1981; Koprowski et al., 1982). Similarly, an anti-teratoma monoclonal antibody has been shown to recognize a stage-specific embryonic antigen that is an isomer of the Lewis[a] structure (Gooi et al., 1981).

Markers of normal adult cells are potentially of use in identifying tumours that lack normal antigen expression. Examples of monoclonal antibodies to normal antigens are those that identify differentiated fibroblasts, liver and kidney cells. Edwards et al. (1980b) have reported the production of monoclonal antibodies to human breast fibroblasts, and have shown by autoradiography that these antibodies bind to fibroblasts in tissue sections, but very little binding occurred to epithelial cells. One of the anti-fibroblast antibodies has also been used to suppress growth of fibroblasts in primary cultures of human squamous carcinoma (Edwards et al., 1980a).

In some cases tumours lose the expression of an antigen expressed by the tissue of origin, and this has been detected by the use of monoclonal antibodies in at least two instances. Fossati et al. (1982) have reported production of monoclonal antibodies to renal carcinoma and normal kidney, and have shown that antibody specific for normal renal tissue did not react with renal carcinomas. In another study, Holmes et al. (1982) prepared monoclonal antibodies to adult rat hepatocytes and showed that the antigens detected were not expressed by hepatomas or preneoplastic lesions induced by liver carcinogens. Although raised against rat hepatocytes, one antibody was found to react also with human hepatocytes but not with human hepatoma tissue (Holmes et al., 1983), and it has been used to demonstrate metastatic foci of other tumours within the liver.

Finally, there are antibodies that recognize a general cell type or product rather than cells of a specific tissue. The prime example is the use of polyclonal and monoclonal antibodies to milk fat globule membrane (also known as epithelial membrane antigen) prepared from delipidated human milk. These antibodies bind to breast epithelial cells, as expected, but also bind to epithelial cells of other organs showing glandular differentiation (Arklie et al., 1981; Foster et al., 1982). They also react with adenocarcinomas and have been used to demonstrate metastatic cells in non-glandular tissues in a diagnostic context. Cell products that can be detected by antibodies and may have diagnostic potential also include hormones (e.g. chorionic gonadotrophin), and a comprehensive list of these is given in a workshop report by De Lellis et al. (1979).

IV. Techniques for identifying tumour cells

A. Biopsy specimens

There are many ways of demonstrating reactions between intact cells and antibodies. Some of these, for example complement-dependent cytotoxicity and antiglobulin binding assays, are applicable primarily to homogeneous cell populations. For identification of cells in biopsy specimens, techniques are needed that can identify subpopulations within a mass of tissue. The best methods for this are immunofluorescence and immunohistochemistry, which can be carried out both on tissue sections and on cell smears.

When using solid biopsies it is important to consider that many of the antigenic components recognized by antibodies may be destroyed by fixation or by dehydration and wax-embedding, so it is necessary initially to use cryostat sections. However, after establishing the utility of a particular antibody on frozen sections, it may be worth comparing its activity on fixed paraffin sections of the same tissue because, if the antigen is stable to this treatment, paraffin sections give a clearer picture of cell morphology than the thicker cryostat sections.

Immunofluorescence techniques suitable for frozen tissue sections are fully discussed by Nairn (1976) and Table 1 gives a brief indication of the procedure and reagents needed. The principal disadvantages of immunofluorescence are the need for a specialized fluorescence microscope and the non-permanent nature of the stained specimens, but in general it is a rapid and simple technique. Immunohistochemical techniques rely essentially on the conversion of a substrate into a coloured product by the action of an enzyme, and this requires a little more expertise. However, no specialist equipment is needed and permanent preparations are obtained. The most widely used enzyme and substrate are peroxidase and hydrogen peroxide/diaminobenzidine. There are two basic methods of applying this system, by using a complex of peroxidase and antiperoxidase antiserum (PAP), or by using a biotin-labelled antibody and biotin-labelled peroxidase complexed with avidin (ABC). PAP procedures are described by De Lellis et al. (1979) and Holmes et al. (1982), and the ABC method is described by Hsu et al. (1981). The basic processes (for murine monoclonal antibodies) are also outlined in Table 1. Immunoperoxidase sections treated with hydrogen peroxide and diaminobenzidine display deposition of brown pigment in areas to which the primary antibody has bound, and following counterstaining (e.g. with haematoxylin) they give excellent visualization of individual antigen-positive cells. Other immunohistochemical staining techniques are available, and Foster et al. (1982) have described one using alkaline phosphatase.

Table 1 Some methods to detect reactivity of murine monoclonal antibodies against human cells and tissues.

Immunofluorescence	Immunoperoxidase staining		Radioisotopic antiglobulin binding
	PAP	ABC	
Test material			
Frozen sections, smears, monolayers and cell suspensions	Frozen sections, smears and monolayers	Frozen sections, smears and monolayers	Cell suspensions
Application of reagents			
1. Primary monoclonal antibody	Primary monoclonal antibody	Primary monoclonal antibody	Primary monoclonal antibody
2. Fluorescein isothiocyanate conjugated rabbit anti-mouse Ig	Rabbit anti-mouse Ig	Rabbit anti-mouse Ig	^{125}I-Labelled rabbit anti-mouse Ig
3. —	Swine anti-rabbit Ig	Biotin-labelled swine anti-rabbit Ig	—
4. —	PAP complex (peroxidase/rabbit anti-peroxidase)	ABC complex (avidin/biotin-peroxidase)	—
5. —	Diaminoben-zidine–H_2O_2 reaction	Diamino-benzidine–H_2O_2 reaction	—
Examination			
Fluorescence microscope	Counterstain; conventional microscope	Counterstain; conventional microscope	Gamma spectrometer

This table briefly summarizes the principal steps and reagents in four techniques for detecting cells reacting with monoclonal antibodies. The types of specimen suitable for use with each technique are indicated as "Test material" and the immunochemical reagents required are listed in their order of application to the specimen. The specimen is incubated for varying periods of time with each reagent in turn, with intermediate washes at each step to remove any excess. Final examination of the specimen or measurement of antibody binding in some cases requires specialized equipment as indicated in "Examination". Immunoperoxidase-stained sections should be counter-stained with haematoxylin to aid visualization of unreactive cells. The table is intended for guidance only, and further details and protocols for the listed techniques are given in the following references: Nairn, 1976 (immunofluorescence); DeLellis et al., 1979 (PAP immunoperoxidase); Hsu et al., 1981a (ABC immunoperoxidase); Embleton et al., 1981a (isotopic protein A or anti-Ig assay).

B. Cell cultures

Identification of tumour cells in mixed cultures is best accomplished using immunofluorescence or immunoperoxidase staining, by which it is possible to examine cells on an individual basis. Cells for this purpose may be smeared onto slides or grown as monolayers on glass coverslips, and the staining procedure is the same as that used for tissue sections. Usually some kind of mild fixation is required for smears or monolayers (to prevent cell loss), and here it is necessary to determine empirically which fixatives do or do not destroy antigenicity.

To confirm the identity of established cultures known to be homogeneous it is possible to use isotopically labelled antiglobulin or *Staph. aureus* protein A binding assays (Embleton *et al.*, 1981a) which can be employed either on adherent or suspended target cells (the procedure for this type of assay is outlined in Table 1). Autoradiographic visualization of labelled cells may also allow use of radiolabelled antibodies in identification of cells in mixed cultures, but the time required for development renders this less practical than immunofluorescence or immunoperoxidase methods.

V. Cell separation and enrichment

Apart from visual identification of tumour cells in biopsies and cell cultures, bound antibodies can be used in the separation of different cell populations. Perhaps the most elegant way of sorting antibody-labelled cells is by using a fluorescence-activated cell sorter (FACS). This instrument, combined with appropriate fluorescent antibody staining, allows a precise analysis of mixed cell populations (Greaves and Janossy, 1978) and has been used to separate normal hepatocytes from hepatoma cells in a rat system (Holmes *et al.*, 1982). However, such sophisticated equipment is not readily available to everyone, and there are two alternative published methods of cell enrichment.

One possibility is to use cytotoxic antibodies in the presence of added complement to deplete mixed cells of a specific subpopulation. Edwards *et al.* (1980a) have used a monoclonal antibody to fibroblasts, together with complement, to deplete primary human squamous carcinoma cell cultures of fibroblasts, thereby promoting growth of epithelioid cells. However, this approach is not universally applicable since not all monoclonal antibodies can fix complement and mediate cell lysis. The other possibility is to use a sheep red blood cell (SRBC) rosetting technique to deplete or enrich mixed cells with respect to a specific subpopulation. This technique has been described in detail (Parish and Hayward, 1974) and can be summarized as follows. Cells are incubated first with antibody, then with SRBC coated with antiglobulin. The

SRBC form rosettes around cells bearing the bound primary antibody, and the rosettes and free SRBC are removed by centrifugation over a Ficoll–sodium metrizoate (or similar) gradient. Cells freed of rosettes (and thus of antigen-positive cells) can be harvested from the interface between the supernatant medium and the gradient, and considerable purification can be achieved by this form of negative selection. Alternatively, if the antigen-positive cells are required they can be recovered from the bottom of the gradient and the SRBC can be lysed by brief exposure to ammonium chloride or hypotonic lysis, which does not harm nucleated cells if properly performed.

VI. Concluding comments

It is readily apparent that monoclonal antibodies offer the best means of identifying human tumour cells by immunological methods. Some are specific for particular tumour types so far as can be determined, hence a positive reaction can be taken as a probable positive identification. Others which are not specific for individual tumour types may nevertheless react preferentially against tumour cells rather than normal cells. This is probably an adequate distinction in most instances, and in appropriate circumstances monoclonal antibodies to normal differentiation antigens can also lead to identification of tumour cells. It is already possible therefore to identify human tumours with a high degree of certainty using panels of existing monoclonal antibodies. (It should be emphasized that panels of antibodies give much more reliable identification than single antibodies.)

Production of monoclonal antibodies is time-consuming and labour-intensive, and should not be undertaken lightly by the inexperienced. Those wishing to pursue use of monoclonal antibodies without already having the capability of producing them would therefore be best advised to obtain them from other sources. Increasing numbers of monoclonal antibodies are becoming commercially available and, bearing in mind that this trend is still relatively in its infancy, it is reasonable to predict that panels of suitable reagents will become widely available in the near future. Immunological identification of human tumours will then be practicable for any laboratory equipped for standard serological assays.

References

Abelev, G. I., Parova, S. D., Kramkova, N. I., Postrikova, Z. A. and Irlin, I. S. (1963). Production of embryonal α-globulin by transplantable mouse hepatomas. *Transplantation* **1,** 174–180.

Arklie, J., Taylor-Papadimitriou, J., Bodmer, W., Egan, M. and Millis, R. (1981). Differentiation antigens expressed by epithelial cells in the lactating breast are also detectable in breast cancers. *Int. J. Cancer* **28**, 23–29.

Ashall, F., Bramwell, M. E. and Harris, H. (1982). A new marker for human cancer cells. 1. The Ca antigen and the Ca1 antibody. *Lancet* **ii**, 1–6.

Breard, J., Reinherz, E. L., Kung, P. C., Goldstein, G. and Schlossman, S. F. (1980). A monoclonal antibody reactive with human peripheral blood monocytes. *J. Immunol.* **124**, 1943–1948.

Brockhaus, M., Magnani, J., Blaszczyk, M., Steplewski, Z., Koprowski, H., Karlsson, K., Larson, G. and Ginsburg, V. (1981). Monoclonal antibodies directed against the human Le^b blood group antigen. *J. Biol. Chem.* **256**, 13223–13225.

Brown, J. P., Wright, P. W., Hart, C. E., Woodbury, R. G., Hellstrom, K. E. and Hellstrom, I. (1980). Protein antigens of normal and malignant human cells identified by immunoprecipitation with monoclonal antibodies. *J. Biol. Chem.* **255**, 4980–4983.

Carrel, S., Accolla, R. S., Carmagnola, A. L. and Mach, J.-P. (1980). Common human melanoma-associated antigen(s) detected by monoclonal antibodies. *Cancer Res.* **40**, 2523–2528.

Ceriani, R. L., Thomson, K., Peterson, J. A. and Abraham, S. (1977). Surface differentiation antigens of human mammary epithelial cells carried on the human milk fat globule. *Proc. Nat. Acad. Sci.* **74**, 582–586.

Colcher, D., Hand, P. H., Nuti, M. and Schlom, J. (1981). A spectrum of monoclonal antibodies reactive with human mammary tumor cells. *Proc. Nat. Acad. Sci.* **78**, 3199–3203.

Cuttitta, F., Rosen, S., Gazdar, A. F. and Minna, J. D. (1981). Monoclonal antibodies that demonstrate specificity for several types of human lung cancer. *Proc. Nat. Acad. Sci.* **78**, 4591–4595.

De Lellis, R. A., Sternberger, L. A., Mann, R. B., Banks, P. M. and Nakane, P. K. (1979). Immunoperoxidase techniques in diagnostic pathology. *Am. J. Clin. Path.* **71**, 483–488.

Deng, C., Terasaki, P. I., El-Awar, N., Billing, R., Cicciarelli, J. and Lagrasse, L. (1981). Cytotoxic monoclonal antibody to a human leiomyosarcoma. *Lancet* **ii**, 403–405.

Edwards, P. A., Easty, D. M. and Foster, C. S. (1980a). Selective culture of epithelioid cells from a human squamous carcinoma using a monoclonal antibody to kill fibroblasts. *Cell. Biol. Int. Rep.* **4**, 917–922.

Edwards, P. A., Foster, C. S. and McIllhinney, R. A. (1980b). Monoclonal antibodies to teratomas and breast. *Transplant. Proc.* **12**, 398–402.

Embleton, M. J., Gun, B., Byers, V. S. and Baldwin, R. W. (1981a). Anti-tumour reactions of monoclonal antibody against a human osteogenic sarcoma cell line. *Br. J. Cancer* **43**, 582–587.

Embleton, M. J., Gunn, B., Byers, V. S. and Baldwin, R. W. (1981b). Antigens on naturally-occurring animal and human tumors defined by monoclonal antibodies. *Transplant. Proc.* **13**, 1966–1969.

Fossati, G., Canevari, S., Balsari, A., Menard, S., Tagliabue, E. and Colnaghi, M. I. (1982). Generation of murine monoclonal antibodies to human kidney. In *Tumour Progression and Markers* (ed. K. Lapis, A. Jeney and M. R. Price), pp. 411–413. Kugler, Amsterdam.

Foster, C. S., Edwards, P. A. W., Dinsdale, E. and Neville, A. M. (1982). Monoclonal antibodies to the human mammary gland. I. Distribution in non-neoplastic mammary and extra-mammary tissues. *Virchows Arch. (Pathol. Anat.)* **394**, 279–293.

Goding, J. W. (1980). Antibody production by hybridomas. *J. Immunol. Methods* **39**, 285–308.

Gold, P. and Freedman, S. O. (1965). Specific carcinoembryonic antigens of the human digestive system. *J. Exp. Med.* **122**, 467–481.

Gooi, H., Feizi, T., Kopaida, A., Knowles, B., Salter, D. and Evans, H. (1981). Stage-specific embryonic antigen involves $\alpha 1 \rightarrow 3$ fucosylated type 2 blood group chains. *Nature* **292**, 156–158.

Greaves, M. F. and Janossy, G. (1978). Patterns of gene expression and the cellular origins of human leukaemias. *Biochim. Biophys. Acta* **516**, 193–230.

Greaves, M. F., Verbi, W., Kemshead, J. and Kennet, R. (1980). A monoclonal antibody identifying a cell surface antigen shared by common acute lymphoblastic leukemias and B lineage cells. *Blood* **56**, 1141–1144.

Herlyn, M., Steplewski, Z., Herlyn, D. and Koprowski, H. (1979). Colorectal carcinoma-specific antigen: detection by means of monoclonal antibodies. *Proc. Nat. Acad. Sci.* **75**, 1438–1442.

Holmes, C. H., Gunn, B., Austin, E. B., Embleton, M. J. and Baldwin, R. W. (1982). Expression of a monoclonal antibody-defined liver-associated antigen in normal rat hepatocytes and hepatocellular carcinoma cells. *Int. J. Cancer* **29**, 559–565.

Holmes, C. H., Hawkey, C. J., Gunn, B., Austin, E. B., Fisk, A., Smith, P. G., Embleton, M. J., Baldwin, R. W. and Toghill, P. J. (1983). A monoclonal antibody reactive with human hepatocytes. *Liver* (in the press).

Hosoi, S., Nakamura, T., Higashi, S., Yamamuro, T., Toyama, S., Shinomiya, K. and Mikawa, H. (1982). Detection of human osteosarcoma-associated antigen(s) by monoclonal antibodies. *Cancer Res.* **42**, 654–659.

Howe, A. J., Seeger, R. C., Molinaro, G. A. and Ferrone, S. (1981). Analysis of human tumor cells for Ia-like antigens with monoclonal antibodies. *J. Nat. Cancer Inst.* **66**, 827–829.

Hsu, S. M., Raine, L. and Fanger, H. (1981). Use of avidin–biotin–peroxidase complex (ABC) in immunoperoxidase techniques. *J. Histochem. Cytochem.* **29**, 577–580.

Imai, K., Natali, P. G., Kay, N. E., Wilson, B. S. and Ferrone, S. (1982). Tissue distribution and molecular profile of a differentiation antigen detected by a monoclonal antibody (345.134S) produced against human melanoma cells. *Cancer Immunol. Immunother.* **12**, 159–166.

Kennet, R. H. and Gilbert, F. (1979). Hybrid myelomas producing antibodies against a human neuroblastoma antigen present on fetal brain. *Science* **203**, 1120–1121.

Kohler, G. and Milstein, C. (1975). Derivation of specific antibody-producing tissue culture and tumor lines by cell fusion. *Eur. J. Immunol.* **6**, 511–519.

Koprowski, H., Steplewski, Z. and Herlyn, D. (1978). Study of antibodies against human melanoma produced by somatic cell hybrids. *Proc. Nat. Acad. Sci.* **75**, 3405–3409.

Koprowski, H., Brockhaus, M., Blaszczyk, M., Magnani, J., Steplewski, Z. and Ginsburg, V. (1982). Lewis blood-type may affect the incidence of gastrointestinal cancer. *Lancet* **ii**, 1332–1333.

Kung, P. C., Goldstein, G., Reinherz, E. L. and Schlossman, S. F. (1979). Monoclonal antibodies defining distinctive human T cell surface antigens. *Science* **206**, 347–349.

McGee, J. O'D., Woods, J. C., Ashall, F., Bramwell, M. E. and Harris, H. (1982). A new marker for human cancer cells. 2. Immunohistochemical detection of the Ca antigen in human tissues with the Ca1 antibody. *Lancet* **ii**, 7–11.

Nairn, R. C. (1976). *Fluorescent Protein Tracing*, 4th edn. Churchill Livingstone, Edinburgh.

Nuti, M., Teramoto, Y. A., Mariani-Constantini, R., Horan Hand, P., Colcher, D. and Schlom, J. (1982). A monoclonal antibody (B72.3) defines patterns of distribution of a novel tumor associated antigen in human mammary carcinoma cell populations. *Int. J. Cancer* **29**, 539–545.

Old, L. J. (1981). Cancer immunology: search for specificity. Clowes Memorial Lecture. *Cancer Res.* **41**, 361–375.

Parish, C. and Hayward, J. (1974). The lymphocyte surface. I. Relation between F_c receptors, $C^1 3$ receptors and surface immunoglobulin. *Proc. Roy. Soc.* **B187**, 47–63.

Reinherz, E. L., Moretta, L., Roper, M., Breard, J. M., Mingari, M. C., Cooper, M. D. and Schlossman, S. F. (1980). Human T lymphocyte subpopulations defined by F_c receptors and monoclonal antibodies. *J. Exp. Med.* **151**, 969–974.

Steplewski, Z. (1980). Monoclonal antibodies to human tumor antigens. *Transplant. Proc.* **12**, 384–387.

Steplewski, Z., Herlyn, M., Herlyn, D., Clark, W. H. and Koprowski, H. (1979). Reactivity of monoclonal anti-melanoma antibodies with melanoma cells freshly isolated from primary and metastatic melanoma. *Eur. J. Immunol.* **9**, 94–96.

Thorpe, W. P., Parker, G. A. and Rosenburg, S. A. (1977). Expression of fetal antigens by normal human skin cells grown in tissue culture. *J. Immunol.* **119**, 818–823.

Trucco, M. M., Stocker, J. W. and Ceppellini, R. (1978). Monoclonal antibodies against human lymphocyte antigens. *Nature* **273**, 666–668.

Yeh, M.-Y., Hellstrom, I., Brown, J. P., Warner, G. A., Hansen, J. A. and Hellstrom, K. E. (1979). Cell surface antigens of human melanoma identified by monoclonal antibody. *Proc. Nat. Acad. Sci.* **76**, 2927–2931.

Part II
Tumour Cell Growth for Drug Sensitivity Measurements

6. Short Term Assay Using Radioactive Nucleic Acid Precursors

J. MATTERN, M. KAUFMANN and M. VOLM

I. Introduction

Although the statistical probability of successful treatment is now known from clinical studies for large groups of patients, the response of the individual patient remains uncertain. Certain conclusions regarding the sensitivity of a given tumour to a specific antitumour agent can be reached from histopathology by determining the degree of proliferation and the degree of cellular differentiation. However, the response of tumours is not governed solely by specific histopathologic criteria. Frequently chemotherapy is initiated but has to be discontinued several weeks later because the drug proves to be ineffective. In addition to the loss in time, the patient is subjected unnecessarily to the side effects of chemotherapeutic agents.

During the past three decades various procedures have been used to test the sensitivity of tumour cells to antitumour drugs prior to therapy. A number of methods use fresh tumour material and can be carried out in a few hours (Bickis *et al.*, 1966; Kummer, 1970; Volm *et al.*, 1970, 1979; Wüst and Matthes, 1970; Possinger *et al.*, 1980). Others require culturing of the tumour cells for 1–3 days (Wright *et al.*, 1957; Limburg and Krahe, 1964; Tanneberger and Bacigalupo, 1970; Dendy *et al.*, 1973; Holmes and Little, 1974; Ebeling and Spitzbart, 1977), or require 2–4 weeks (Hamburger *et al.*, 1978; Salmon *et al.*, 1978; Meyskens *et al.*, 1981; Von Hoff *et al.*, 1981), or even 2–3 months (Fujita *et al.*, 1980; Shorthouse *et al.*, 1980). However, none of the test methods described has acquired widespread clinical use, although certain procedures have achieved clinical importance in some centres (Limburg and Krahe, 1964; Tanneberger and Bacigalupo, 1970; Salmon *et al.*, 1978; Volm *et al.*, 1979).

Our own research group has described a simple *in vitro* test in which a cell suspension is prepared from tumours, and the uptake of radioactive nucleic acid precursors into the cells is determined after addition of the drugs. During

10 years' experience this test has shown good reproducibility and predictive value in animal tumours (Volm *et al.*, 1974, 1975a) as well as in various human tumours (Mattern *et al.*, 1976; Volm *et al.*, 1979; KSST, 1981).

II. Short-term test methodology

Tumour material freed from fat, muscle, and necrotic parts is placed in a plastic Petri dish and cut into small pieces with scissors under sterile conditions. Tissue pieces are suspended in Hanks balanced salt solution (HBSS), pipetted several times using a sharp-edged glass pipette, and the resultant cell suspension is filtered through gauze (pore size 200 μm). Cells are collected in culture tubes, centrifuged for 5 min at 200 g, and washed with HBSS. After centrifugation the HBSS is decanted and the pellet resuspended in tissue culture medium (TCM) 199. The cell count is adjusted to 500 000 cells ml^{-1} using a Neubauer counting chamber. With non-sterile tumours, a broad spectrum antibiotic such as streptomycin/penicillin is added to the cell suspension. Cells are then distributed into test tubes in aliquots of 0.9 ml. After pre-incubation at 37°C for 15 min in a shaking water bath, the chemotherapeutic agents are added to the cell suspensions in 50 μl aliquots per test tube.

The agents that are suitable for investigation *in vitro* in this short-term test are listed in Table 1. Drugs are dissolved in TCM 199 and are usually tested over a 4 × log concentration range. After incubation for 2 h, the appropriate radioactive nucleic acid precursors are pipetted into the test tubes (2.5 μCi ml^{-1} cell suspension) and incubation is continued for 1 h. At the end of incubation 100 μl aliquots are pipetted from each test tube onto round filter papers and dried in a stream of warm air for 1 min. The non-incorporated radioactivity is extracted with ice-cold 5% trichloroacetic acid (TCA) twice for 30 min (100 filters to 1 l TCA). The filters are then washed in ethanol–ether (1 : 2) for 20 min, ether for 10 min, and air-dried. Scintillation fluid (5 ml) is added to each filter in a vial and the incorporated radioactivity (counts min^{-1}) is determined by liquid scintillation counting. Uptake values for the individual concentrations are expressed as percentages of controls.

III. Results

A. Detection of acquired resistance and cross-resistance

Clinical experience shows that many previously sensitive tumours become resistant during treatment. In order to determine whether acquired resistance

Table 1   Radioactive precursor and dose range for various agents in the *in vitro* short-term test.

Agent	Nucleic acid precursor			Dose range *in vitro* for 3 h incubation (μg ml^{-1} medium)
	TdR	UdR	dUdR	
Alkylating agents				
Trenimon	●	●		0.05–0.5
Cyclophosphamide:				
Metabolite urine	●	●		Dil. 1 : 2–1 : 64
4-Hydroperoxy-CTX	●	●		0.1–100
Antibiotics				
Adriamycin	●	●		0.1–100
Daunorubicin	●	●		0.1–100
Actinomycin D		●		0.1–100
Antimetabolites				
Methotrexate			●	0.01–10
5-Fluorouracil			●	0.1–100
Ftorafur			●	100–10 000
Miscellaneous				
Hydroxyurea	●			1–10
Procarbazine	●			10–300
Cis-platinum		●		0.5–500

TdR = ^{3}H-thymidine; UdR = ^{3}H-uridine; dUdR = ^{3}H-deoxyuridine; CTX = cyclophosphamide.

is detectable by means of this *in vitro* short-term test, we have developed animal tumour cell lines that are resistant to cyclophosphamide (Volm *et al.*, 1977), adriamycin (Volm and Lindner, 1978), cytosine arabinoside (ara-C) (Volm *et al.*, 1980), and daunomycin (Volm *et al.*, 1981). After treatment of the cell lines with drugs over many passages, resistance to the appropriate drug could be observed and was detectable both in animal experiments and in the short-term *in vitro* test.

The possibility that adriamycin-resistant tumour cells had developed cross-resistance to other cytostatics was also investigated using the short-term test. This might be expected with the structurally similar daunomycin. It was observed that the short-term test did indeed detect cross-resistance to daunomycin in adriamycin-resistant cells, whereas no resistance was detected against cyclophosphamide and methotrexate. Results of these short-term tests were confirmed in animal experiments which demonstrated that adriamycin-resistant tumour cells were insensitive to treatment *in vivo* with daunomycin, but not to treatment with the other two agents (Volm *et al.*, 1979).

An attempt was also made to follow the development of resistance with time by means of the short-term test. For example, when trying to induce ara-C resistance, cells of the original tumour and of the ara-C-pretreated line were incubated *in vitro* in short-term tests. Results of this investigation for an *in vitro* dose level of 3 μg ml^{-1} ara-C are shown in Fig. 1. Thymidine incorporation in both untreated and pretreated tumour cells was inhibited by this concentration of ara-C until the 9th passage, but thymidine incorporation subsequently increased in the pretreated tumour cells until by the 15th passage they showed no further reaction to treatment with 3 μg ml^{-1} ara-C. It is therefore possible, using the short-term test, to carry out resistance tests during the course of treatment with cytostatics with a view to identifying and eliminating those drugs that have become inactive.

B. Measurement of the proliferative activity of tumours

Often one wishes to establish whether resistance to treatment is likely to be exhibited in non-pretreated tumours. It is considered that tumours with a low rate of proliferation often show no response to treatment with antitumour agents. Using the short-term test it is possible to assess the proliferative activity of tumours.

^{3}H-Thymidine is incorporated into all cells that are in the DNA synthetic

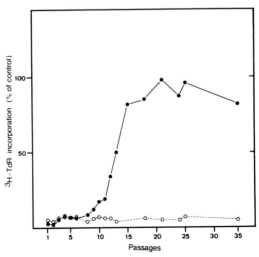

Fig. 1 Effect of ara-C in the short-term test on untreated (sensitive) (O) and ara-C-pretreated (resistant) (●) leukaemia L1210 cell lines at different passages.

phase during the incubation period. Incorporation can be measured by autoradiography or liquid scintillation counting. In the *in vitro* short-term test the effect of drugs on DNA synthesis is investigated over a period of 3 hours and during this short period the proliferative state of the tumour is largely maintained (Helpap and Maurer, 1969). Thus rapidly proliferating tissues, i.e. tissues with many cells in S-phase, can easily be recognized by high labelling indices or high incorporation rates of ³H-thymidine. In earlier investigations with animal transplanted tumours it was shown that the faster growing tumours also had higher levels of ³H-uridine incorporation than tumours with slower growth rates (Wayss *et al.*, 1974; Mattern *et al.*, 1981).

Studies with human tumours show that great variations exist in the levels of nucleoside incorporation for tumours at the same primary site and between different tumour types (Figs 2 and 3). Thus, measurement of nucleic acid metabolism by using radioactive precursors allows us to distinguish between malignant tissues with a low rate of proliferation, which may be unresponsive to drug treatment, and tissues with a high rate of proliferation where drug treatment could be successful.

C. Detection of proliferation-dependent drug effects

It is unsatisfactory just to take the amount of incorporation of radioactive nucleic acid precursor as a measure of the rate of proliferation of the tumour. The absolute value for this incorporation can be influenced by various factors, for example varying degrees of damage to the tumour cells during isolation or differences in nucleotide pool sizes of individual tumours. Thus tumours that have similar proliferative activities *in vivo* can demonstrate different

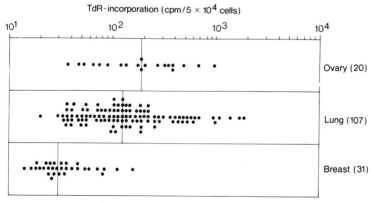

Fig. 2   Incorporation of ³H-thymidine in cell suspensions of different human tumour types.

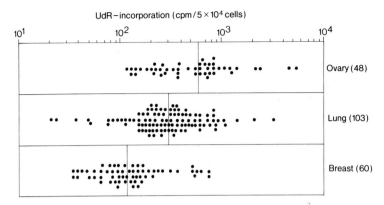

Fig. 3 Incorporation of ^{3}H-uridine in cell suspensions of different human tumour types.

incorporation rates for radioactive precursors *in vitro*. However, these considerations can, to a large extent, be ignored if inhibitory effects of a drug are expressed as percentage values.

In our short-term test, adriamycin (ADM), a substance that acts mainly on proliferating cells, is used as a test drug. Thus, the proliferation rate of a tumour can also be measured in an indirect way.

In order to show how the rate of ^{3}H-uridine incorporation and the dose–response relationship of ADM are influenced by different proportions of dead cells, ascites cells of the Walker carcinosarcoma 256 were mixed with varying numbers of cells which were killed by exposure to 50°C. The incorporation rate depends on the proportion of living cells, and the dose–response curves for ADM are different (Fig. 4). However, the differences disappear if the inhibitory effects of ADM are presented as a percentage of control values, and, with the exception of 0% and 10% proportion of living cells, all corrected dose–response curves exhibit similar patterns. This means that proportions of up to 70–80% dead cells do not influence the dose–response relationship to ADM provided that inhibitory effects of ADM *in vitro* are expressed as percentage values of untreated controls.

Tests *in vitro* on various human lung and ovarian carcinomas using an ADM concentration of 10^{-2} mg ml^{-1} show that when the inhibitory effects of ADM on ^{3}H-uridine incorporation are compared with control untreated values, in general, tumour cells that show high rates of uridine incorporation also show more pronounced inhibitory effects on treatment with ADM (Fig. 5).

A significant correlation exists between the inhibitory effect of ADM on lung tumours and the corresponding effects of daunomycin, 5-fluorouracil,

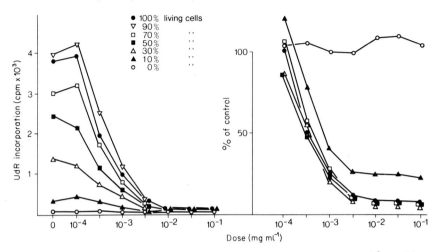

Fig. 4 Dose–response curves of ADM derived from measurement of ³H-uridine incorporation into cell suspensions of the Walker carcinosarcoma 256 in ascites form containing different proportions of living cells.

actinomycin D, and cyclophosphamide (Volm *et al.*, 1979). In other words, if a rapidly proliferating tumour responds to ADM treatment *in vitro*, in most cases a similar effect can be detected with the other agents tested. In addition, tumours that are insensitive to ADM are also usually unaffected by other drugs. This fact makes it possible to conduct tumour tests with drugs not included in the therapy schedule. According to our investigations on human tumours (see Chapter 20) a test using ADM would appear to be sufficient to detect proliferation-dependent tumour resistance. Therefore this short-term test is not used in order to find the most effective compound but merely to determine whether the tumour responds to any chemotherapy at all.

IV. Discussion

Use of radioactive isotopes to analyse metabolic processes in tissues has received extensive attention (Wüst and Matthes, 1970; Kummer, 1970; Volm *et al.*, 1970, 1979; Freshney *et al.*, 1975; Livingston *et al.*, 1977; Willnow, 1979; Possinger *et al.*, 1980; Sanfilippo *et al.*, 1981). Initially, incorporation of DNA and RNA precursors was measured by autoradiography since that method was particularly advantageous for assessing the proliferative activity of specific, morphologically defined cells. However, only a limited number of cells can be counted using this technique which can lead, particularly in tissue

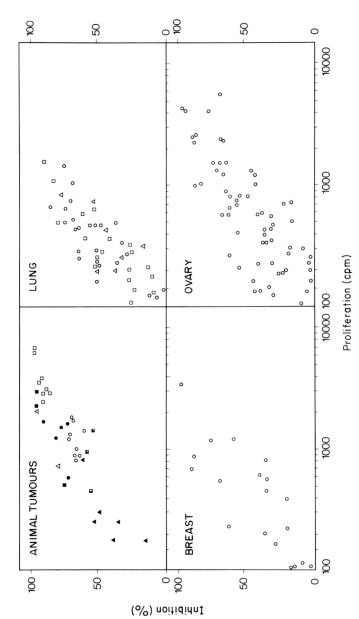

Fig. 5 Relationship between ^{3}H-uridine incorporation *in vitro* and the inhibitory effect of ADM in the short-term test with animal tumours and human tumours of the lung, breast, and ovary.
Abscissa: ^{3}H-uridine incorporation with no cytostatic drug (control values).
Ordinate: ^{3}H-uridine incorporation after adriamycin treatment (10^{-2} mg ml −1; % inhibition).
Symbols for animal tumours: (on the rat) □ Walker carcinosarcoma 256, ■ adenocarcinoma; (on the mouse) △ sarcoma 180, ▲ spontaneous tumours; (on the hamster) ○ plasmocytoma, ● melanoma Fortner III. Symbols for human lung tumours: ○ small cell, △ adenocarcinoma, □ epidermoid.

having a very low labelling index, to a significant statistical error. Furthermore, since tissue preparations or explants are comprised of several cell layers, a difference in oxygen supply can result in a variable degree of labelling (Rajewski, 1966). Moreover, evaluation of the preparations is very time-consuming.

The problem of regional variations in the proportion of DNA-synthesizing cells in tumours can be avoided by the use of liquid scintillation spectrometry. This technique measures the mean incorporation value of the entire tissue, yielding an average of the proliferative activity. Consequently, measurement of ^{3}H-thymidine or ^{3}H-uridine incorporation can provide an index of the proliferative activity of a tumour (Volm et al., 1979). In a clinical study it was shown that faster growing tumours had higher levels of ^{3}H-thymidine or ^{3}H-uridine incorporation than tumours with slower growth rates (Kofman et al., 1960; Kummer and Mildenberger, 1974). The principal advantage of biochemical short-term testing is the opportunity of using the original tumour cells in the test procedure. Cells need not be cultured beforehand and the test is comprehensive, i.e. practically all tumour types, including solid tumours, can be tested if adequate cells can be isolated. Thus, even tumour types that can seldom be grown successfully in tissue culture, e.g. breast carcinomas, can be included. A further advantage is the limited time required since an experienced technician can complete testing of several tumours within 1 day. Test results can be available within 1 day, thereby avoiding delay in initiating therapy. The short contact time of tumour cells with the drug enables only those cells to react that are proliferating and in a sensitive phase of their cell cycle. Since cellular metabolism in vitro can be maintained for at least 3 hours (Helpap and Maurer, 1969), in vitro results may mirror the proliferation of the original tumour.

Various limiting factors associated with the culture conditions, mechanisms of drug action and methods of investigating metabolic processes, lead to the exclusion of specific drugs from this short-term test. Since cells continue DNA synthesis initiated in vivo but do not enter a new cell cycle (Rajewski, 1966), mitotic blocking agents such as vincristine or vinblastine cannot be included. Also excluded are substances such as cyclophosphamide, which require metabolic activation, although the metabolite 4-hydroperoxycyclophosphamide considered to be the active form of the drug (Voelcker et al., 1974; Kaufmann et al., 1975) can be used in vitro. Results of in vitro tests may be misleading when substances such as podophyllic acid ethylhydrazine are used, since they reduce the entry of ^{3}H-uridine into the cell (Volm et al., 1975b). For each substance to be tested, the most suitable radioactive precursor and the optimal concentration of the substance must be used. Owing to the diverse mechanisms of drug action, it cannot be expected that a simple nucleic acid precursor could be comprehensively employed for all anticancer drugs.

V. Conclusions

Measurement of nucleic acid metabolism of tumours by radioactive precursors using an *in vitro* short-term test permits both (1) identification of tumours that fail to respond to a specific agent after prior treatment with chemotherapeutic agents (acquired resistance to one or more agents), and (2) identification of tumours that will not respond to chemotherapy (e.g. tumours with a slow proliferation rate).

References

Bickis, I. J., Henderson, I. W. D. and Quastel, J. H. (1966). Biochemical studies of human tumors. II. In vitro estimation of individual tumor sensitivity to anticancer agents. *Cancer* **19**, 103–113.

Dendy, P. P., Dawson, M. P. A. and Honess, D. J. (1973). Studies on the drug sensitivity of human tumor cells in short term culture. In *Aktuelle Probleme der Therapie maligner Tumoren* (ed. G. Wüst), pp. 34–45. Thieme Verlag, Stuttgart.

Ebeling, K. and Spitzbart, H. (1977). Zur Erfassung zytostatischer Effekte an Zellkulturen in vitro und deren gegenwärtige Bedeutung für einer individualisierte Tumortherapie des fortgeschrittenen Ovarialkarzinoms. *Zbl. Gynäkol.* **99**, 1041–1054.

Freshney, R. I., Paul, J. and Kane, I. M. (1975). Assay of anticancer drugs in tissue culture; conditions affecting their ability to incorporate ^{3}H-leucine after drug treatment. *Br. J. Cancer* **31**, 89–99.

Fujita, M., Hayata, S. and Taguchi, T. (1980). Relationship of chemotherapy on human cancer xenografts in nude mice to clinical response in donor patient. *J. Surg. Oncol.* **15**, 211–219.

Hamburger, A. W., Salmon, S. E., Kim, M. B., Trent, J. M., Soehnlein, B. J., Alberts, D. S. and Schmidt, H. J. (1978). Direct cloning of human ovarian carcinoma cells in agar. *Cancer Res.* **38**, 3438–3444.

Helpap, B. and Maurer, W. (1969). Autoradiographische Untersuchung zur Frage der Vergleichbarkeit des Einbaus von markiertem Thymidin unter in vivo Bedingungen und bei Inkubation von Gewebsproben. *Virchows Arch.* (B) (*Zellpathol.*) **4**, 102–118.

Holmes, H. L. and Little, J. M. (1974). Tissue-culture microtest for predicting response of human cancer to chemotherapy. *Lancet* **ii**, 985–987.

Kaufmann, M., Mattern, J. and Volm, M. (1975). In vitro testing of cyclophosphamide on tumors. *Naturwiss.* **62**, 446–447.

Kofman, S., Sky-Peck, H. H., Perlia, C. P., Economou, S. G., Winzler, R. J. and Taylor, S. G. (1960). A correlation between the incorporation of formate-^{14}C in tumors and the clinical course of patients with disseminated breast cancer. *Cancer* **13**, 425–431.

KSST—Group for Sensitivity Testing of Tumors (1981). In vitro short-term test to determine the resistance of human tumors to chemotherapy. *Cancer* **48**, 2127–2135.

Kummer, D. (1970). Cytostatika- und Röntgenstrahleneffekte im Nukleinsäurestoffwechsel von soliden, malignen Tumoren in vitro. *Z. Krebsforsch.* **74**, 76–90.

Kummer, D. and Mildenberger, H. (1974). Messungen im Nukleinsäurestoffwechsel des Neuroblastoms und Nephroblastoms in vitro und deren Bedeutung für die Cytostatikatherapie. *Z. Kindershir.* **14**, 121–131.

Limburg, H. and Krahe, M. (1964). Die Züchtung von menschlichem Krebsgewebe in der Gewebekultur und seine Sensibilitätstestung gegen neuere Zytostatika. *Deutsch. Med. Wochenschr.* **89**, 1938–1946.

Livingston, R. B., Sulkes, A., Thirlwell, M. P., Murphy, W. K. and Hart, J. S. (1977). Cell kinetic parameters: correlation with clinical response. In *Growth Kinetics and Biochemical Regulation of Normal and Malignant Cells* (ed. B. Drewinko and R. M. Humphrey), pp. 767–785. Williams and Wilkins, Baltimore.

Mattern, J., Kaufmann, M., Wayss, K., Volm, M., Kleckow, M., Mostaghi, M. and Vogt-Moykopf, I. (1976). Clinical correlates of in vitro effect of adriamycin on advanced lung carcinoma. *Klin. Wochenschr.* **54**, 665–670.

Mattern, J., Haag, D., Wayss, K. and Volm, M. (1981). Growth kinetics of human lung tumours in nude mice. *Exp. Cell Biol.* **49**, 34–40.

Meyskens, F. L., Moon, T. E., Gilmartin, B. D. E., Casey, W. J., G-Chen, H. S., Franks, D. H., Young, L. and Salmon, S. E. (1981). Quantitation of drug sensitivity by human metastatic melanoma colony-forming units. *Br. J. Cancer* **44**, 787–797.

Possinger, K., Hartenstein, R. and Ehrhardt, H. (1980). In vitro Resistenztestung von Tumoren gegenüber Zytostatika. 2. Untersuchungen an menschlichen Malignomen. *Onkologie* **6**, 297–300.

Rajewski, M. F. (1966). Zellproliferation in normalen und malignen Geweben: ^{3}H-Thymidin Einbau in vitro unter Standardbedingungen. *Biophysik* **3**, 65–93.

Salmon, S. E., Hamburger, A. W., Soehnlein, B., Durie, B. G. M., Alberts, D. S. and Moon, T. E. (1978). Quantitation of differential sensitivity of human-tumor stem cells to anticancer agents. *New Engl. J. Med.* **298**, 1321–1327.

Sanfilippo, O., Daidone, M. G., Costa, A., Canetta, R. and Silvestrini, R. (1981). Estimation of differential in vitro sensitivity of non-Hodgkin lymphomas to anticancer drugs. *Eur. J. Cancer* **17**, 217–226.

Shorthouse, A. J., Smyth, J. F., Steel, G. G., Ellison, M., Mills, J. and Peckham, M. J. (1980). The human tumour xenograft—a valid model in experimental chemotherapy? *Br. J. Surg.* **67**, 715–722.

Tanneberger, S. and Bacigalupo, G. (1970). Einige Erfahrungen mit der individuellen zytostatischen Behandlung maligner Tumoren nach prätherapeutischer Zytostatika Sensibilitätsprüfung in vitro (Onkobiogramm). *Arch. Geschwulstforsch.* **35**, 44–53.

Voelcker, G., Draeger, U., Peter, G. and Hohorst, H. J. (1974). Studien zum Spontanzerfall von 4-Hydroxycyclophosphamid und 4-Hydroxyperoxycyclophosphamid mit Hilfe der Dünnschichtchromatographie. *Arzneim. Forsch.* **24**, 1172–1176.

Volm, M. and Lindner, E. (1978). Detection of induced resistance in short-term tests. *Z. Krebsforsch.* **91**, 1–10.

Volm, M., Kaufmann, M., Hinderer, H. and Goerttler, K. (1970). Schnellmethode zur Sensibilitätstestung maligner Tumoren gegenüber Zytostatika. *Klin. Wochenschr.* **48**, 374–376.

Volm, M., Mattern, J. and Wayss, K. (1974). Effect of cytostatic drugs on transplanted tumours: investigation of the correlation between in vivo and in vitro results. *Arch. Geschwulstforsch.* **43**, 137–144.

Volm, M., Kaufmann, M., Mattern, J. and Wayss, K. (1975a). Möglichkeiten und Grenzen der prätherapeutischen Sensibilitätstestung von Tumoren gegen Zytostatika im Kurzzeittest. *Schweiz. Med. Wochenschr.* **105**, 74–82.

Volm, M., Kaufmann, M., Mattern, J. and Wayss, K. (1975b). Sensibilitätstestung maligner Tumoren gegen Zytostatika in vitro und in vivo: untersuchungen am Sarkom 180 der Maus. *Arzneim. Forsch.* **25**, 1042–1048.

Volm, M., Mattern, J. and Wayss, K. (1977). Detection of induced tumour-resistance for cyclophosphamide by the in vitro short term test. *Arch. Gynäkol.* **223**, 249–257.

Volm, M., Wayss, K., Kaufmann, M. and Mattern, J. (1979). Pretherapeutic detection of tumour resistance and the results of tumour chemotherapy. *Eur. J. Cancer* **15**, 983–993.

Volm, M., Maas, E. and Mattern, J. (1980). Detection of induced resistance to cytosine-arabinoside with a short-term test. *Eur. J. Cancer* **16**, 733–736.

Volm, M., Maas, E. and Mattern, J. (1981). In vivo and in vitro detection of induced resistance to daunorubicin in murine leukemia L1210. *Arzneim. Forsch.* **31**, 300–302.

Von Hoff, D. D., Casper, J., Bradley, E., Sandbach, J., Jones, D. and Makuch, R. (1981). Association between human tumor colony-forming assay results and response of an individual patient's tumor to chemotherapy. *Am. J. Med.* **70**, 1027–1032.

Wayss, K., Mattern, J., Volm, M. and Zimmerer, J. (1974). Der Einbau von radioaktiv markiertem Thymidin als Mass für die Wachstumsgeschwindigkeit von Tumoren. *Arch. Geschwulstforsch.* **44**, 307–311.

Willnow, U. (1979). Die Zytostatikum-Sensibilitätstestung solider Tumoren des Kindesalters mit einer autoradiographischen in vitro Methode (Kurzzeittest). *Arch. Geschwulstforsch.* **49**, 201–210.

Wright, J. C., Cobb, J. P., Gumport, S. A., Golomb, F. M. and Safadi, D. (1957). Investigation of the relation between clinical and tissue-culture: response to chemotherapeutic agents on human cancer. *New Engl. J. Med.* **257**, 1207–1211.

Wüst, G. P. and Matthes, K. J. (1970). In vitro Messung des Einbaues von ^{3}H-Thymidin in Jensen Sarkom unter Cytostatikaeinwirkung mit Hilfe der Flüssigkeits-Szintillations-Spektrometrie. *Z. Krebsforsch.* **73**, 204–214.

7. Culture Methods for Assays of Intermediate Duration

R. I. FRESHNEY and P. P. DENDY

I. Introduction

In this chapter we shall discuss critically some of the methods developed using cultures of human tumour cells grown for a matter of days, rather than hours or weeks, to assess the cytotoxicity of antineoplastic drugs. The requirements of a predictive test system that suggest such an approach may be desirable are as follows.

1. For individual patients, the duration of the test is of paramount importance. It may not be necessary for the result to be available within a few hours, especially if a period of post-operative convalescence is required, but the oncologist will wish to draw up a treatment plan reasonably quickly and may need the result within 1–2 weeks.

2. In many cases only a small amount of material is available for culture, and sometimes, even when the specimen is larger, the degree of cellularity is poor. Many of the culture methods discussed here are applicable to relatively small numbers of cells, and special emphasis will be placed on developments that allow the cellular requirement to be reduced. Limitation on cell numbers is generally less of a problem for pleural or ascites specimens although biochemical assays requiring in excess of 10^6 cells per replicate will not be feasible even for these samples.

3. Technical feasibility is important and may be considered from two viewpoints. First is the need for a high percentage of successes, and for certain tumour types, notably ovarian cancer, glioma, and most melanomas, the methods discussed here are very successful. The second is the level of technical expertise required of the operators; methods that require "green fingers" are notoriously bad travellers when transferred from one laboratory to another. The basic ideas described here have been applied successfully, with minor variations, in many laboratories.

4. The cost must also be considered. Although in the longer term the

purchase of equipment is not a significant consideration, the cost of highly skilled technical staff and of lengthy training of replacement staff is important. Most of the methods discussed here require an appreciable degree of technical skill but are generally adaptations of methods used widely for continuous cell lines, so a substantial corpus of knowledge and expertise already exists (Kruse and Patterson, 1973; Paul, 1975; Dendy, 1976; Jakoby and Pastan, 1979; Freshney, 1983).

5. Finally, the problem of *in vivo* relevance must be kept in mind. Pharmacological problems associated with predictive drug sensitivity testing will be discussed in Chapter 17 but questions relating to adaptation of cells to an *in vitro* environment, and possible consequent changes in their drug sensitivity spectrum, are appropriate to this chapter.

II. Disaggregation and culture methods

Many disaggregation methods have been employed (Fig. 1) and only brief details will be given. For solid tumours, mechanical disaggregation will always be necessary and, depending on the degree of fibrosity, crossed scalpel blades or scissors may be preferable. Further mechanical disaggregation by mincing has been used but most groups have preferred enzymatic methods.

Trypsin, at concentrations in the range 0.1–1%, has frequently been used, and provided that certain precautions are taken, for example the pH must be carefully controlled and the action of trypsin on disaggregated cells must be stopped as soon as possible by the addition of serum-containing medium, good yields of viable cells may be obtained. However, less aggressive enzymatic methods are now generally preferred, for example the use of 0.1% type II collagenase in complete growth medium at 37°C, sometimes supplemented with pronase and/or deoxyribonuclease (Warenius and Bleehen, 1982). Length of exposure can be adjusted to the degree of fibrosity of the specimen, and may range from a few hours to 5 days (Freshney, 1976). Overnight exposure is frequently chosen because, from a practical viewpoint, it is convenient.

Primary monolayer cultures have been established both on glass and on treated plastic surfaces, for example culture bottles, coverslips, inclined test-tubes, and microtitration plates. The choice is dictated by the amount of biopsy material available, the method of analysis to be used, the number of replicates required, and the cost. Microtitration plates are probably the most suitable when testing several drugs at different concentrations with a minimum of cells.

The physical shape of the container must be suitable for the method of assay to be used. For example, microtitre trays are readily adapted to many

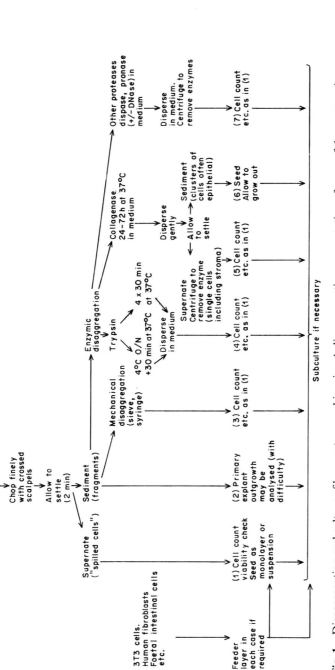

Fig. 1 Disaggregation and culture of human tumour biopsies. A diagrammatic representation of some of the routes taken to produce primary cultures and cell lines from human tumours. Seeding the primary disaggregate on to a feeder layer or adding irradiated or mitomycin C treated cells later often enhances tumour survival and inhibits fibroblastic overgrowth (see text).

automatic pipetters and diluters. Since these dishes have a very small culture volume, they must be protected against evaporation and loss of dissolved CO_2. Various self-adhesive plate sealers are available (e.g. Mylar film, Flow Laboratories) and are generally satisfactory. However, the advent of oxygen/CO_2 diffusible membranes may provide better conditions for cultures maintained either in sealed plastic boxes or in CO_2 incubators.

Low cell densities, which obtain sometimes during the initial phase of monolayer culture and particularly in cloning experiments, are very sensitive to CO_2 deprivation. It is therefore essential to supplement the gas phase of such cultures with CO_2; 5% is usual but 2% is optimal for some cells and enables 20 mM HEPES to be incorporated in the medium. This is useful in preventing rapid fluctuation in pH experienced in microtitration plates during medium change and drug addition. A low O_2 tension may also be beneficial for some tumour cells (see Chapter 9).

III. Heterogeneity and purification

Production of a pure culture of tumour cells comprises two stages. First, we require methods that will maximize the number of tumour cells, as a percentage of all cell types, in the primary suspension obtained from the surgical specimen. Secondly, we require culture procedures that will either maintain or improve that percentage.

A. Composition of cell suspension

A number of techniques have been described including the "spillage" technique (Lasfargues, 1973) where cells are teased out with a scalpel from slices of tumour, or selection by differential sensitivity to collagenase (Lasfargues, 1973). In many carcinomas tumour cells occur in clusters or cords surrounded by stroma. Disaggregation in collagenase preferentially disperses the stroma, and nodules of tumour cells may remain intact and can be collected by allowing them to settle through the more finely dispersed stroma (Freshney, 1972).

Many physical cell separation techniques have been applied to heterogeneous cell suspensions obtained from tumours (Freshney *et al.*, 1982) (Table 1). Briefly, these depend largely on differences in size or density between tumour cells and normal stromal elements. Fractionation of the primary disaggregate by velocity sedimentation at unit gravity (Miller and Phillips, 1969) has the advantage of simplicity and low cost, but the diversity in cell size often observed in a tumour reduces the value of this technique. The potential of sedimentation analysis has benefitted greatly from the development of

Table 1 Physical cell separation techniques that have been applied to heterogeneous cell suspensions obtained from tumours

Basis for separation	Technique	References
Cell size	Unit gravity sedimentation	Miller and Phillips (1969)
Cell size, density and surface configuration	Isokinetic centrifugation Centrifugal elutriation	Brattain et al. (1977) Meistrich et al. (1977)
Density	Isopycnic gradient centrifugation	Sykes et al. (1970)
Cell surface area, fluorescence	Flow cytophotometry	Herzenberg et al. (1976)

centrifugal elutriation (Meistrich et al., 1977), enabling high cell yields to be obtained rapidly, but cellular heterogeneity remains a problem. Pretlow and others (Brattain et al., 1977) found isokinetic sedimentation in Ficoll gradients in a zonal rotor to be effective, and Sykes et al. (1970) separated colon carcinoma cells from stroma by isopycnic centrifugation on density gradients of Ficoll. Percoll (Pharmacia) has provided a useful sedimentation medium of appropriate density, low viscosity, and low toxicity.

All physical separation techniques currently available are of limited value because tumour cell populations are heterogeneous and therefore some elements of the population coincide in their physical properties with normal cells. It may be possible to obtain nearly pure tumour cell populations if fairly stringent discrimination criteria are adopted but an appreciable proportion of the cells will be lost. To gain a reasonably high yield some stromal cells must be tolerated and these will tend to overgrow the culture rapidly. Physical cell separation might be better employed after drug exposure and recovery, i.e. immediately prior to making an assay measurement. At this time overgrowth ceases to be a problem but handling a large number of replicates is difficult.

Undoubtedly development of selective culture conditions (see below) will provide easier and more effective purification of tumour cells, and the use of cell sorting in conjunction with flow cytophotometry as discussed in Chapter 3 has considerable future potential.

Assessment of the quality of cellular material at this stage is important although not always easy. The percentage of viable cells can usually be estimated using trypan blue or some other viability stain (Kaltenbach et al., 1958) but there is no guarantee that all viable cells will survive. For example they may be unable to attach and proliferate in monolayer culture. The proportion of cells that are present as clumps is also important because migration of cells from clumped material during an assay could seriously alter both the number and type of cells exposed to drugs and their capacity to proliferate. Clumping also impairs the uniform distribution of cells between replicate samples, particularly in microtitration assays where the sample volume and cell number are low. Finally, some indication of the proportion of normal and stromal cells is required. This can normally be obtained retrospectively by one or other of the methods particularly suitable for freshly disaggregated cells discussed in Chapter 3.

B. Selective maintenance of tumour cells

The ideal would be a culture medium that was totally selective in favour of neoplastic cells, and work on growth of cells in chemically defined media (Sato et al., 1982) may help to achieve this. There have been many recent reports of media formulations that are selective for certan cell types. For example Carney et al. (1981) have reported a serum-free medium (HITES) that supports the selective growth of tumour cells from patients with small cell carcinoma of the lung. Successful growth and replication of tumour cells increased from 67% (10 out of 15 cases) when serum-supplemented medium was used, to 93% (14 out of 15 cases) when HITES medium was used, and stromal cell growth was inhibited. Whether this finding is unique to small cell carcinoma, which is known to produce a number of trophic peptides, or will apply also to other tumours remains to be seen. Preliminary results with other lung tumours (Brower et al., 1982) and recent success with breast carcinoma (Lan et al., 1981) suggest that serum-free selective media for other cell types may be possible (see also Sato et al., 1982). For optimal growth, a particular medium formulation may be required for each tumour type.

Attempts have been made to develop media containing selective inhibitors such as ethylmercurithiosalicylate (Braaten et al., 1974), D-valine (Gilbert and Migeon, 1975), cis-OH-proline (Kao and Prockop, 1977), and phenobarbitone (Fry and Bridges, 1979) to suppress fibroblastic overgrowth, or selective substrates such as polyacrylamide (Jones and Haskill, 1973) or PTFE (Parenjpe et al., 1975) to favour tumour cell growth. While many are effective with virally transformed cells or transplantable animal tumours, success with freshly explanted human tumour cells seems to be limited. Perhaps the most promising approach is that of Edwards et al. (1980) who removed epithelial cells from cultures of human squamous carcinomas of the head and neck by using a monoclonal antiserum which was toxic to human mesenchymal cells. Hallowes (personal communication) has had some success using this method in the prolonged treatment of explant growth from fragments of mammary tumour.

Clonal growth of tumour cells in agar is another selective culture technique, which is discussed in detail in Chapters 9 and 10. It requires care in its application since some normal cells, e.g. glia or embryonic skin fibroblasts, grow in suspension in agar or methocel as well (or as poorly) as glioma or melanoma (Freshney and Hart, 1982).

Aaronson et al. (1970) showed that cultures from human fibrosarcoma could be propagated selectively on confluent monolayers of normal fibroblasts. Foetal human intestinal cells were first used by Hackett (personal communication) to cultivate breast epithelium, and Freshney et al. (1982) showed that, when this technique was used to clone cells from primary cultures of breast carcinoma containing different cell types, the cloning efficiency was higher and colonies were predominantly epithelial-like. However, culture of normal breast also gave similar epithelial colonies and this technique appears to select epithelial cells against stroma rather than tumour against normal. Recent results (Freshney and Macdonald, in preparation) suggest that a homologous cell type used as a feeder may be more effective in selecting tumour cells from normal. Thus confluent normal glial feeder layers prevent growth of normal glia in glioma cultures, while foetal human intestine and skin fibroblasts may allow some lines of normal glia to grow. Iype (1980) has shown that normal rat hepatocytes, seeded onto a confluent monolayer of hepatocytes, will not proliferate, while hepatoma cells will do so.

C. Subculture

Primary cultures are more representative of the tumour from which they were derived than cell lines as less time has elapsed since explantation, and the opportunity for selective overgrowth and alteration of phenotype properties is less. Subculturing of many carcinomas often results in loss of the epithelial component and accelerated overgrowth by stromal cells.

However, subculture may be necessary when (i) insufficient biopsy material is available, (ii) fractionation and further characterization of the culture is required, and (iii) a high growth fraction is essential.

With some tumours this is less of a problem than with others. For example, melanoma cells can be maintained for extended periods (Whitehead, 1976), are often recognizable by their melanotic properties, and, if derived from lymph-node secondaries, are reasonably "pure" cultures. Cultures that are free from fibroblastic stroma are readily obtained from glial tumours. The cells appear to be aneuploid (Guner et al., 1977) and can be maintained with a high growth fraction for many passages. On the other hand, Ling et al. (1981) obtained variable results with ovarian tumour cells that were maintained and subcultured in vitro (see Chapter 3), and it has been extremely difficult to maintain breast tumour cells in anything approaching exponential growth after subculture. Recent results of Lan et al. (1981) suggest that this may be possible with the correct medium.

When subculture is successful it will usually provide a population that is more uniform in terms of cell type and proliferative capacity and has a higher growth fraction (90–100%) than the primary culture. Estimates of drug sensitivity which showed major fluctuations when performed on primary cultures behaved much more predictably when repeated on secondary or tertiary cultures (Morgan *et al.*, 1983). Subculture also provides more cells to perform replicates and parallel samples for characterization studies and makes cloning easier. The most obvious disadvantages are the increased time interval between receipt of the surgical material and the drug sensitivity test, the increased possibility that cell properties may change in response to the culture environment, and further selection in favour of those cells adaptable to culture.

In summary, the need to subculture is governed by two main requirements: (i) to increase cell numbers to provide sufficient replicates; and (ii) to provide greater uniformity of cell type and growth capacity essential for most types of assay with a biochemical endpoint to measure survival.

IV. Cell density, cell interaction, and growth fraction

It has been assumed in much of the foregoing discussion that proliferating cells are the main target for cytotoxic drugs, that a high growth fraction is desirable during drug exposure, and that a method that measures growth capacity is the best measure of response. It is true that, as cell density increases, sensitivity in terms of cell survival to most cytotoxic drugs decreases, but there are certain exceptions. For example, Barranco *et al.* (1973) suggested that nitrosourea may be more effective at high cell densities and glucocorticoids only exert a cytostatic effect on glioma when the cells are at a high density (Freshney *et al.*, 1980a).

When cells are cultured at a high cell density ($> 10^5$ cm^{-2}) the growth fraction falls to around 10% or less, the potential for functional communication and other forms of cell interaction increases, phenotypic alteration may occur, e.g. the percentage of differentiated cells may increase (Freshney *et al.*, 1980b), and the production of plasminogen activator (a putative tumour marker) decreases (Frame, personal communication). Thus high density cultures may respond quite differently to cytotoxic drugs, both quantitatively (owing to a lower growth fraction) and qualitatively (owing to phenotypic alteration).

Low-density cultures with a high growth fraction give data that are more readily interpreted and probably more relevant to the drug sensitivity of the proliferative compartment of the tumour. High-density cultures, on the other hand, reflect more accurately both cell growth kinetics and phenotypic expression of the tumour *in vivo*. Whilst these cultures may present some handling difficulties which limit their use in a predictive test, they provide a valuable model for investigations of drug action, drug penetration, and development of resistance (see Chapter 20).

The action of cytostatic drugs and steroids on low-density cultures is readily assessed by cell survival. Survival may also be measured in high-density cultures by assaying clonogenicity, but precursor studies may be difficult to interpret owing to restoration of saturation density within the recovery period at all but the highest drug concentrations.

Cell survival after cloning is not necessarily the only criterion for drug effects. Cells at high density may respond in other ways, e.g. by reduction in cell motility, increase in expression of differentiated properties, or increased sensitivity to density limitation of growth. None of these responses will kill tumour cells but they may halt tumour progression, inhibit invasion and metastasis, or otherwise bring cells back within the realm of normal homeostatic control. Therefore a distinction should be made between a cell kinetic response such as growth and a physiological response indicated by a more subtle, but perhaps equally important, phenotypic alteration.

V. Assay methods

The design of a suitable assay can be divided into two components.

A. Exposure

If the integral exposure is described by the product of time of exposure and concentration, a short exposure at a high drug concentration should in theory be equivalent to a long exposure at a low concentration. However, in practice this is not the case since duration of exposure also governs the number of cells that will complete one or more mitotic cycles in the presence of drug. Furthermore the use of a short exposure period may require a drug concentration that cannot be attained *in vivo*.

1. *Drug concentrations*

The concentrations used *in vitro* cannot readily be matched to those achieved *in vivo* in the tumour. The latter will vary both from one patient to another and from one time to another within the same patient. Perhaps the best way to solve this problem *in vitro* is to make observations on chemosensitivity at a range of concentrations and to plot a dose response curve. It may be useful to describe the curve by a single numerical parameter, e.g. the concentration required to cause 50% inhibition (ID_{50}), but the shape of the curve should also be examined for evidence of particular sensitivity or resistance.

2. Duration of exposure

This is important, particularly when dealing with antimetabolites such as methotrexate and mercaptopurine which show little effect following short exposure but may show a pronounced increase in effect following completion of one or two cell cycles (Freshney *et al.*, 1975, and Fig. 2). Most drugs show an increase in effect with prolonged exposure; for example glioma cultures only approach maximum sensitivity after exposure for 72 hours to 5-fluorouracil (Morgan *et al.*, 1983, and Fig. 3).

There is some conflict in available data here, however, since effective drug exposures *in vivo* are often quite short ($\frac{1}{2}$–2 h) for pharmacokinetic reasons. If the ability of cells to concentrate drug is lost *in vitro*, longer exposure times would be required to achieve the same integral exposure.

A prolonged assay presents certain practical problems. For example, since the sensitivity to some drugs changes as the cell population moves from subconfluent exponential growth to confluent density-limited growth (Cass, 1971; Freshney *et al.*, 1975), it is necessary to monitor cell density and to

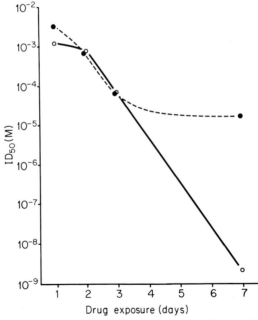

Fig. 2 Effect of increasing length of drug exposure on HeLa cells. Microtitration plates were set up at 2×10^3 cells/well (10^4 ml^{-1}). Drugs were added after 3 days and replaced with fresh drug at 24, 48, and 72 hours. After removal of the drugs at the times specified the cultures were allowed to recover for 22 hours and residual viability was determined by measuring incorporation of ^{3}H-leucine. (O) Methotrexate. (●) 6-mercaptopurine.

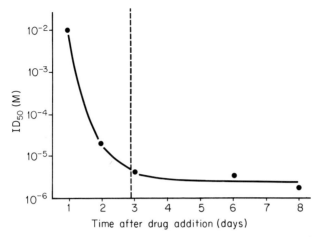

Fig. 3 Time course of the development of sensitivity to 5-fluorouracil (5-FU). A microtitration plate culture of MWA human glioma cells set up at 2000 cells/well $(2 \times 10^4 \, ml^{-1})$ was treated with a range of concentrations of 5-FU, replaced daily for 3 days. 5-FU was removed at day 3 (vertical line on graph) and culture continued for a further 5 days. ID_{50} values were calculated from the ^3H-leucine incorporated at the times indicated. On days 1, 2, and 3 the drug was removed and the cells allowed to recover for 4 hours before labelling.

ensure that the culture remains in exponential growth throughout the assay. Results from over 200 subconfluent primary cultures of human tumours showed a wide variation in $^{125}IUdR$ uptake per cell, indicating a variation in growth fraction. However, when cultures become confluent, typically above about 5×10^5 cells cm^{-2}, uptake of $^{125}IUdR$ was consistently low, indicating that cells had stopped cycling (Fig. 4; Dendy and Dawson, personal communication).

A further problem is that many drugs are unstable *in vitro* and will need frequent replacement. Ideally the replacement time should be related to the half-life of the drug, but in practice this would introduce too much complexity in the assay and daily replacement is often employed.

It will also prove difficult to simulate the scheduling given *in vivo* since drug concentrations, plasma clearance times, and cell cycle times may all be different. Cells in culture generally receive a much longer exposure than is possible *in vivo* but it should be noted that it is often not possible to demonstrate irreversible cytotoxicity in monolayer cultures when the exposure time is reduced to the *in vivo* exposure time (Freshney *et al.*, 1975).

3. *Recovery period*
Since the purpose of a cytotoxicity assay is to measure survival rather than metabolic inhibition, it is important that the assay for viability follows drug

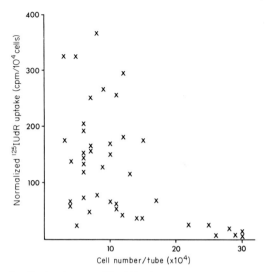

Fig. 4 Effect of cell density on ^{125}IUdR incorporation. Observations were on untreated controls of short-term cultures from many different patients. Cells growing as monolayers in inclined test tubes were exposed to 0.06 μCi ml^{-1} ^{125}I-iododeoxyuridine in complete medium for 24 hours. After thorough washing the ^{125}I incorporation was measured with a NaI well counter. A single cell suspension was then prepared from each tube using trypsin/versene and the cell number per tube was measured on a Coulter counter. The large variation in normalized uptake for sub-confluent cultures ($< 1.5 \times 10^5$ cells/tube) demonstrates the variability of the fraction of the cell population in cycle. Above about 1.5×10^5 cells/tube, growth is density limited and ^{125}I uptake is consistently low.

exposure. After the drug is removed, lethal damage may continue to accumulate with alkylating agents and some antimetabolites such as methotrexate and 6-mercaptopurine (see Fig. 2). With other drugs such as the vinca alkaloids, drug is released from the cell and partial or complete recovery may ensue. It is important to allow a period for these processes to stabilize, although the precise time interval required may depend on the assay endpoint adopted.

B. Endpoint

Assays should measure variations in survival rather than changes in metabolism which may be reversible. For example, although ^{3}H-thymidine, ^{3}H-leucine, and cell morphology will react differently to methotrexate treatment in a short exposure (< 24 h), the final common pathway following prolonged exposure (2–3 cell cycles) and prolonged recovery (a further 2–3 cell cycles) will be cell death and hence will be depicted similarly regardless of method of measurement.

This problem is minimized if a period of growth is permitted following drug exposure before an assay is attempted. The choice of endpoint then becomes a matter of reproducibility and technical convenience, but it should be emphasized that, in the selection of drugs for individual patients, a quantitative assay method provides a more objective form of analysis than morphological examination and reduces operator variability. Radionuclide methods in particular are more readily automated both for processing and for data reduction, and this becomes critical when large numbers of samples are handled. Hence, although morphological examination may have certain advantages when cell recognition is required, with a defined population it is not essential and radiolabelled precursors may be more useful.

^{125}I-Iododeoxyuridine, ^{3}H-thymidine, and other nucleotide precursors have been used extensively because of their involvement in replication. They provide useful additional information when the growth fraction is variable but may be prone to error where the respective pathways and transport mechanisms have been the sites of action of nucleotide analogues; for example, 5-fluorouracil and methotrexate can both stimulate incorporation of exogenous thymidine, while bromodeoxyuridine resistant mutants will not incorporate exogenous thymidine at all owing to a deficiency of thymidine kinase. In situations where the growth fraction is known to be high and constant, ^{3}H-precursors of protein synthesis may be preferable.

The most direct measurement of proliferation can be gained by daily counts *in situ* (Lickiss *et al.*, 1974; Holmes and Little, 1974) when changes in growth rate can be related to the drug concentration to derive an ID_{50}. Major problems here are that visual counting is time-consuming and leads to significant operator variation whilst large numbers of cells are required for accurate measurements by electronic particle counting.

Clonogenic assay, the most generally accepted method for measuring cell survival by proliferative ability, may of course be applied. After drug treatment the cells are passaged and diluted so that they will form discrete colonies when plated out. However, there are a number of drawbacks:

(i) Even after a period of growth in monolayer culture, cells tend to clone with a very low efficiency which varies greatly from one culture to another (0.1–20%). This means that even in untreated controls there is low survival and implied selection.

(ii) Cloning requires a very low cell density which is far removed from the *in vivo* situation. This may produce additional trauma, and may fail to detect cells that may be drug resistant at higher cell densities.

(iii) The time required for clonal growth frequently will be 15 days or longer for tumour biopsy cultures.

(iv) Colony counting is time-consuming and difficult to automate, and can therefore be prone to variation due to subjective interpretation. Automated colony counters go some way towards solving this problem but only operate effectively with uniform, dense colonies. Diffuse, irregular colonies can give multiple counts.

Nevertheless cloning has considerable advantages. For example, since each colony is a clone, provided that a cytological, histochemical, or fluorescent technique is available to identify the cells, only tumour colonies need be scored. Furthermore survival (cloning efficiency) and proliferative capacity (colony size) can be measured in the same assay. Interpretation of survival curves is also easier and a more accurate determination of the surviving fraction is possible (Fig. 5). However, it should be noted that small, resistant fractions may be lost unless steps are taken to guard against the additional trauma induced by growth at such low cell densities. The presence of an irradiated or mitomycin C treated feeder layer of homologous cells is one way to deal with this problem (Fig. 6).

Attempts to assay reversibility of damage must distinguish between cellular recovery after the drug is removed, and apparent reversibility caused by overgrowth of a resistant population. Cells may also be spared because of their position in the cell cycle at the time of drug exposure. For example, a short exposure to a drug that is S-phase specific will never demonstrate total irreversible cytotoxicity because cells in the G_1 and G_2 phases during drug exposure will be spared. Non-cycling cells will also be spared and constitute a threat if they are able to re-enter the cell cycle.

It is difficult to determine the surviving fraction accurately by a biochemical assay. However, such assays are quicker, more objective to analyse, and can clearly indicate reversibility of drug sensitivity by the cell population. If the duration of exposure is long enough to eliminate phase-specific resistance, reversibility will indicate that all the cells have recovered partially or that some cells have recovered completely. It will not be possible to distinguish between these alternatives without cloning the cells and counting and sizing the colonies.

Comparison of ID_{50} values obtained by cloning immediately after drug exposure or scintillation autofluorography 5 days later show good correlation (correlation coefficient $= 0.96$; $p < 0.001$; gradient of regression line $= 0.90$). Ranking 5 cultures in order of sensitivity with 6 different drugs showed good overall agreement (Freshney et al., 1983).

A number of other criteria of viability have either been used or proposed. Dye-exclusion tests have been used for many years (Kaltenbach et al., 1958) but doubts have frequently been expressed over the relevance of the measurements. This approach has recently been revived by the work of Weisenthal and Marsden (1981) who used fast green. Results obtained by

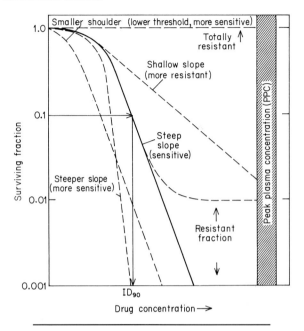

Fig. 5 Interpretation of survival curve. The solid-line curve represents a typical survival curve for a sensitive culture. Changes in slope, shoulder, resistant fraction, and ratio of the ID_{90} (90% inhibitory dose, 10% survival) to the peak plasma concentration will all influence sensitivity. Frequently the curve is complex and comparison by one of the above parameters alone is difficult, so the area under the survival curve is taken in an attempt to combine all of them. It should be realized, however, that this is only a rough measurement and may obscure important information, such as the presence of a small resistant fraction on a steep curve.

Bosanquet *et al.* (1983) using this method on cells from chronic lymphocytic leukaemia have been promising but more data are required before a full evaluation is made. ^{51}Cr release, as used for lymphocyte toxicity experiments, is only of value in short-term assay (2–4 h) owing to the spontaneous release of ^{51}Cr which may be particularly high in early passaged cultures.

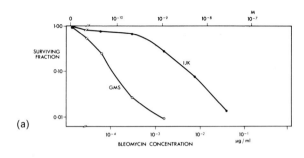

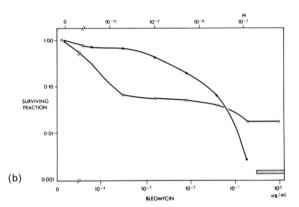

Fig. 6 Effect of feeder layer on shape of survival curve. Two early passage cell lines from human anaplastic astrocytoma were treated with bleomycin for 3 days, replacing the drug daily at the concentrations shown. Survival was determined by plating the cells at 250 cells ml^{-1} (125 cells cm^{-2}) in 9-cm Petri dishes (b) with and (a) without a feeder layer of the same cells previously treated with mitomycin C (2 μg/10^6 cells, overnight) to prevent growth in the feeder layer. GMS appears more sensitive than IJK when plated in the absence of a feeder layer, but in the presence of a feeder layer GMS displays a resistant fraction (Freshney et al., 1983).

Two new assays suggested recently involve biophysical methods based on changes in electrical properties of cells. The first is an extension of the observation by Walliser and Redmann (1981) that addition of cytotoxic drugs to suspensions of cells caused rapid and characteristic changes in their transmembrane potentials (TMP). In the past this approach has always been suspect because of the mechanical damage frequently caused by using microelectrodes to measure TMP, but the development of fluorescent probes for this purpose (see, for example, Philo and Eddy, 1978; Rink et al., 1980) provides a promising alternative approach. The second new technique involves changes in electrical impedance of cells in culture, first developed to measure bacterial growth and recently applied successfully to measure sensitivity of cancer cells to anticancer drugs (Khan and Ommaya, 1981). Both methods are very quick and may be readily automated (see below) but it remains to be determined how well changes in these electrical properties after drug treatment correlate with long-term survival.

VI. Automation

Radioactive counting remains the most widely adopted method of assay for monolayer cultures, and where the endpoint requires measurement of different levels of tracer incorporation, scintillation counting provides an accurate and readily computerized source of digital information. However, this often involves labour-intensive steps in sample preparation and it may be preferable to develop *in situ* scanning techniques such as autoradiography with gamma emitters, e.g. ^{125}I, and hard beta emitters, e.g. ^{32}P. A similar method can be extended to soft beta emitters such as ^{3}H by *in situ* treatment of cultures in microtitration plates with scintillant, followed by autofluorography on high-speed X-ray film (Freshney and Morgan, 1978). Both autoradiography and scintillation autofluorography can be assessed directly from the image on the X-ray film or it can be scanned on a simple densitometer to give more precise inhibition values and an ID_{50} (Fig. 7).

General acceptance of a clonal growth assay method may also require automated colony counting and scanning densitometry for colony sizing. This may be within the scope of computerized image analysis systems already available, but further development of staining techniques and recognition criteria is required.

Measurement of electrical impedance of cells in culture may be readily automated, for example by using the Mathus Microbiological Growth Analyser which measures conductance between two platinum electrodes immersed in the culture and is sensitive to changes of 0.1 microsiemens. Khan and Ommaya (1981) have used a similar system to measure responses of human gliomas, human melanomas, and two mouse leukaemic cell lines to 8-azoguanine, methotrexate, BCNU, and CCNU. The system is fully automated and changes in electrical impedance may be measured at different times after drug exposure.

VII. Conclusions

If it can be demonstrated that tumour cells from a biopsy sample can be plated with a high efficiency, with normal cells either absent or clearly distinguished

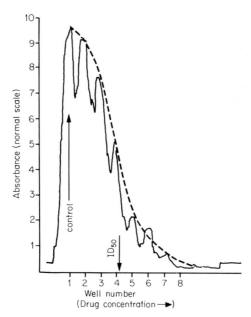

Fig. 7 Densitometric scan of autofluorograph from one row of a microtitration experiment. A microtitration plate culture of human glioma was treated with drug for 3 days, allowed to recover for 5 days, and then labelled for 3 hours with ^{35}S-methionine at 10 μCi ml^{-1}. The labelled cultures were fixed with methanol, dried, and treated with 50 μl scintillation fluid (Instagel, Packard). The scintillation fluid was dried off by centrifuging the plate, and the dried plate was bound up with X-ray film, placed at −70°C for 3 days, and then developed. The trace shown is a scan of density of one row of the plate, performed on a Helena Autoscanner with a modified 1 mm × 5 mm slit.

from them, and within a time acceptable to the clinician, clonogenic assays of survival have considerable advantages over other methods. If, as is more often the case, clonogenic survival is very low in primary culture, making interpretation difficult, there may be considerable advantage in using a biochemical assay such as isotopically labelled precursor incorporation. This may require cells to be subcultured to obtain a high and uniform growth fraction, but it will yield results quickly and objectively if contamination with stromal cells can be kept to a minimum.

Acknowledgment

This work was supported by the Cancer Research Campaign.

References

Aaronson, S. A., Todaro, G. J. and Freeman, A. E. (1970). Human sarcoma cells in culture: identification by colony-forming ability on monolayers of normal cells. *Exp. Cell Res.* **61**, 1–5.

Barranco, S. C., Novak, J. K. and Humphrey, R. M. (1973). Response of mammalian cells following treatment with bleomycin and 1,3-bis-(2-chloroethyl)-1-nitrosourea during plateau phase. *Cancer Res.* **33**, 691.

Bosanquet, A. G., Bird, M. C., Price, W. J. P. and Gilby, E. D. (1983). An assessment of short-term tumour chemosensitivity assay on chronic lymphocytic leukaemia. *Br. J. Cancer* **47**, 781–789.

Braaten, J. T., Lee, M. J., Schewk, A. and Mintz, D. H. (1974). Removal of fibroblastoid cells from primary monolayer cultures of rat neonatal endocrine pancreas by sodium ethylmercurithiosalicylate. *Biochem. Biophys. Res. Comm.* **61**, 476–482.

Brattain, M. G., Kimball, P. M., Pretlow, T. G. and Pitts, A. M. (1977). Partial purification of human colonic carcinoma cells by sedimentation. *Br. J. Cancer* **35**, 850–857.

Brower, M., Carney, D., Oie, H., Matthews, M. and Minna, J. (1982). Growth of human adenocarcinoma of the lung: cell lines and clinical specimens in serum-free defined medium. American Society for Clinical Oncology (Abstract) meeting at St. Louis, MO, April 1982. *Proc. Am. Soc. Clin. Oncol.* **1**, 140.

Carney, D. N., Bunn, P. A., Jr, Gazdar, A. F., Pagan, J. A. and Minna, J. D. (1981). Selective growth in serum-free hormone-supplemented medium of tumor cells obtained by biopsy from patients with small cell carcinoma of the lung. *Proc. Nat. Acad. Sci.* **78**, 3185–3189.

Cass, C. E. (1971). Density-dependent resistance to puromycin in cell cultures. *J. Cell Physiol.* **79**, 139–146.

Dendy, P. P. (ed.) (1976). *Human Tumours in Short Term Culture*. Academic Press, London.

Edwards, P. A. W., Easty, D. M. and Foster, C. S. (1980). Selective culture of epithelioid cells from a human squamous carcinoma using a monoclonal antibody to kill fibroblasts. *Cell Biol. Int. Rep.* **4**, 917–922.

Freshney, R.I. (1972). Tumour cells disaggregated in collagenase. *Lancet* **ii**, 488–489.

Freshney, R. I. (1976). Preparation of primary cultures. In *Human Tumours in Short Term Culture* (ed. P. P. Dendy), pp. 20–24. Academic Press, London.

Freshney, R. I. (1983). *Culture of Animal Cells: Manual of Basic Technique*. Alan Liss Inc., New York.

Freshney, R. I. and Hart, E. (1982). Clonogenicity of human glia in suspension. *Br. J. Cancer* **46**, 459.

Freshney, R. I. and Morgan, D. (1978). Radioisotope quantitation in microtitration plates by an autofluorographic method. *Cell Biol. Int. Rep.* **2**, 375–380.

Freshney, R. I., Paul, J. and Kane, I. M. (1975). Assay of anticancer drugs in tissue culture: conditions affecting their ability to incorporate ^{3}H-leucine after drug treatment. *Br. J. Cancer* **31**, 89–99.

Freshney, R. I., Sherry, A., Hassanzadah, N., Freshney, M., Crilly, P. and Morgan, D. (1980a). Control of cell proliferation in human glioma by glucocorticoids. *Br. J. Cancer* **41**, 857–866.

Freshney, R. L., Morgan, D., Hassanzadah, N., Shaw, R. and Frame, M. (1980b). Glucocorticoids, proliferation and the surface. In *Tissue Culture in Medical*

Research (ed. R. J. Richards and K. T. Rajan), pp. 125–132. Pergamon Press, Oxford.

Freshney, R. I., Hart, E. and Russell, J. M. (1982). Isolation and purification of cell cultures, from human tumours. In *Cancer Cell Organelles* (ed. E. Reid, G. M. W. Cook and D. J. Morre), Methodological Surveys (B): Biochemistry, Vol. 11. Horwood, Chichester, England.

Freshney, R. I., Celik, F. and Morgan, D. (1983). Analysis of cytotoxic and cytostatic effects. In *The Control of Tumor Growth and its Biological Base* (ed. W. Davis, C. Maltoni and St. Tanneberger). Fortschritte in der Onkologie, Band 10. Akademie-Verlag, Berlin.

Fry, J. and Bridges, J. W. (1979). The effect of phenobarbitone on adult rat liver cells and primary cell lines. *Toxicol. Lett.* **4,** 295–301.

Gilbert, S. F. and Migeon, B. R. (1975). D-Valine as a selective agent for normal human and rodent epithelial cells in culture. *Cell* **5,** 11–17.

Guner, M., Freshney, R. I., Morgan, D., Freshney, M. G., Thomas, D. G. T. and Graham, D. I. (1977). Effects of dexamethasone and betamethasone on in vitro cultures from human astrocytoma. *Br. J. Cancer* **35,** 439–447.

Herzenberg, L. A., Sweet, R. G. and Herzenberg, L. A. (1976). Fluorescence-activated cell sorting. *Sci. Amer.* **234,** 108–117.

Holmes, H. L. and Little, J. M. (1974). Tissue-culture microtest for predicting response of human cancer to chemotherapy. *Lancet* **ii,** 985–987.

Iype, P. T. (1980). Interaction between normal and malignant rat liver epithelial cells in culture. In *Cell Movement and Neoplasia* (ed. M. de Brabander, M. Mareel and L. de Ridder). Pergamon Press, Oxford.

Jakoby, W. B. and Pastan, I. H. (1979). *Cell Culture Methods in Enzymology* (ed. S. P. Colowick and N. O. Kaplan), Vol. 58. Academic Press, New York.

Jones, T. L. and Haskill, J. S. (1973). Polyacrylamide: an improved surface for cloning of primary tumours containing fibroblasts. *J. Nat. Cancer Inst.* **51,** 1575–1580.

Kaltenbach, J. P., Kaltenbach, M. H. and Lyons, W. B. (1958). Nigrosin as a dye for differentiating live and dead ascites cells. *Exp. Cell Res.* **15,** 112.

Kao Whei-Yang, W. and Prockop, D. J. (1977). Proline analogue removes fibroblasts from cultured mixed cell populations. *Nature* **266,** 63–64.

Khan, W. H. and Ommaya, A. K. (1981). Rapid measurement of cancer cell sensitivity to anticancer drugs by an electrical impedance method. Abstract for 3rd Int. Symp. on Rapid Methods and Automation in Microbiology.

Kruse, P. F. and Patterson, M. K. (eds) (1973). *Tissue Culture Methods and Applications.* Academic Press, New York and London.

Lan, S., Smith, H. S. and Stampfer, M. R. (1981). Clonal growth of normal and malignant human breast epithelia. *J. Surg. Oncol.* **18,** 317–322.

Lasfargues, E. Y. (1973). Human mammary tumours. In *Tissue Culture Methods and Applications* (ed. P. Kruse and M. K. Patterson), pp. 45–50. Academic Press, New York and London.

Lickiss, J. N., Cane, K. A. and Baikie, A. G. (1974). In vitro drug selection in antineoplastic chemotherapy. *Eur. J. Cancer* **10,** 809–814.

Ling, C. R., Dendy, P. P. and Abramovich, D. R. (1981). The use of quantitative cytochemistry to monitor human tumour cells in culture. *Arch. Geschwulstforsch.* **51,** 80–86.

Meistrich, M. L., Grdina, D. J., Meyn, R. E. and Barlogie, G. (1977). Separation of cells from mouse solid tumours by centrifugal elutriation. *Cancer Res.* **37,** 4291–4296.

Miller, R. G. and Phillips, R. A. (1969). Separation of cells by velocity sedimentation. *J. Cell. Phys.* **73**, 191–201.

Morgan, D., Freshney, R. I., Darling, J. L., Thomas, D. G. T. and Celik, F. (1983). Assay of anticancer drugs in tissue culture: cell cultures of biopsies from human astrocytoma. *Br. J. Cancer* **47**, 205–214.

Parenjpe, M. S., Boone, C. W. and Ande Eaton, S. del (1975). Selective growth of malignant cells by in vitro incubation on Teflon. *Exp. Cell Res.* **93**, 508–512.

Paul, J. (1975). *Cell and Tissue Culture,* 5th edn. Livingstone, Edinburgh.

Philo, R. D. and Eddy, A. A. (1978). The membrane potential of mouse ascites tumour cells studied with the fluorescent probe 3,3-dipropylthiodicarbocyanine. *Biochem. J.* **174**, 801.

Rink, T. J., Montecucco, C., Heskett, T. R. and Tsien, R. Y. (1980). Lymphocyte membrane potential assessed with fluorescent probes. *Biochem. Biophys. Acta* **595**, 15–30.

Sato, G. H., Pardee, A. B. and Sirbasku, D. A. (1982). Growth of cells in hormonally defined media. *Cold Spring Harbor Conf. Cell Prolif.* **9**.

Sykes, J. A., Whitescarver, J., Briggs, L. and Anson, J. H. (1970). Separation of tumor cells from fibroblasts with use of discontinuous density gradients. *J. Nat. Cancer Inst.* **44**, 855–864.

Walliser, S. and Redmann, K. (1981). Effects of cytostatic drugs on the transmembrane potential and surface charge of cultured cells. *Arch. Geschwulstforsch.* **51**, 125–132.

Warenius, H. M. and Bleehen, N. M. (1982). In vivo-in vitro clonogenic assays in a human tumour xenograft with a high plating efficiency. *Br. J. Cancer* **46**, 45–50.

Weisenthal, L. M. and Marsden, J. (1981). A novel dye exclusion assay for predicting response to cancer chemotherapy. *Proc. Am. Assoc. Cancer Res.* **22**, 155.

Whitehead, R. H. (1976). The culture of tumour cells from human tumour biopsies. *Clin. Oncol.* **2**, 131–140.

8. An Overview of Clonogenic Assays for Human Tumour Biopsies

B. T. HILL

I. Introduction

Clonogenic assays have been widely used in experimental laboratory studies employing animal tumours and cell lines since Puck and Marcus first described their methodology in 1955. However, attempts to extend these procedures to human tumour biopsy specimens generally proved fruitless or were rejected since such low colony-forming efficiencies were obtained. In the mid-1970s, however, two independent groups published details of successful assay procedures for use with human tumour material (Hamburger and Salmon, 1977b; Courtenay and Mills, 1978). Although colony-forming efficiencies obtained frequently remained low, Salmon and his colleagues (1978) provided preliminary evidence that for certain tumours their *in vitro* assay could be used to quantitate differential sensitivities of these human tumour "stem" cells to anticancer drugs and hence predict clinical responses. The pioneering work provided the impetus for other groups to try both to confirm and to extend these studies. It is disappointing that more of the effort put into attempting to invalidate these claimed clinical correlations has not been channelled into optimizing growth conditions to improve colony-forming efficiencies and to extend the tumour types that can be studied. It is only in this way that the potential of these methodologies for expanding our knowledge of the biology of human tumours can be appreciated fully.

II. Current status of assays

Colony growth has been achieved with a variety of tumour types; examples are listed in Table 1. Using present methodologies approximately one colony-

Table 1 Progenitor/stem cell assays available for human neoplasms and their specific growth requirements.

Tumour type	References	Specific growth conditions defined for "stem" cell assays	Chemically defined (serum-free) media available for cell lines	References
Haematopoietic				
AML	Buick *et al.* (1977)	Yes	No	—
	Spitzer *et al.* (1978)			
Myeloma	Hamburger and Salmon (1977a)	Yes	No	—
	Izaguirre *et al.* (1980)			
	Shimizu *et al.* (1982)			
Lymphoma	Jones *et al.* (1979)	Yes	Yes	Darfler and Insel (1982)
	Izaguirre *et al.* (1980)			
"Solid" tumours				
Ovary	Hamburger *et al.* (1978)	No	No	—
	Ozols *et al.* (1980)			
	Von Hoff *et al.* (1981)			
	Bertoncello *et al.* (1982)			
Bladder	Buick *et al.* (1979)	No	Yes	Messing *et al.* (1982)
	Von Hoff *et al.* (1981)			
Melanoma	Pavelic *et al.* (1980)	No	No	—
	Meyskens *et al.* (1981)			
	Von Hoff *et al.* (1982)			
Neuroblastoma	Von Hoff *et al.* (1980)	No	Yes	Bottenstein (1980)
Breast	Von Hoff *et al.* (1981)	No	Yes	Barnes and Sato (1980)
Colon	Buick *et al.* (1980a)	No	No	—
	Von Hoff *et al.* (1981)			
	Kern *et al.* (1982)			
	Agrez *et al.* (1982)			
	Laboisse *et al.* (1981)			
Lung	Pavelic *et al.* (1980)	Yes	Yes	Simms *et al.* (1980)
	Carney *et al.* (1981a)			
	Von Hoff *et al.* (1981)			
Head and neck	Mattox and Von Hoff (1980)	No	No	—

Brain	Rosenblum *et al.* (1978)	No	No	—
Pancreas	Von Hoff *et al.* (1981)	No	No	—
Prostate	Von Hoff *et al.* (1981)	No	Yes	Kaign *et al.* (1981)
Testicular	Von Hoff *et al.* (1981)	No	No	—
Renal	Von Hoff *et al.* (1981) Kovach and Lieber (1981)	No	No	—
Sarcoma	Pavelic *et al.* (1980)	No	No	—

forming cell is found per 10^3–10^4 nucleated cells. This frequency appears relatively consistent for most tumour cell populations. It is envisaged, however, that this figure can be increased as culture conditions are improved and specific growth factors are identified for individual tumours (as discussed below). Whilst specific growth conditions for these clonogenic assays have been defined for the haematopoietic neoplasms, as pointed out by Buick *et al.* (1980a), apart from lung carcinomas, such information is still not available for most "solid" tumours. However, this may soon be rectified, at least for certain tumours including those of the bladder, breast, prostate, and neuroblastomas, since chemically defined, serum-free or serum-depleted media have now been described that allow growth of cell lines from these tumour types.

In the major centres clonogenic cell growth is reported in at least 50–75% of specimens tested, although a figure of 20–50% is more frequently the experience of smaller groups of investigators. These differences are most likely to be related to the suitability of specimens received for study and variabilities in collection and storage procedures. It is generally reported that success rates are highest using cells from bone marrow, pleural effusions, or ascites, rather than "solid" tumours (Salmon and Von Hoff, 1981; Von Hoff *et al.*, 1981).

III. Methodologies

The most widely used procedure, that described by Hamburger and Salmon, is described in Chapter 10. Full details of the Courtenay procedure are given in Chapter 9. Few significantly modified methods have been published, although a procedure considered optimal for gastrointestinal adenocarcinomas, based on original work by Macpherson (1973), is described in Chapter 11. Other variations in these procedures which have been adopted by certain groups are discussed below.

A. Processing of tumour specimens

1. *Tumour collection and storage*
Effusions, ascites, and bone marrow samples are collected in preservative-free heparin or EDTA, whilst "solid" tumours are placed in complete medium. The consensus is that specimens should be processed at the earliest opportunity but, if stored, a temperature of 4° is preferred, except by two groups who found storage of effusions at room temperature superior (Mackintosh *et al.*, 1981; Von Hoff *et al.*, 1981). Cryopreservation appears generally to result in reduced viability after thawing and a marked decrease in colony-forming efficiencies, although the occasional tumour specimen has proved an exception.

2. *Tumour disaggregation*
The choice of either mechanical or enzymatic disaggregation appears not to be related to tumour type. In general, laboratories tend to favour one particular procedure, with certain groups employing almost exclusively mechanical procedures (Buick *et al.*, 1979; Meyskens *et al.*, 1981; Von Hoff *et al.*, 1981, 1982; Hamburger, 1983, Chapter 10), whilst other groups report increased viable cell yields with enzymatic methods (Rosenblum *et al.*, 1978; Mackintosh *et al.*, 1981; Slocum *et al.*, 1981; Courtenay, 1983, Chapter 9). Interestingly, however, Slocum *et al.* (1981) report that the proportions of clonogenic cells in populations obtained after either mechanical or enzymatic disruption are similar. Indeed this serves to highlight consensus opinion that dye-excluding cells cannot be equated with clonogenic cells (Mattox and Von Hoff, 1980; Hamburger, 1983, Chapter 10).

3. *Elimination of unwanted cells*
Red blood cell contamination, depending on its degree, can be reduced by sedimentation in linear density gradients of Ficoll. This procedure appears superior to using buffered NH_4Cl (Mackintosh *et al.*, 1981) although Hamburger (Chapter 10) describes an alternative lysis buffer. However, further separation techniques must be approached with caution in view of the finding that removal of phagocytic cells from ovarian cancer cell preparations may decrease colony-forming efficiencies (Hamburger *et al.*, 1978). Buick *et al.* (1980b) similarly have demonstrated that adherent cells enhance colony-forming efficiencies of tumour cells derived from patients with other types of cancer, and recently Hamburger and White (1981) have shown that autologous macrophages enhance growth of human tumour cells in soft agar.

4. *Preparation of single-cell suspensions*

There is clearly an essential requirement for obtaining single-cell suspensions for use in drug sensitivity assays that require quantitation. However, it has been our experience that colonies form more readily from cell doublets and triplets. Furthermore, where a minimum number of manipulations aimed at obtaining a single-cell suspension fail, further attempts generally result only in a drastic reduction in cell viability.

B. Culture conditions

1. *Media and sera*

These vary from laboratory to laboratory, and data proving definite superiority for a particular type or serum concentration are not available.

2. *Semi-solid matrix*

Agar is employed both in the Courtenay and in the Hamburger and Salmon methods. Buick *et al.* (1979) reported substitution of methyl cellulose for agar in the plating layer for bladder tumours, and a similar modification has been employed by Pavelic *et al.* (1980) for a range of tumours, whilst Carney *et al.* (1981a) use agarose for lung cancer specimens. Definite superiority for one or the other of these substances has not been reported.

3. *Oxygen tension*

This is considered a major factor in the Courtenay methodology (see Chapter 9). In one of the few published comparative studies Tveit *et al.* (1981a,b) emphasized that low oxygen concentration was one of the factors associated with the increased colony-forming efficiencies obtained using the Courtenay as opposed to the Hamburger and Salmon procedure, working with melanomas. Clearly this condition could readily be incorporated into the Hamburger and Salmon methodology, as recently reported in xenograft studies by Gupta and Krishan (1982) who showed elevated colony-forming efficiencies using an atmosphere of 5% oxygen.

4. *"Feeders"*

The Hamburger and Salmon technique does not employ feeder cells, and they are included in the Courtenay methodology only when less than 10^4 tumour cells are used per assay, an unusual situation if working directly with biopsy specimens on account of their low colony-forming efficiencies. However, lung fibroblasts are a constituent of Laboisse's methodology for gastrointestinal tumours (see Chapter 11). Attempts to improve colony-forming efficiencies in general will require further investigation of the potential value of feeders in particular tumour types, as well as the specific additions discussed below.

5. *"Additional factors"*

The "conditioned" medium originally defined by Hamburger and Salmon (1977a) for growth of myeloma colonies is now considered unnecessary for other tumour types by most groups. Many workers also omit the 2-mercaptoethanol, although this has been routinely employed by Von Hoff's group. Several of the other additions, including DEAE-dextran and tryptic soya broth, have been reported as toxic by certain groups, and there may be problems of batch or source variability. However, it would also appear that their presence is not essential for colony formation. The importance of the growth-promoting effect of lysed red blood cells in the Courtenay method has been emphasized in the comparative studies of Tveit *et al.* (1981a,b) and confirmed by Hill and Whelan (1983). These groups have also demonstrated, in xenografts and cell lines respectively, increased colony-forming efficiencies when red blood cells were incorporated into the Hamburger and Salmon methodology. This approach should now be tested with fresh tumour specimens, although Pavelic *et al.* (1980) reported no benefit from red blood cell additions using the Pluznik and Sachs assay system.

Other additions that have proved beneficial for certain tumour types include epidermal growth factor (Hamburger *et al.*, 1981) and insulin (Mackintosh *et al.*, 1981).

IV. Colony counting and calculation of colony-forming efficiencies

Discriminating between clusters and true colonies remains a controversial topic but is clearly a critical issue. It appears intimately related to the time between cell plating and the scoring of colonies. The introduction of computerized, automated colony counting has permitted scoring within 7–14 days of setting up the assay, contrasting with the longer periods of 3–8 weeks when manual microscopic evaluation is used. The automated procedures frequently utilize a much lower cut-off point for defining colony size, i.e. $\geqslant 20$ or 30 cells per colony, but the majority of groups, scoring by eye, utilize the higher value of $\geqslant 50$ cells per colony. This problem of cluster versus colony also must be remembered if counting is replaced by the suggested measurement of ^{3}H-thymidine incorporation by cells plated in soft agar (Tanigawa *et al.*, 1982). The question as to whether different cell populations are being scored by these two procedures also remains to be answered, particularly in relation to drug sensitivity evaluations. Similarly, the dependence of colony-forming efficiency on the number of cells plated must be clearly established. Whilst this has been reported for ovarian carcinomas, melanomas by certain groups, and transitional cell carcinomas of the bladder (e.g. Hamburger *et al.*,

1978; Buick *et al.*, 1979; Pavelic *et al.*, 1980; Meyskens *et al.*, 1981), it may too frequently be taken for granted. Tveit *et al.* (1981a) emphasized that for melanomas, whilst the number of colonies formed was proportional to the number of cells plated using the Courtenay assay, this was not so using the Hamburger and Salmon methodology. Recently we have demonstrated that it is not proportional with all ovarian samples (Rupniak, unpublished data), even using the Courtenay assay.

V. Characterization of cells in the colonies

There are three main aspects to be considered. The first is to document that the cells growing in the semi-solid matrix are tumour cells. The second requires establishing that these colony-forming cells are representative of the tumour in the patient from which they were derived. The third aspect concerns the relationship of these cells to tumour stem cells.

Growth of cells in soft agar is cited frequently as evidence for cell transformation, but this is clearly an oversimplification. It is known that haematopoietic precursor cells may form colonies in agar and their presence must be monitored by suitable histochemical staining procedures (Hamburger and Salmon, 1977a). It has also been reported that attempts to grow breast cancer cells as colonies in agar medium containing phytohaemagglutinin-stimulated human lymphocyte-conditioned medium resulted in the development of colonies of T-lymphocytes (Asano and Mandell, 1981). Further evidence that malignancy of tissue *in vivo* is not necessary for colony formation in agar is provided by the report of direct cloning of non-malignant fresh human parathyroid hyperplasia cells in agar culture (Bradley *et al.*, 1980). Full identification of cells within the colonies is therefore essential.

Attempts to ensure that the colony-forming cells have characteristics consistent with the tumour of origin have centred on histologic comparisons, production of similar tumour markers (Von Hoff and Johnson, 1979), and karyotypic analyses (Trent and Salmon, 1982). Table 2 summarizes some published data for particular tumour types. The development of monoclonal antibodies directed towards tumour-specific or differential antigens may also prove valuable in this respect.

Establishment of self-renewal capacity, the distinguishing property of stem cells, is a more difficult problem to tackle and will be aided by achieving optimal conditions for colony growth. Several groups have reported that colonies pooled from a single plate produced tumours in nude mice with, for example, some melanomas, sarcomas, and ovarian carcinomas (Pavelic *et al.*, 1980; Slocum *et al.*, 1981). Carney *et al.* (1981b) have reported similar successes with lung tumours and have been able to establish continuous cell

Table 2 Characterization of cells in colonies in semi-solid matrix.

Tumour type	Light and/or electron microscopy	Tumour markers	Karyo-typic analysis	Growth in nude mice	Self-renewal potency	References
Melanoma	●	●	●		●	Meyskens et al. (1981) Thomson and Meyskens
	●	●		●		Von Hoff et al. (1982)
Myeloma	●	●	●			Hamburger and Salmon (1977a)
	●	●	●			Von Hoff and Johnson (1979)
Neuroblastoma	●	●	●			Von Hoff et al. (1980)
Ovary	●	●	●		●	Hamburger et al. (1978) Buick and MacKillop (1981)
Bladder	●		●			Buick et al. (1979)
Lung	●			●	●	Carney et al. (1981b)
Colon	●	●				Buick et al. (1980a)
Gastrointestinal (general)	●	●		●	●	Laboisse (1983) (this volume)

cultures in this way, which they consider confirms the "stem cell" nature of these clonogenic cells. Both human leukaemic clonogenic cells (Buick et al., 1981) and some human ovarian tumours have been shown to have a capacity for self-renewal (Buick and MacKillop, 1981), and recently a procedure to measure directly the self-renewal capacity of clonogenic cells from biopsies of metastatic melanomas has been described (Thomson and Meyskens, 1982). This recent study leads the way for further work with other tumour types.

VI. Overall summary and future prospects

The ability to grow human tumours successfully *in vitro* should have enlarged the horizons of all cell biologists, and if tumour stem cells can be identified from these clonogenic populations the impact should be even greater. It is therefore disappointing that more effort has not already been directed towards optimizing tissue disaggregation procedures and conditions for colony growth for all the various tumour types. This remains a challenge. Whilst the prognostic significance of employing these culture techniques for drug sensitivity testing has to be fully evaluated and the limitations clearly appreciated, as discussed in Chapters 18, 19, 24, and 25, the potential applications for *in vitro* biological studies should not be overlooked. These include identification of the nutritional and hormonal requirements for cells of different histological types, investigations of cell–cell interactions and factors that modulate growth and differentiation of clonogenic cells, analyses of their self-renewal properties, establishment of continuous cell lines, and studies of clonal heterogeneity and cytogenetics of human "solid" tumours.

References

Agrez, M., Lieber, M. M. and Kovach, J. S. (1982). *In vitro* drug sensitivity testing of human colorectal carcinomas. *Stem Cells* **1,** 319.

Asano, S. and Mandel, T. E. (1981). Colonies formed in agar from human breast cancer and their identification as T-lymphocytes. *J. Nat. Cancer Inst.* **67,** 25–32.

Barnes, D. and Sato, G. (1980). Serum-free cell culture: a unifying approach. *Cell* **22,** 649–655.

Bertoncello, I., Bradley, T. R., Campbell, J. J., Day, A. J., McDonald, I. A., McLeish, G. R., Quinn, M. A., Rome, R. and Hodgson, G. S. (1982). Limitations of the clonal agar assay for the assessment of primary human ovarian tumour biopsies. *Br. J. Cancer* **45,** 803–811.

Bottenstein, J. E. (1980). Serum-free culture of neuroblastoma cells. In *Advances in Neuroblastoma Research* (ed. A. E. Evans), pp. 161–170. Raven Press, New York.

Bradley, E. C., Reichert, C. M., Brennan, M. F. and Von Hoff, D. D. (1980). Direct cloning of human parathyroid hyperplasia cells in soft agar culture. *Cancer Res.* **40,** 3694–3696.

Buick, R. N. and MacKillop, W. J. (1981). Measurement of self-renewal in culture of clonogenic cells from human ovarian carcinoma. *Br. J. Cancer* **44,** 349–355.

Buick, R. N., Till, J. E. and McCulloch, E. A. (1977). Colony assay for proliferative blast cells circulating in myeloblastic leukaemia. *Lancet* **i,** 862–863.

Buick, R. N., Fry, S. E., Salmon, S. E. and Stanisic, T. (1979). Development of an agar–methyl cellulose clonogenic assay for cells in transitional cell carcinoma of the bladder. *Cancer Res.* **39,** 5051–5056.

Buick, R. N., Fry, S. E. and Salmon, S. E. (1980a). Application of *in vitro* soft agar techniques for growth of tumour cells to the study of colon cancer. *Cancer* **45,** 1238–1242.

Buick, R. N., Fry, S. E. and Salmon, S. E. (1980b). Effect of host–cell interactions on clonogenic carcinoma cells in human malignant effusions. *Br. J. Cancer* **41,** 695–704.

Buick, R. N., Chang, J.-A. L., Messner, H. A., Curtis, J. E. and McCullouch, E. A.

(1981). Self-renewal capacity of leukemic blast progenitor cells. *Cancer Res.* **41**, 4849–4952.

Carney, D. N., Bunn, P. A., Gazdar, A. F., Pagan, J. A. and Minna, J. D. (1981a). Selective growth of small cell carcinoma of the lung obtained from patient biopsies in serum-free hormone supplemented medium. *Proc. Nat. Acad. Sci.* **78**, 3185–3189.

Carney, D. N., Gazdar, A. F., Bunn, P. A. and Guccion, J. G. (1981b). Demonstration of the stem cell nature of clonogenic tumour cells from lung cancer patients. *Stem Cells* **1**, 149–164.

Courtenay, V. D. and Mills, J. (1978). An *in vitro* colony assay for human tumours grown in immune-suppressed mice and treated *in vivo* with cytotoxic agents. *Br. J. Cancer* **37**, 261–268.

Darfler, F. J. and Insel, P. A. (1982). Serum-free culture of resting, PHA-stimulated, and transformed lymphoid cells, including hybridomas. *Exp. Cell Res.* **138**, 287–295.

Gupta, V. and Krishan, A. (1982). Effect of oxygen concentration on the growth and drug sensitivity of human melanoma cells in soft-agar clonogenic assay. *Cancer Res.* **42**, 1005–1007.

Hamburger, A. W. and Salmon, S. E. (1977a). Primary bioassay of human myeloma stem cells. *J. Clin. Invest.* **60**, 846–854.

Hamburger, A. W. and Salmon, S. E. (1977b). Primary bioassay of human tumor stem cells. *Science* **197**, 461–463.

Hamburger, A. W. and White, C. P. (1981). Interaction between macrophages and human tumor clonogenic cells. *Stem Cells* **1**, 209–223.

Hamburger, A. W., Salmon, S. E., Kim, M. B., Trent, J. M., Soehnlen, B. J., Alberts, D. S. and Schmidt, H. J. (1978). Direct cloning of human ovarian carcinoma cells in agar. *Cancer Res.* **38**, 3438–3444.

Hamburger, A. W., White, C. P. and Brown, R. W. (1981). Effect of epidermal growth factor on proliferation of human tumor cells in soft agar. *J. Nat. Cancer Inst.* **67**, 825–830.

Hill, B. T. and Whelan, R. D. H. (1983). Attempts to optimize colony-forming efficiencies using three different survival assays and a range of continuous human tumour cell lines. *Cell Biol. Int. Rep.* in press.

Izaguirre, C. A., Minden, M. D., Howatson, A. F. and McCulloch, E. A. (1980). Colony formation by normal and malignant human B-lymphoblasts. *Br. J. Cancer* **42**, 430–437.

Jones, S. E., Hamburger, A. W., Kim, M. B. and Salmon, S. E. (1979). Development of a bioassay for putative human lymphoma stem cells. *Blood* **53**, 294–303.

Kaign, M. E., Kirk, D., Szalay, M. and Lechner, J. F. (1981). Growth control of prostatic carcinoma cells in serum-free media: interrelationship of hormone response, cell density and nutrient media. *Proc. Nat. Acad. Sci.* **78**, 5673–5676.

Kern, D. H., Campbell, M. A., Worth, G. D. and Morton, D. L. (1982). Techniques for cloning colorectal carcinomas in soft agar. *Stem Cells* **1**, 319.

Kovach, J. S. and Lieber, M. M. (1981). Drug sensitivity testing of primary cancers with the human tumor stem cell colony assay. Proc. 3rd NCI-EORTC Symp. on New Drugs in Cancer Therapy, Brussels, Belgium. Abstract No. 29.

Laboisse, C. L., Ougeron, C. and Potet, F. (1981). Growth and differentiation of human gastrointestinal adenocarcinoma stem cells in soft agarose. *Cancer Res.* **41**, 310–315.

Mackintosh, F. R., Evans, T. L. and Sikic, B. I. (1981). Methodologic problems in clonogenic assays of spontaneous human tumours. *Cancer Chemother. Pharmacol.* **6**, 205–210.

Macpherson, I. (1973). Soft agar techniques. In *Tissue Culture Methods and Applications* (ed. P. F. Kruse, Jr, and M. K. Patterson, Jr), pp. 276–280. Academic Press.

Mattox, D. E. and Von Hoff, D. D. (1980). *In vitro* stem cell assay in head and neck squamous carcinoma. *Am. J. Surg.* **140**, 527–530.

Messing, E. M., Fahey, J. L., deKernion, J. B., Bhuta, S. M. and Bubbers, J. E. (1982). Serum-free medium for the *in vitro* growth of normal and urinary bladder epithelial cells. *Cancer Res.* **42**, 2392–2397.

Meyskens, F. L., Soehnlen, B. J., Saxe, D. F., Casey, W. J. and Salmon, S. E. (1981). *In vitro* clonal assay for human metastatic melanoma cells. *Stem Cells* **1**, 61–72.

Ozols, R. F., Willson, J. K. V., Grotzinger, K. R. and Young, R. C. (1980). Cloning of human ovarian cancer cells in soft agar from malignant effusions and peritoneal washings. *Cancer Res.* **40**, 2743–2747.

Pavelic, Z. P., Slocum, H. K., Rustum, Y. M., Creaven, P. J., Nowak, N. J., Karakousis, C., Takita, H. and Mittelman, A. (1980). Growth of cell colonies in soft agar from biopsies of different human solid tumours. *Cancer Res.* **40**, 4151–4158.

Puck, T. T. and Marcus, P. I. (1955). A rapid method for viable cell titration and clone productions with HeLa cells in tissue culture: the use of X-irradiated cells to supply conditioning factors. *Proc. Nat. Acad. Sci.* **41**, 432–437.

Rosenblum, M. L., Vasquez, D. A., Hoshimo, T. and Wilson, C. B. (1978). Development of a clonogenic cell assay for human brain tumours. *Cancer* **41**, 2305–2314.

Salmon, S. E. and Von Hoff, D. D. (1981). *In vitro* evaluation of anticancer drugs with the human tumour stem cell assay. *Semin. Oncol.* **8**, 377–385.

Salmon, S. E., Hamburger, A. W., Soehnlen, B. J., Durie, B. G. M., Alberts, D. S. and Moon, T. E. (1978). Quantitation of differential sensitivity of human tumour stem cells to anticancer drugs. *New Engl. J. Med.* **298**, 1321–1327.

Shimizu, T., Motoji, T., Oshimi, K. and Mizoguchi, H. (1982). Proliferative state and radiosensitivity of human myeloma stem cells. *Br. J. Cancer* **45**, 679–683.

Simms, E., Gazdar, A. F., Abrams, P. G. and Minna, J. D. (1980). Growth of human small cell (oat cell) carcinoma of the lung in serum-free growth factor-supplemented medium. *Cancer Res.* **40**, 4356–4363.

Slocum, H. K., Pavelic, Z. P., Kanter, P. M., Nowak, N. J. and Rustum, Y. M. (1981). The soft agar clonogenicity and characterisation of cells obtained from human solid tumours by mechanical and enzymatic means. *Cancer Chemother. Pharmacol.* **5**, 219–225.

Spitzer, G., Verma, D. S., Dicke, K. A. and McCredie, K. B. (1978). Culture studies *in vitro* in human leukaemia. *Semin. Hematol.* **15**, 352–378.

Tanigawa, N., Kern, D. H., Hikasa, Y. and Morton, D. L. (1982). Rapid assay for evaluating the chemosensitivity of human tumours in soft agar culture. *Cancer Res.* **42**, 2159–2164.

Thomson, S. P. and Meyskens, F. L. (1982). A method for measurement of self-renewal capacity of clonogenic cells from biopsies of metastatic human malignant melanoma. *Cancer Res.* **42**, 4606–4613.

Trent, J. M. and Salmon, S. E. (1982). Human tumour karyology: marked analytic enhancement via short-term agar culture. *Br. J. Cancer* **41**, 867–874.

Tveit, K. M., Endresen, L., Rugstad, H. E., Fodstad, O. and Pihl, A. (1981a).

Comparison of two soft-agar methods for assessing chemosensitivity of human tumours *in vitro*: malignant melanomas. *Br. J. Cancer* **44,** 539–544.

Tveit, K. M., Fodstad, O. and Pihl, A. (1981b). Cultivation of human melanomas in soft-agar: factors influencing plating efficiency and chemosensitivity. *Int. J. Cancer* **28,** 329–334.

Von Hoff, D. D. and Johnson, G. E. (1979). Secretion of tumour markers in the human tumour stem cell system. *Proc. Am. Assoc. Cancer Res* **20,** 51.

Von Hoff, D. D., Casper, J., Bradley, E., Trent, J. M., Hodach, A., Reichart, C., Makuch, R. and Altman, A. (1980). Direct cloning of human neuroblastoma cells in soft agar culture. *Cancer Res.* **40,** 3591–3597.

Von Hoff, D. D., Cowan, J., Harris, G. and Reisdorf, G. (1981). Human tumour cloning: feasibility and clinical correlations. *Cancer Chemother. Pharmacol.* **6,** 265–271.

Von Hoff, D. D., Forseth, B., Metelmann, H.-R., Harris, G., Rowan, S. and Coltman, C. A. (1982). Direct cloning of human melanoma in soft agar culture. *Cancer* **50,** 696–701.

9. The Courtenay Clonogenic Assay

D. COURTENAY

I. Introduction

The ability to form colonies in soft agar is one criterion of cell transformation. Growth in soft agar is a convenient means of discriminating between tumour and stromal cells which readily grow in monolayer culture but, being anchorage dependent, do not normally form colonies in agar. Experience so far has shown that by no means all tumour cells form colonies in agar; among those that do, plating efficiency (PE) is usually low. There may be a number of reasons for this. One of the most important is that cells may be irreparably damaged during tumour disaggregation, and it may be no coincidence that tumours giving the highest PE in agar tend to be most readily disaggregated. Both enzymatic and mechanical methods have been used successfully but the choice of method must depend on the characteristics of the individual tumour. Another factor influencing PE is the proportion of non-tumour cells in the final cell suspension, which can be high in disaggregated tumours or in effusions. Also it is widely believed that not all tumour cells are stem cells capable of continued division although, in rapidly growing highly anaplastic tumours, the proportion of stem cells is likely to be high. Finally, PE may be low because of inadequacy of culture conditions. The Courtenay soft agar system represents an attempt to improve PE of tumour cells by simulating more closely growth conditions *in vivo*.

II. Detailed methodology

A. Preparation of cell suspensions

Biopsy specimens should be processed as soon as possible and within 24 hours of excision from the patient. The tumour tissue should be transferred to culture medium at 4°C and transported in water-tight containers in iced water.

Mechanical disaggregation

Solid tumours should be finely chopped using crossed scalpels rather than scissors which can cause bruising of the tissue. From certain tumours, e.g. some melanomas and small cell lung tumours, a good cell yield may be obtained simply by shaking the tumour pieces in phosphate-buffered saline (PBS) and collecting the shed cells. More vigorous mechanical treatments can irreparably damage cells.

METHOD
1. Remove all extraneous tissue from tumour and rinse in PBS.
2. Chop into pieces of < 1 mm diameter in a 90-mm Petri dish using crossed scalpels.
3. Add PBS and pipette pieces into a sterile tube and allow to settle.
4. Remove supernatant and examine microscopically as a guide to nature of treatment required.
5. Incubate tumour pieces in 5 ml PBS for 5 min at 37°C, give two or three sharp shakes by hand to dislodge any loose tumour cells, then allow pieces to settle and remove supernatant.
6. Stain non-viable cells by ejecting 1 drop of supernatant from a Pasteur pipette onto a spot of lissamine green dye solution (2%) previously dried on a microscope slide; mix and transfer to a haemocytometer.
7. Estimate viable cell yield under phase contrast. (If cell yield is low, i.e. less than 10^6 viable cells, the enzymatic method should then be used.)
8. Add 1 ml foetal calf serum to cell suspension, spin, re-suspend in Ham's F12 medium and 15% foetal calf serum, filter through a 20-μm or 30-μm polyester mesh (Henry Simon, Stockport, U.K.).
9. Count viable cell number, keeping cell suspension at 4°C to prevent cell re-aggregation.

Enzymatic disaggregation

Most solid tumours require some form of enzymatic treatment. Various methods have been used as detailed below.

METHOD
(a) *Collagenase–pronase cocktail* (Brown *et al.*, 1980)
Stock cocktail. Dissolve, in Ham's F12 medium, 20 mg collagenase (ex *Clostridium histolyticum*; Boehringer), 50 mg pronase (protease ex *Strep. griseus*; Calbiochem-Behring), and 20 mg DNase (Sigma). Pass through 0.45-μm filter and store at 4°C.
1. To 250 mg tumour pieces add 5 ml cocktail diluted 1/10 with medium without serum.
2. Incubate for 10 min at 37°C on a blood suspension mixer, allow pieces to settle, and discard supernatant.
3. Add 10 ml diluted cocktail and incubate on mixer for 30 min, finally giving two or three sharp shakes to dislodge loose cells.
4. Allow pieces to settle and estimate viable cell yield in supernatant (as described in step 6 above).
5. Repeat enzyme treatment to harvest more cells.

(b) *Trypsin alone*
1. Add 5 ml 0.25% trypsin to 250 mg tumour pieces and incubate at 37°C for 10 min, agitating gently.

2. Allow pieces to settle and discard supernatant.
3. Replace with 5 ml prewarmed 0.25% trypsin and continue incubation until cells begin to detach.
4. Allow pieces to settle in vertical tube and remove supernatant.
5. Add 5 ml medium and incubate at 37°C for 5 min, giving two or three sharp shakes to dislodge cells.
6. Add 1 ml serum and estimate viable cell yield as described above.

(c) *Collagenase followed by trypsin*
1. To 250 mg tumour pieces add 5 ml collagenase (2 mg ml^{-1} in Ham's F12+15% serum), and incubate for 30 min in a horizontal tube (test tube or flat-sided tube; Nunc).
2. Allow pieces to settle (tube vertical) and remove supernatant.
3. Gently rinse tumour pieces twice with warmed PBS.
4. Add 5 ml warmed 0.05% trypsin (Bacto-Difco) in PBS and incubate for 8–10 min, agitating just sufficiently to prevent pieces sticking together.
5. Allow pieces to settle in vertical tube and proceed as in (b)5 above.

In each case the resultant suspension should be passed through a 20–30-μm mesh to exclude clumps.

B. Assay procedures

The Courtenay procedure involves the use of a low O_2 concentration in the gas phase to provide a more physiological oxygen tension in the medium, and the addition of rat red blood cells (RBC) to supply labile growth factors lacking in culture medium. The addition of a replenishable liquid phase permits continued growth of colonies which would otherwise be limited by depletion of the agar medium (see Fig. 1).

Molten 0.5% agar in culture medium is added to a suspension of tumour cells plus RBC. Aliquots (1 ml) of the 0.3% agar mixture are allowed to set in replicate tubes and incubated in an atmosphere with 3% O_2. To maintain the cells in active growth, liquid medium is added at weekly intervals. Colonies of more than 50 cells are counted usually after 3–4 weeks.

Medium
Medium used as the liquid phase and in the agar is Ham's F12. This medium was originally developed for the growth of cells at low cell densities. We have found it superior to basal MEM, alpha medium, or RPMI 1640, but little different from McCoy's medium, in a limited number of tests. Foetal bovine serum at a concentration of 15% or the much cheaper special bobby calf serum (Gibco) have given equally good results. The antibiotics penicillin, streptomycin, and neomycin are added at concentrations of 250, 50, and 100 mg l^{-1}.

Rat RBC
The growth-promoting effect of lysed red blood cells was first demonstrated

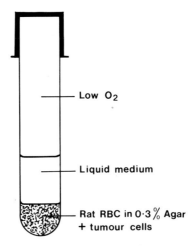

Fig. 1   The replenishable soft agar assay.

by Bradley *et al.* (1971) who showed that growth of colonies from normal mouse bone marrow in agar was greatly enhanced by addition of washed RBC. We have found a similar effect on colony formation by human tumour cells in primary culture. In our soft agar system, addition of washed August rat RBC has consistently improved plating efficiency in virtually all tumours tested and has increased colony growth rate. The effect is most marked in tumours with very low PE.

Growth factors in RBC, some of which have been shown by Kriegler *et al.* (1981) to be related to haemoglobin, are released only after lysis. In culture the active substances are evidently partly labile, since suspensions of whole RBC, which lyse after addition to the agar, were more effective in promoting colony formation than lysates (Bertoncello and Bradley, 1977). Growth-promoting activity declined on storage after 3 weeks. We have had similar experience using RBC to promote growth of tumour cell colonies (Courtenay, 1976); August rat RBC, which conveniently lyse after about 5 days in agar, have given the best results. Human RBC or RBC from other rat strains, including Wistar and Marshall, do not readily lyse in agar and were found unsuitable. RBC are prepared from fresh whole blood rinsed three times with PBS and finally re-suspended to the original volume in medium with serum. Remaining viable nucleated rat blood cells can be toxic to human tumour cells, so these are inactivated by storage at 4°C for 1 week or by heating for 1 hour at 44°C. RBC are used at a final dilution of 1/80 in 0.3% agar. Higher concentrations may initially give greater growth enhancement but their breakdown products may reach levels toxic to tumour cells.

Liquid phase

In general, human tumour cells proliferate less rapidly than those from experimental animal tumours, so starting from a single cell suspension there is a need to maintain cultures longer before colonies of comparable size are obtained. After 10–14 days at 37°C there is some deterioration of the medium and nutrients may become depleted. The use of capped test tubes has made it a simple matter to add liquid medium above the agar and change it when necessary (Courtenay and Mills, 1978). Another advantage of tubes over dishes is that individual caps with tight closure help to maintain stable O_2 concentrations, prevent drying out of agar, and prevent cross infection by moulds or fungi. We have examined the possibility of using 24-mm multidishes (Linbro) as an alternative, but under otherwise identical culture conditions PE was lower.

Oxygen concentration

The need for low oxygen tensions for growth of unadapted tumour cells has become evident only recently. The fact that established cell lines in culture give high PE when gassed with air has been misleading, since such lines have been selected and conditioned to grow under these artificial culture conditions.

In man, toxicity from continued breathing of high oxygen concentrations is well known and normal cells of the body are rarely exposed to O_2 tensions equivalent to that in air. Improved growth of normal cells grown at low O_2 tensions was demonstrated by Richter *et al.* (1972) culturing recently explanted mouse embryonic cells with a gas phase containing 3% O_2 instead of air.

For tumour cells, the importance of low O_2 tensions first became apparent when attempting to grow Lewis lung mouse tumour cells taken directly from the passaged mouse tumour (Courtenay, 1976). It is generally accepted that high cell concentrations are necessary for growth of tumour cells in primary culture, and we also found that the ability to establish viable cultures from mouse tumours depended critically on the number of cells plated. In monolayer cultures, using 35-mm Petri dishes gassed with air + 5% CO_2, continued growth was obtained from 5000 cells but not from 2000 cells. Whilst adding conditioned medium from crowded cultures or increasing the CO_2 concentration to 10% had no effect, reducing the O_2 concentration to 5% yielded viable cultures from 2000 cells or less. Similar results were obtained with the B16 mouse melanoma.

These results suggested that, at high cell concentrations, the rate of oxygen consumption by cell metabolism reduces local oxygen concentration, creating a microenvironment with an oxygen tension significantly lower than at the surface of the medium. However, with a low cell concentration, O_2

consumption will also be low and the O_2 tension in the medium surrounding the cells will approach that in the gas phase. When this is air, cultures may fail owing to O_2 toxicity.

These observations led us to test the effect of low O_2 tensions for growth of human tumour cells. In soft agar cultures we found a consistent improvement in PE of cells taken directly from human biopsy specimens. In our earlier studies we used a 5% O_2 concentration, and some results obtained are shown in Table 1.

Table 1 Plating efficiencies of colonies grown *in vitro* from cell suspensions prepared from tumour biopsies (Courtenay *et al.*, 1978)

Tumour type	Form	Treatment of suspension	Plating efficiency (%)
Melanoma	sc deposit	m	0
	sc deposit	m	15
	sc deposit	m	0.5
	sc deposit	m	3.0
	sc deposit	m	5.6
	sc deposit	m	0
	sc deposit	m	0.2
	node deposit	m	0
	node deposit	m	0
	node deposit	m	0.5
	node deposit	m	0.25
	primary	m	0
	ascites	u	0
Ovarian carcinoma	ascites	u	2.7
	ascites	u	0.25
	ascites	u	0.02
	ascites	u	0.2
	ascites	u	1.0
	ascites	u	1.0
	primary	t	0.4
	secondary dep.	t	1.3
	peritoneal dep.	m	4.5
Colorectal cancer	primary	t+c	0
	primary	t+c	0
	primary	t	0.03
	primary	t	0
	secondary dep.	t+c	0.3
Pancreatic carcinoma	primary	t+c	0.17
Uterine ca. (body)	secondary dep.	m	12
Hypernephroma	secondary dep.	t	0.1
Orchioblastoma	primary	t	0.04

u = untreated; m = mechanical separation; t = trypsin; t+c = trypsin + collagenase.

Subsequently we have found that a further improvement in PE can be obtained, for most tumours, by gassing with 3% oxygen (3% O_2+5% CO_2+92%N_2). For example, with human melanoma biopsies 8/12 tumours tested gave a PE > 1% and 4/12 gave a PE > 5%. Cell concentration is also important since PE generally falls when more than 10 000 tumour cells are plated. This is the standard number of cells plated per assay, and when the number of viable cells is below this the total cell number is made up to 10 000 with heavily irradiated cells of the same tumour type.

Colony counting
Colonies in agar decanted onto a slide or dish are readily counted using a dissecting microscope. For radiation studies a colony size of 50 cells is the minimum acceptable since abortive colonies of up to 30 cells may be produced after low radiation doses. For most drugs the number of abortive divisions is smaller than for radiation and 30-cell colonies may be acceptable. Nevertheless even here there are dangers in counting colonies as small as 30 cells because of the practical difficulty of preparing single cell suspensions from some tumour biopsy specimens. Even when filtered through a 30-μm mesh, clumps of 8 or more cells often pass through, and after 1 or 2 abortive divisions they may be confused with colonies unless a rigorous size standard is maintained.

PRACTICAL METHODS

A. *Preparation of RBC*

(a) *Materials*
August rats; 10 ml syringe with No. 12 needle; heparin (preservative free); PBS; Ham's F12 medium with 15% serum and antibiotics; Universal containers.

(b) *Procedure*
1. With sterile precautions, take up sufficient heparin into syringe to fill the needle.
2. Anaesthetize rat with ether and soak fur of thorax with methylated spirit.
3. Withdraw blood by cardiac puncture; eject blood into a universal container.
4. Mark level of meniscus and centrifuge at 3000 rpm for 15–20 min.
5. Remove buffy coat together with supernatant and discard.
6. Rinse RBC twice with PBS and re-suspend to original blood volume in medium.
7. RBC may be stored for up to 3 weeks at 4°C.
8. Blood used within 7 days of collection must be heat-inactivated for 1 hour at 44°C.

B. *Assay technique*

(a) *Materials*
17×100 mm sterile test tubes (Falcon 2051); metal racks in tray containing iced water; water baths at 37°C and 44°C; culture medium, Ham's F12 + 15% foetal or special bobby calf serum; 5% agar (Difco Agar Noble) in PBS; washed August rat RBC

suspended in culture medium to original blood volume; human tumour cell suspension.

(b) *Procedure in setting up cultures*
1. Dilute tumour cell suspension with culture medium to $5 \times$ required final concentration.
2. Dilute washed RBC 1/8 with medium.
3. Heavily irradiated tumour cells (HR) (added only when less than 1×10^4 tumour cells per tube) are exposed to 40 Gy of X- or γ-radiation, and diluted to 1×10^5 cells ml^{-1}.
4. To set up 5 replicate tubes, measure out in a test tube: 1.2 ml tumour cell suspension $+0.6$ ml RBC $+0.6$ ml HR cells (A).
5. Prepare agar:
  (i) To make 50 ml 0.5% agar medium weigh 250 mg agar in a bijou bottle and add 5 ml PBS.
  (ii) Warm culture medium in 44°C water bath (45 ml to make 50 ml agar medium).
  (iii) Sterilize 5% agar solution by boiling in water bath for 10 min.
  (iv) Remove, tighten cap, swirl to mix, and cool to 60°C.
  (v) Stand in water bath at 44°C for 1 min and then mix with medium at 44°C to make 0.5% agar medium. (0.5% is a nominal concentration. A small amount of agar remaining in the bottle can be ignored. Provided that the agar is firm enough to remain intact with careful handling, colony growth is generally better at final agar concentrations below 0.3%.)
6. Warm mixed cells (A) to 37°C; add 3.6 ml of 0.5% agar medium.
7. Mix by inverting capped tube and then pipette out 1 ml aliquots into 5 vertical Falcon tubes in rack in ice bath.
8. When agar has set (5 min), loosely capped tubes in racks are placed in an incubator at 37°C and gassed with $3\% O_2 + 5\% CO_2 + 92\% N_2$.
9. Caps are tightened 24 hr later to prevent evaporation.

(c) *Alternative gassing systems*
Culture tubes may be incubated in gas-tight containers such as polystyrene lunch boxes (Stewart Plastics) or modular incubator chambers (Flow Laboratories). For this method, both individual culture tubes and containers are gassed.
1. Uncap vertical tubes in racks, and gas individual tubes at a rate of 2 litres min^{-1} for 4 s using a vertical Pasteur pipette.
2. Immediately press on caps in the "gas tight" position.
3. Transfer tubes, which must be kept within 45° of vertical, to lunch boxes and seal box lids with polythene sellotape.
4. Gas boxes at 2 litres min^{-1} for 10 min via 2 holes on opposite sides of the box, and then seal holes with polythene sellotape.

(d) *Maintenance of cultures*
1. After 5–7 days gently pipette 1 ml medium on top of agar and re-gas.
2. Repeat at 14 days.
3. At 21 days withdraw 1 ml "old" medium and replace with 1 ml "new" medium.

(e) *Colony counting* (usually at 21–28 days)
1. Discard medium and decant agar onto a slide or shallow dish.
2. Cover with a 25 mm × 50 mm cover glass and count colonies of more than 50 cells under an inverted microscope.

References

Bertoncello, I. and Bradley, T. R. (1977). The physicochemical properties of erythrocyte derived activity which enhances murine bone marrow colony growth in agar culture. *Aust. J. Exp. Biol. Med. Sci.* **55,** 281–292.

Bradley, T. R., Telfer, P. A. and Fry, P. (1971). The effect of erythrocytes on mouse bone marrow colony development *in vitro*. *Blood* **38,** 353–359.

Brown, J. M., Twentyman, P. R. and Zamvil, S. S. (1980). Response of the RIF-1 tumor *in vitro* and in C3H/Km mice to X-radiation (cell survival, regrowth delay, and tumor control), chemotherapeutic agents and activated macrophages. *J. Nat. Cancer Inst.* **64,** 605–611.

Courtenay, V. D. (1976). A soft agar colony assay for Lewis lung tumour and B16 melanoma taken directly from the mouse. *Br. J. Cancer* **34,** 39–45.

Courtenay, V. D. and Mills, J. (1978). An *in vitro* colony assay for human tumours grown in immune-suppressed mice and treated *in vivo* with cytotoxic agents. *Br. J. Cancer* **37,** 261–268.

Courtenay, V. D., Selby, P. J., Smith, I. E., Mills, J. and Peckham, M. J. (1978). Growth of human tumour cell colonies from biopsies using two soft-agar techniques. *Br. J. Cancer* **38,** 77–81.

Kriegler, A. B., Bradley, T. R., Hodgson, G. S. and McNiece, I. K. (1981). Identification of the "factor" in erythrocyte lysates which enhances colony growth in agar cultures. *Exp. Hematol.* **9,** 11–21.

Richter, A. J., Sanford, K. A. and Evans, V. J. (1972). Influence of oxygen and culture media on plating efficiency of some mammalian tissue cells. *J. Nat. Cancer Inst.* **49,** 1705–1712.

10. The Salmon–Hamburger "Stem" Cell Assay

A. W. HAMBURGER

I. Introduction

Data collected during the past 20 years indicate that only a small percentage of the total tumour cell population is made up of effective stem cells, capable of repopulating a tumour (Steel, 1977). At present descendants of a particular tumour stem cell cannot be counted *in situ*. However, the capacity of cells to form a clone under artificial conditions can be assçessed. Results of a large body of work on animal and human tumours and haematopoietic cells indicate that cells that are clonogenic under test conditions may be the stem cells *in vivo* (Bruce *et al.*, 1966).

Current active interest in the use of cloning techniques in predictive cancer chemotherapy arose from the work of Park *et al.* (1971) at the Ontario Cancer Institute. They devised an *in vitro* system for cloning cells from transplantable murine myeloma and demonstrated *in vitro* that cells from different myeloma sublines responded differently to a number of anticancer drugs. *In vitro* predictions were confirmed by long-term survival tests (Ogawa *et al.*, 1971). Later Steel *et al.* (1977) measured survival of clonogenic B16 melanoma cells, by lung colony assays, endpoint dilution techniques, and growth of cells in soft agar. Results from the three methods agreed well and predicted *in vivo* responses, supporting the biological validity of these *in vitro* methods.

The University of Arizona group was impressed by the success of investigators at the Ontario Cancer Institute in predicting response of mice bearing myelomas to drugs using *in vitro* assays. We hoped to extend their work by developing an assay for human myeloma colony-forming cells. Park had been able to do this but the number of colonies formed was not linearly related to the number of cells plated and the assay could not be used to measure drug effects.

In 1975, when our work began, Courtenay *et al.* (1976) had begun to culture human tumour cells from xenografts in immune-suppressed mice. This system

113

offered the advantage that mice could be treated with appropriate drugs *in vivo*, and thus drugs needing metabolic activation could be tested. However, we believed that the relative simplicity and economy of a Petri dish assay might lead more easily to clinical application of the assay.

The soft agar cloning method as currently practised in our laboratory is now described.

II. Materials

For preparation of conditioned media
BALB/c AnN mice (Charles River Laboratories, Wilmington, Massachusetts). Tissue culture dishes, 60-mm (Falcon 2001). Medium, RPMI 1640 (Gibco, Grand Island, New York). Horse serum and foetal bovine serum (KC Biologicals, Kansas City, Missouri). Penicillin–streptomycin solution (Penicillin 10 000 IU ml^{-1}; streptomycin 10 000 μg ml^{-1}. Glutamine (200 mM), 100 × stock. Filter units, sterile 0.22- and 0.45-μm (Nalgene, Rochester, New York).

For preparation of overlayer
Medium, CMRL 1066 (Gibco). CaCl$_2$ analysed reagent (Baker Chemical, Phillipsburg, New Jersey). Insulin, zinc-crystalline (Elanco, Indianapolis, Indiana). 2-Mercaptoethanol (Sigma). Petri dishes, plastic 35-mm; Gentran 6% (Travenol Laboratories, Deerfield, Illinois). Bacto-Agar (Difco, Detroit, Michigan). Trypan blue, 0.4% solution (Gibco).

For preparation of underlayers
McCoy's 5A medium (Gibco). Sodium pyruvate (tissue culture tested), L-ascorbic acid, L-asparagine (anhydrous), and L-serine (Gibco).

For preparation of tumour cells
Hank's balanced salt solution (10 ×) (Gibco). Heparin, sodium salt, preservative-free (Sigma). Hyaluronidase, Type I (Sigma). Collagenase, Type I (Sigma). DNase, Type I (Sigma). Nylon gauze, various meshes (Tekto, Elmsford, New York). Percoll (Pharmacia, Piscataway, New Jersey).

III. Procedure

A. *Preparation of conditioned media*

1. Inject one BALB/c mouse with 0.2 ml mineral oil intraperitoneally using a 1-ml tuberculin syringe and a 22-ga needle.
2. Kill mouse 8–12 weeks later by cervical dislocation.
3. Under aseptic conditions, make a small incision midpoint of the left side and remove spleen.
4. Place spleen in a 60-mm tissue culture dish and tease with 22-ga needles in 5 ml RPMI 1640 medium without serum.
5. Transfer resultant cell suspension to a 50-ml centrifuge tube and allow large debris and clumps to settle (2–4 min).
6. Pass supernatant through 18-, 22-, and 25-ga needles in 5-ml syringes; this should result in a single cell suspension.

7. Check viability by trypan blue staining and count cells in a haemocytometer.
8. Adjust cell concentration to 1×10^6 cells ml^{-1} in RPMI 1640 medium and 15% foetal bovine serum (FBS).
9. Distribute 5 ml to each 60-mm tissue culture dish to deliver 5×10^6 per plate. (One spleen usually yields enough cells for 15 plates.)
10. Place dishes in incubator for 2–4 h to allow cells to adhere, then aspirate medium and non-adherent cells and rinse dishes 3 times in cold phosphate-buffered saline (pH 7.4).
11. To each dish, add 5 ml RPMI 1640 medium supplemented with 15% FBS, 1% penicillin–streptomycin solution, and 1% glutamine solution.
12. Three days later, examine dishes with an inverted phase microscope. Each $20 \times$ field should be at least half confluent.
13. Collect medium and centrifuge at 800g for 20 min.
14. Pass supernatant through a 0.22-μm Nalgene filter, aliquot, and store for up to 6 months at $-20°C$. NOTE Do *not* freeze–thaw.

B. *Preparation of cell-free underlayers*

1. Prepare Bacto-Agar in double glass distilled water as 3% stock.
   (a) Place 1.5 g agar in 50 ml distilled water in 100-ml bottles.
   (b) Autoclave for 15 min on slow exhaust to dissolve and sterilize agar.
2. Prepare enriched McCoy's 5A medium.
   (a) Make up all supplements: L-serine (21 mg ml^{-1}), penicillin–streptomycin, and sodium pyruvate (2.2%) in glass distilled water.
   (b) Sterilize by filtration in Nalgene units with 0.22-μm grids.
   (c) Add to 500-ml bottle of McCoy's 5A medium the following: 50 ml of FBS, 25 ml horse serum, 1 ml L-serine, 5 ml penicillin–streptomycin, 5 ml sodium pyruvate.
3. Dilute agar to 0.5% in either enriched McCoy's 5A medium or BALB/c spleen cell conditioned medium.
4. Prepare plates containing BALB/c spleen cell conditioned medium.
   (a) Prepare 10 ml of final mixture by adding 2.5 ml BALB/c spleen cell conditioned medium, 1.7 ml 3% agar stock, and 5.8 ml enriched McCoy's. Thus the conditioned medium is present at a final concentration of 1/4. The final concentration of agar is 0.5%.
   (b) Keep agar in water bath at 42°C and medium at 37°C before mixing.
   (c) Vortex the mixture or pipette vigorously.
   (d) Distribute 1 ml final mixture to each 35-mm plastic Petri dish.
   (e) Allow agar to gel for about 10–20 min before applying the second layer containing tumour cells.

NOTE Only myeloma cells required this conditioned media. Blank underlayers consist of 0.83 ml enriched McCoy's 5A medium and 0.17 ml agar stock. These plates are prepared as in steps 1–4. Other growth factors may be added to this underlayer (see Discussion).

C. *Collection and preparation of tumour cells*

1. *Bone marrow cells*
   (a) Collect cells in a syringe containing heparin (10 U ml^{-1}).
   (b) Mix cells with an equal volume of 3% Gentran-saline and allow to sediment at room temperature for 45 min. Red blood cells and mature granulocytes will sediment.

(c) Draw off the supernatant containing cells with a sterile plugged Pasteur pipette and centrifuge at 200g for 20 min.

(d) Wash cells twice in Hank's saline (HBSS) without divalent cations and 10% FBS.

(e) Determine the viable nucleated cell count in a haemocytometer using 3% acetic acid to lyse residual red blood cells.

(f) Determine viability by trypan blue staining.

(g) Prepare enriched CMRL 1066 medium: To a 100-ml bottle of CMRL 1066 medium, add 15 ml horse serum, 1 ml penicillin–streptomycin solution, 1 ml glutamine stock, 4 ml $CaCl_2$ stock (stock = 100 mM), 2 ml insulin stock (stock = 200 U ml^{-1}), and 1 ml L-ascorbic acid stock (stock = 30 mM).

NOTE Prepare all supplements in double-distilled water and sterilize by filtration. Enriched medium may be keep at 4°C for 3–4 weeks.

(h) Re-suspend cells at a concentration of 5×10^6 cells ml^{-1} in enriched CMRL medium.

(i) Prepare slides of bone marrow cells for differential counts.

2. *Cells from pleural effusions*
(a) Collect pleural effusions in bottles containing heparin (10 U ml^{-1}).

(b) Remove cells from pleural effusions by centrifuging at 200g for 10 min.

(c) Lyse excess red blood cells if necessary as follows. Prepare lysing buffer by dissolving 8.29 g NaCl, 1.0 g $KHCO_3$, and 0.037 g EDTA in 1 litre distilled water. Add 2 ml lysing buffer to 0.5 ml packed cell pellet in a 50-ml centrifuge tube. Incubate for 2–5 min at room temperature, rotating tube gently and monitoring for haemolysis. Wash cells twice in HBSS and 10% FBS at 400g for 7 min.

(d) Count cells in a haemocytometer and determine viability.

(e) Re-suspend cells at 5×10^6 cells ml^{-1} in enriched CMRL medium.

(f) Prepare slides for morphologic studies.

3. *Cells from solid tumour biopsies*
(a) Mince solid tumour biopsies with scissors into 3–6 mm pieces and place in a 25-ml trypsinizing flask containing enzyme solution. Add approximately 1 g tissue to 7 ml collagenase (1800 U ml^{-1}), 7 ml hyaluronidase (1220 U ml^{-1}), and 0.14 ml 0.2% DNase (3800 kU ml^{-1} protein). Prepare all enzymes in HBSS and store in appropriate size aliquots at −40°C. Incubate tissue pieces in a shaking water bath at 37°C for 1.5–3 h. Filter cells released into the enzyme solution through 22-μm Nitex gauze to remove cell clumps. Wash cells twice in HBSS with 10% FBS.

(b) Draw filtrate up and down pipette to break up any remaining cell clumps.

(c) Count in a haemocytometer for viability and cell number.

(d) Re-suspend to 5×10^6 cells ml^{-1} in enriched CMRL 1066 medium.

(e) Remove a small aliquot for morphological studies.

(f) We have obtained successful cultures from effusions or bone marrows kept at 4°C for as long as 48 h after collection. Solid tumours are more susceptible to cell death and those cultured within 4 h of collection have provided the highest degree of success. However, if solid tumours are minced into 3–6 mm pieces, stored in complete medium, and gassed to proper pH, cells may be successfully cultured up to 36 h after excision. Although trypan blue viability cannot predict cloning efficiency, we have found it useful to enrich for viable cells. When cell suspensions contain excess debris or viability is less than 10%, cells (2×10^6 ml^{-1} in RPMI 1640 medium without serum) are placed on an equal volume of 25% Percoll in HBSS and spun at 400*g* for 15 min at 15°C. Viable cells pellet and debris remains in the supernatant. Cells are then washed twice with HBSS.

D. *Preparation of overlayers*

1. Prepare enriched CMRL.
2. Prepare 2-mercaptoethanol (2-ME) fresh each week as 5×10^{-3} M stock in double-distilled water. Dispense aliquots in tubes (fill to top) and discard immediately after use. (2-ME is used only to culture myeloma cells.)
3. For each 10 ml final mixture, add 1 ml 3% agar stock to 8 ml enriched CMRL medium and 0.1 ml 2-ME stock.
   (a) Vortex or pipette vigorously.
   (b) Add 1 ml tumour cell suspension when the agar medium mixture has cooled to about 39°C.
   (c) Pipette 1 ml resultant mixture onto 1 ml feeder layers in 35-mm Petri dishes. Each plate should contain 5×10^5 cells.

E. *Evaluation of colony growth*

1. Incubate cultures at 37°C in 5% CO_2 in a humidified atmosphere with no additional feeding. Incubators should be kept very humid to prevent cultures from drying out.
2. Examine cultures twice weekly with an inverted phase microscope at $100 \times$ and $200 \times$.
3. Make final colony counts when colonies reach maximum size (10–21 days after plating). Both colonies (aggregates of 40 or more cells) and clusters (3–40 cells) should be scored. Colonies may be counted using an inverted phase microscope or an automated image-analyser such as the Bausch and Lomb FAS-II. The automated instrument provides a histogram of colony size versus frequency.
4. Dried slides may be prepared from agar cultures to maintain permanent records of colony growth.
   (a) Carefully fill each Petri dish with HBSS and incubate for 15 min at room temperature to elute most of the extracellular proteins and reduce background staining. Aspirate supernatant.
   (b) Fill each dish with fixative solution consisting of 90% absolute ethanol and 10% formaldehyde, and stand at room temperature. Remove fixative.
   (c) Fill each dish with distilled water, agitate, and submerge in a tray containing at least 50 ml distilled water. Incubate for 10 min. Agitate plates to displace the plating layer from Petri dish so that it floats in the water. Introduce a clean microscope slide into an undrained tray and allow the plating layer to spread on the slide.
   (d) Carefully place a prewetted cellulose acetate electrophoresis membrane on the slide. This strip provides for uniform evaporation of water from the agar. Dry the slide for 4–12 h and remove the strip carefully.
   (e) Stain the slide. Papanicolau staining is used for routine purposes, using standard staining times. Colonies can be stained for peroxidase activity prior to fixation. Non-specific esterase and Luxol blue stains performed after the slides have been prepared have proved useful in identifying haematopoietic colonies.

F. *Drug sensitivity assay studies*

1. For routine studies three plates are used per point. Re-suspend cells at 3×10^6 cells

ml^{-1} in McCoy's medium. Add 0.5 ml cell suspension (1.5×10^6 cells) to 0.15 ml drug solution (containing the required drug for three plates) and 0.85 ml McCoy's 5A medium and 10% FBS. Appropriate controls contain 1.0 ml media only.
2.   Incubate for 1 h at 37°C. Wash twice by centrifugation at 600g with HBSS and 10% FBS. Add 2.7 ml enriched CMRL to the cell pellet. Add 0.3 ml 3% agar at 39°C to the tube to yield a final concentration of 0.3% agar. Dispense into three Petri dishes.

NOTE Certain drugs, such as cyclophosphamide, need metabolic activation and cannot be used in this system. The use of drugs such as methotrexate is problematical since cells may be rescued by nucleosides in the medium and serum.

IV. Discussion

The soft agar method described here has proved useful in a number of laboratories for studying basic biology of human tumour clonogenic cells and in predictive drug testing. However, problems inherent in this system remain and should become areas of active investigation over the next few years.

The first problem relates to the low cloning efficiencies of cells from many patients' tumours in this assay. Of course, this may accurately reflect the low proportion of stem cells in a given tumour cell population. However, it is more likely that the clonogenic cell fraction underestimates the true number of *in vivo* stem cells, as we have calculated for multiple myeloma (Hamburger and Salmon, 1977). Therefore attention must be focused on preparation of adequate culture conditions to increase cloning efficiencies of many types of tumour cells. The nutritional and hormonal needs of human tumour cells are still largely unknown. However, the present commercial availability of complex culture media and purified growth factors may facilitate the search for optimal culture conditions. We have found that addition of epidermal growth factor increased cloning efficiencies of cells from a subset of patients with epithelial-derived neoplasms (Hamburger *et al.*, 1981). Similarly, Carney *et al.* (1981) demonstrated that tumour cells derived from patients with small cell carcinoma of the lung could clone under serum-reduced conditions with the addition of hydrocortisone, transferrin, selenium, oestradiol, and insulin. Cowan and Graham (1981) have demonstrated that platelet-derived growth factor influences clonogenicity of human tumour cells in soft agar. Approaches such as these may eventually result in optimization of media for individual tumour types.

Other technical problems include incomplete disaggregation of solid tumours, variability in serum batches, and calculation of drug dosages and times of exposure. However, these problems relate to all *in vitro* assays and are discussed elsewhere in this volume. Finally, the need for close cooperation between personnel in the clinical facilities and in the cell culture laboratory must always be stressed.

References

Bruce, W. R., Meeker, B. E. and Valeriote, F. A. (1966). Comparison of the sensitivity of normal hematopoietic and transplanted lymphoma colony-forming cells to chemotherapeutic agents administered *in vivo*. *J. Nat. Cancer Inst.* **37,** 233–245.

Carney, D., Bunn, P., Gazdar, A. *et al.* (1981). Selective growth in serum free hormone supplemented medium of tumor cells obtained by biopsy from patients with small cell carcinoma of the lung. *Proc. Nat. Acad. Sci.* **78,** 3185–3189.

Courtenay, V. D., Smith, I. E., Peckham, M. J. and Steel, G. C (1976). *In vitro* and *in vivo* radiosensitivity of human tumour cells obtained from a pancreatic carcinoma xenograft. *Nature* **263,** 77–79.

Cowan, D. H. and Graham, J. (1981). Effect of platelet-derived growth factors on human tumor colony growth. *Proc. Am. Assoc. Cancer Res.* **22,** 56.

Hamburger, A. W. and Salmon, S. E. (1977). Primary bioassay of human myeloma stem cells. *J. Clin. Invest.* **60,** 846–854.

Hamburger, A. W., White, C. P. and Brown, R. W. (1981). Effects of epidermal growth factor on proliferation of human tumor cells in soft agar. *J. Nat. Cancer Inst.* **67,** 825–830.

Ogawa, M., Bergsagel, D. and McCulloch, E. (1971). Differential effect of melphalan on mouse myeloma (Adj. PC5) and hematopoietic stem cells. *Cancer Res.* **31,** 2116–2119.

Park, C. H., Bergsagel, D. E. and McCulloch, E. A. (1971). Mouse myeloma tumor stem cells: a primary cell culture assay. *J. Nat. Cancer Inst.* **46,** 411–422.

Steel, G. C. (1977). *Growth Kinetics of Tumours*, pp. 217–267. Oxford University Press, London.

Steel, G. G., Adams, K. and Stephens, T. C. (1977). Clonogenic assays in B16 melanoma: response to cyclophosphamide. *Br. J. Cancer* **36,** 618–624.

11. The Agarose Method for Clonogenic Culture of Gastrointestinal Tumours

C. L. LABOISSE

I. Introduction

Cells in a tumour that survive injuries caused by the disaggregation methods and then grow in a "hostile" environment are called clonogenic cells. The exact role played by these cells in tumour growth *in vivo* remains to be elucidated. The prognostic value of the proportion of clonogenic cells in a tumour is not clearly understood (Laboisse *et al.*, 1981; Loesch *et al.*, 1982), and the differentiation properties of many of these cells are not known. When we began studying growth and differentiation of clonogenic cells of human gastrointestinal cancers there was a clear need for a colony assay optimized for these cancers. Pioneering work of Macpherson and Montagnier (1964) and studies of Montagnier (1971) and of Hamburger and Salmon (1977a) on the growth of tumour cells in semi-solid media furnished a firm conceptual framework for our work.

II. Methods

A. Production of monodispersed cell suspensions from human gastrointestinal tumours

Collection of tumour fragments and washings has been described in detail elsewhere (Laboisse *et al.*, 1981). Emphasis here will be on our enzymatic dispersion method. After five washings, tumour fragments are finely minced with a scalpel (No. 23, Feather) in 100 mm diameter Petri dishes containing phosphate-buffered saline (PBS) so that the enzyme solution can penetrate the matrix easily. Collagenase type IV (Sigma or Worthington) is used for tissue

121

disaggregation, and it may be necessary to test several batches to find one suitable. Unlike trypsin, collagenase requires the presence of Ca^{2+} ions and is not inactivated by serum (Lasfargues, 1973). Tumour samples may thus be left for 12–20 hours in a serum-containing medium with gentle agitation. Our protocol involves overnight treatment of tumour fragments at 37°C in 0.07% collagenase in Dulbecco's modified Eagle's medium (DME) buffered with 25 mM Hepes and supplemented with 10% heat-inactivated foetal bovine serum (FBS). The disaggregation process is monitored two or three times and dissociation is completed by gently pipetting the cell suspension with a large bore pipette. The cell suspension is washed twice, filtered through sterile gauze, and cells are then re-suspended in DME containing 20% FBS and 10% tryptose phosphate broth (Flow Laboratories, Rockville, Maryland). The number of cells recovered is counted in haemocytometer chambers and viability is assessed by trypan blue exclusion. The percentage of nucleated cells is determined on haematoxylin-eosin stained smears.

B. Soft agarose clonogenic assay

Culture conditions are very critical for cell growth, so they are reported here in detail.

Agarose and DME stock
To prepare 1.25% agarose stock, 1.25 g of agarose (agarose A37, indubiose; Réactifs IBF, Villeneuve-la-Garenne, France) is added to 100 ml of water in a screw-capped bottle (water used throughout the experiment is passed through ion exchange resin and then twice distilled in quartz glassware). After completely dissolving the agarose, in a boiling water bath, the stock is left for an additional 20 min in the boiling water bath to ensure sterilization. Simple boiling is preferred to autoclaving since it may be less damaging to the agarose. For use, agarose is transferred to a 45° water bath. (A 1.125% agarose stock is prepared similarly.)

DME ($2 \times$) is made up as follows: 20 ml of $10 \times$ DME (Gibco); 4 ml of L-glutamine (200 mM); 66 ml of sterile water; 10 ml of sodium bicarbonate (7.5%).

Complete nutritional medium
Heat inactivated FBS (20 ml) and 20 ml of tryptose phosphate broth are added to 80 ml of $2 \times$ DME. This nutritional medium is placed in a 45°C water bath.

Preparation of 0.5% agarose underlay
Complete nutritional medium (60 ml) is mixed with 40 ml of the 1.25% agarose stock solution. Antibiotics (gentamycin, 40 μg ml^{-1}; amphotericin B, 3 μg

ml^{-1}) and insulin from bovine pancreas (Sigma) (10 μg ml^{-1}, prepared in 0.05 N HCl) are added. 0.5% agarose solution (6 ml) is pipetted into 60-mm Petri dishes which are left to set at room temperature.

Preparation of the cell-containing overlay
A 0.45% agarose solution is made by mixing 60 ml of complete nutritional medium with 40 ml of 1.125% agarose stock solution. Antibiotics and insulin are added as above. One volume of cell suspension in medium at 37°C is mixed with two volumes of 0.45% agarose medium at 45°C. The volume of the top layer is 1.5 ml. The number of cells per culture should be sufficiently high (2–5 × 10^5 nucleated viable cells) to ensure a significant number of colonies. Finally the overlay is allowed to gel at room temperature by placing dishes on a vibration-free support for a few minutes. Cultures are incubated at 37°C in a 5% CO_2 humidified atmosphere. Colonies (aggregates of ⩾40 cells) can be counted 15 days after plating (Fig. 1a).

C. Preparation of the feeder layer

Normal human lung fibroblasts (MRC5 cells strain) are used, between passage numbers 20–30, as feeder cells. Confluent monolayers are trypsinized and the cells added to 0.5% agarose solution. One ml of cell suspension in agarose, containing 4–5 × 10^5 cells, is poured onto a 3 ml agarose underlay and allowed to gel. Cells are then covered with 1.5 ml of 0.5% agarose to isolate feeder cells from the overlay containing tumour cells. Thus feeder cells are suspended in soft agarose just under the overlay.

D. Morphological examination of the colonies

Characterization of colonies grown in agarose is a difficult task. Squash preparations, often employed by haematologists, were found to be unsuitable. In our laboratory, as shown by C. Augeron, adequate processing of colonies for morphological examination as well as for histochemical characterization necessitates glutaraldehyde fixation and Epon embedding. This may be achieved by fixation of the entire content of the Petri dish according to Zucker-Franklin and Grusky (1974), with some modifications (Laboisse *et al.*, 1981). In some cases it is also possible to pick up colonies with a hard gelatin capsule from the agarose and to process each colony separately in embedding moulds. Thereafter routine staining (Fig. 1b) or specific histochemical reactions may be performed on semi-thin sections. Colonies embedded in Epon are also processed for electron microscopy (Fig. 2a).

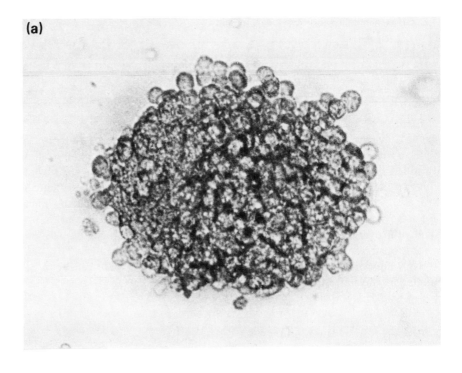

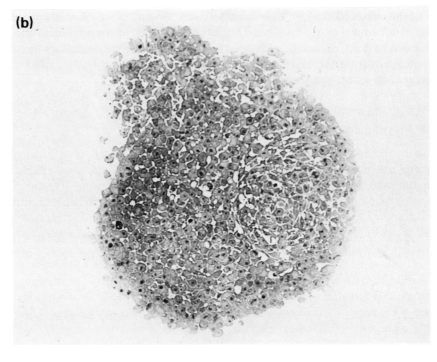

E. Subculturing colonies

In certain cases colonies may be subcultured to establish a continuous cell line. Colonies are removed from agarose with a pipette and resuspended in liquid medium. This suspension is then poured onto a 5 ml underlay of 0.5% agarose containing human fibroblastic feeder cells prepared as above. These colonies can grow in liquid medium, can free themselves from the agarose matrix, and release actively growing cells into the medium. An overlay sample is then transferred to a plastic Falcon flask (25 cm^2) in which colonies can attach to the bottom and grow as a monolayer (Fig. 2b).

III. Discussion

Tissue disaggregation methods and culture conditions are critical for growth of human gastrointestinal clonogenic cancer cells. Enzymatic dissociation of tumours using collagenase (Laboisse et al., 1981), enrichment of the clonogenic cell population by velocity sedimentation (Kimball et al., 1978), and optimization of culture conditions (i.e. agarose preferred over agar, addition of insulin, and use of feeder cells) (Laboisse et al., 1981) were found to improve clonogenic growth of digestive tract tumours. Subsequent reports have indicated that dispersion of cells with collagenase (Besch et al., 1982; Hamburger et al., 1982) as well as culture in agarose instead of agar (Daniels et al., 1981) markedly improved clonal growth of a variety of tumours. Interestingly, Kirk et al. (1981, 1982) have shown that human lung fibroblasts cultured in a non-anchored fashion in soft agar or agarose stimulate growth of numerous cancer cell lines in semi-solid media.

In spite of these efforts to improve growth of clonogenic tumour cells, cloning efficiencies remain low (0–0.8% in our studies with digestive tract tumours), and this represents only a minimum estimate of the clonogenic pool of a tumour. In particular, some cancer cells are clearly anchorage dependent (Dodson et al., 1981), so cloning efficiency, as measured by soft agar or agarose clonogenic assay, does not take this anchorage dependent clonogenic tumour cell pool into account.

The nature of clonogenic cells may be inferred from morphological examination of their progeny, from re-plating experiments or from subculture of colonies and transplantation into nude mice. In our assay the cancerous nature of clonogenic cells is proven by cytological criteria when examining

Fig. 1 (a) Colony composed of numerous tightly packed cells grown from a poorly differentiated gastric adenocarcinoma. (Inverted microscope × 240.) (b) Semi-thin section of a colony arising from a poorly differentiated gastric adenocarcinoma. (Toluidine blue × 200.)

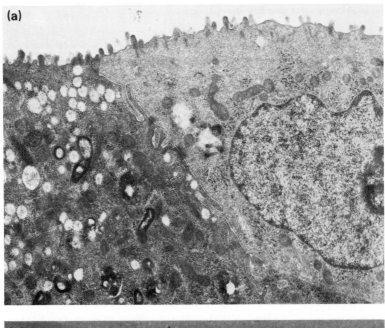

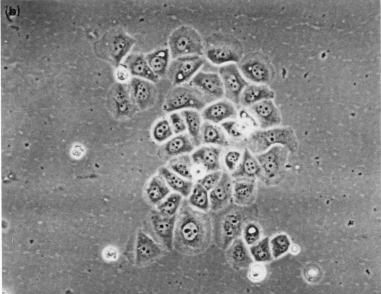

Fig. 2 (a) Electron micrograph showing a portion of a colony arising from a differentiated, mucin secreting colonic adenocarcinoma. Desmosomes are present between the cells. One cell contains many secretory vacuoles. (× 11 600) (b) Subculture of colonies, showing attachment of a tumour colony to the bottom of a plastic flask. Epithelial cells grow in clusters without fibroblastic cell contamination. (Phase contrast × 200.)

semi-thin colony sections. Moreover histochemical staining of colonies that arose from differentiated, mucin secreting tumours revealed secretory vacuoles exhibiting histochemical characters similar to those of the initial tumour. At the ultrastructural level, the occurrence of typical desmosomes between cells was good evidence for the epithelial nature of colonies (Fig. 2a). Further proof of the malignant nature of clonogenic cells was obtained by subculturing colonies from a gastric carcinoma for several passages *in vitro* and then injecting them into nude mice. Tumours formed and they exhibited a histological pattern similar to that of the initial tumour (Laboisse *et al.*, 1982). However, even using all these criteria, we can only assume that a major proportion of colonies arise from cancer cells, since the malignant nature of all colonies is not proven. Contamination of soft agar cultures by normal cells of haematopoietic origin is well documented when bone marrow cells of patients with multiple myeloma are cultured (Hamburger and Salmon, 1977b). Contamination by fibroblasts may also occur. In a recent study Peehl and Standbridge (1981) showed that normal human fibroblasts can be grown in methylcellulose provided that the medium is supplemented with sufficient serum and hydrocortisone. This finding therefore poses a warning to investigators attempting to optimize culture conditions by adding numerous mitogenic factors.

Finally, are clonogenic cells of digestive tract cancers true tumour stem cells? In order to answer this question it would be necessary to test the self-renewal potency of these cells by extensive re-plating experiments. We have not attempted these experiments. However, a gastric carcinoma plated in soft agarose did display a relatively high cloning efficiency, and this feature encouraged us to begin long-term culture of the colonies *in vitro*. Our success in establishing this cell line HGT-1 (Laboisse *et al.*, 1982) was a clear demonstration that many clonogenic cells were in fact true tumour stem cells with extensive proliferative capacity.

References

Besch, G. J., Wolberg, W. H., Gilchrist, K. W. and Gould M. N. (1982). A comparison of methods for the production of monodispersed cell suspensions from human primary breast carcinomas. *Proc. Am. Assoc. Cancer Res.* **23,** 717 (abstract).

Daniels, A. M., Daniels, J. R. and Luck, E. E. (1981). Agarose matrix and enzymatic disaggregation improve efficiency of the soft agar chemosensitivity test. *Proc. Am. Assoc. Cancer Res.* **22,** 616 (abstract).

Dodson, M. G., Slota, J., Lange, C. and Major, E. (1981). Distinction of the phenotypes of *in vitro* anchorage-independent soft-agar growth and *in vivo* tumorigenicity in the nude mouse. *Cancer Res.* **41,** 1441–1446.

Hamburger, A. W. and Salmon, S. E. (1977a). Primary bioassay of human tumor stem cells. *Science* **197,** 461–463.

Hamburger, A. W. and Salmon, S. E. (1977b). Primary bioassay of human myeloma stem cells. *J. Clin. Invest.* **60,**846–854.

Hamburger, A. W., White, C. P. and Tencer, K. (1982). Effect of enzymatic disaggregation on proliferation of human tumor cells in soft agar. *J. Nat. Cancer Inst.* **68,** 945–949.

Kimball, P. M., Brattain, M. G. and Pitts, A. M. (1978). A soft agar procedure measuring growth of human colonic carcinomas. *Br. J. Cancer* **37,** 1015–1019.

Kirk, D., Szalay, M. F. and Kaighn, M. E. (1981). Modulation of growth of a human prostatic cancer cell line (PC-3) in agar culture by normal human lung fibroblasts. *Cancer Res.* **41,** 1100–1103.

Kirk, D., Vener, G. and Kaighn, M. E. (1982). Comparative growth modulation of different human tumor cells in soft agarose by neonatal lung fibroblats. *In Vitro* **18,** 18 (abstract).

Laboisse, C. L., Augeron, C. and Potet, F. (1981). Growth and differentiation of human gastrointestinal adenocarcinoma stem cells in soft agarose. *Cancer Res.* **41,** 310–315.

Laboisse, C. L., Augeron, C., Couturier-Turpin, M. H., Gespach, C., Cheret, A. M. and Potet, F. (1982). Characterization of a newly established human gastric cancer cell line HGT-1 bearing histamine H_2-receptors. *Cancer Res.* **42,** 1541–1548.

Lasfargues, E. Y. (1973). Human mammary tumors. In *Tissue Culture: Methods and Applications* (ed. P. F. Kruse, Jr, and M. K. Patterson, Jr), pp. 45–50. Academic Press, New York.

Loesch, D. M., Von Hoff, D. D., Page, C. P., Rodriguez, V. and the South Texas Cloning Group (1982). Direct cloning of human adenocarcinoma of the colon in soft agar: relationship to negative clinical correlates and level of CEA titer. *Proc. Am. Assoc. Cancer Res.* **23,** 735 (abstract).

Macpherson, I. and Montagnier, L. (1964). Agar suspension culture for the selective assay of cells transformed by polyoma virus. *Virology* **23,** 291–294.

Montagnier, L. (1971). Factors controlling the multiplication of untransformed and transformed BHK 21 cells under various environmental conditions. In *Growth Control in Cell Cultures* (ed. G. E. W. Wolstenholme and J. Knight), pp. 33–44. Churchill Livingstone, Edinburgh.

Peehl, D. M. and Standbridge, E. J. (1981). Anchorage-independent growth of normal human fibroblasts. *Proc. Nat. Acad. Sci.* **78,** 3053–3057.

Zucker-Franklin, D. and Grusky, G. V. (1974). Ultrastructural analysis of hematopoietic colonies derived from human peripheral blood. *J. Cell Biol.* **63,** 855–863.

12. Use of Continuous Human Tumour Cell Lines to Evaluate Drugs by Clonogenic Assays

B. T. HILL

I. Introduction

In the last decade a great deal of progress has been made in culturing human tumour tissues. The establishment of human tumours in continuous culture has provided a further experimental system for cytotoxic drug evaluation, and its potential value in this respect merits full investigation.

This chapter discusses various human tumour cell lines that have been characterized, summarizes results obtained in the relatively few studies where they have been used to evaluate antitumour drugs, comments on their limitations and advantages, and suggests areas for future study.

II. Continuous cell lines established from human tumours

Primary tumours, bone marrow aspirations, pleural effusions, and other metastases have all provided material for developing cell lines. Techniques adopted have involved (i) direct plating of disaggregated tumour cells into primary culture, (ii) outgrowth from tissue explants, (iii) isolation of colonies from semi-solid growth media, and (iv) xenografting tumour specimens. There is no clear-cut evidence specifically favouring one particular source of material or technique. Success rates of 1–10% are most frequently reported for establishing continuous lines from human tumour material (Smith and Dollbaum, 1981). Reasons for this must include inadequate tumour sampling, overgrowth by fibroblasts, suboptimal growth conditions relating to essential concentrations of basal salts or specific growth factors, and use of only plastic or glass substrates. With more research effort it is hoped that these figures will be significantly improved. Detailed characterization of the lines is essential, as discussed in a recent review (Smith and Dollbaum, 1981), particularly ensuring their human origin by chromosome and isoenzyme analyses, and confirming the absence of cell contaminants such as HeLa.

Over the past 10 years cell lines have been established in culture from a variety of human tumours. The major types are listed in Table 1 and some reviews and more recent references are quoted. These data emphasize that certain tumour types have received more attention than others and/or are

Table 1 List of human tumour types from which continuous cell lines have been established and characterized

---

Group I   Reports of at least 20 continuous lines
Bladder (predominantly from transitional cell carcinomas)
Breast (from primary tumours and metastases)
Colon
Head and neck (from squamous cell carcinomas)
Lung (from small cell carcinomas)
Melanoma
Sarcomas

Group II   Reports of at least 10 continuous lines
Brain (predominantly from gliomas)
Kidney (predominantly from renal cell carcinomas)
Lymphoid
Myeloma
Neuroblastoma
Testis

Group III   Reports of less than 10 continuous lines
Cervix
Liver
Lung (from adenocarcinomas)
Ovary
Pancreas
Prostate (predominantly from metastases)
Stomach
Thyroid
Uterus
Vagina
Vulva

Reviews and References: Leibovitz *et al.* (1976); Fogh *et al.* (1977a,b); Engel and Young (1978); Sinkovics *et al.* (1978); Gazdar *et al.* (1980); Pettengill *et al.* (1980); Reid *et al.* (1980); Bottenstein (1981); Brodeur *et al.* (1981); Easty *et al.* (1981); Smith and Dollbaum (1981); Tveit *et al.* (1981b); Yung *et al.* (1982); Rupniak *et al.* (1982); Hepburn and Masters (1983); Metcalfe *et al.* (1983).

more amenable to establishment in culture, whilst more lines are needed particularly from tumours of the ovary, pancreas, prostate, and stomach. The major criticism of these tumour lines is that they represent discrete subpopulations within a heterogeneous tumour specimen, characterized by their capacity for vigorous and maintained growth under the *in vitro* conditions provided. Such selection appears inevitable but perhaps serves only to emphasize the need to examine a whole panel of tumour lines for each tissue type.

III. Assay procedures for drug evaluations

If continuous cell lines are to be used for drug sensitivity testing two major requirements must be met: (i) a single-cell suspension must be readily obtainable; (ii) cells must be capable of forming colonies so that survival can be accurately assessed, since most authors consider clonogenic assays the most reliable predictors of survival (Roper and Drewinko, 1976; Hamburger and Salmon, 1977; Courtenay and Mills, 1978). Colony-forming assays used for human tumours have been described in detail in earlier chapters of this book. Cells from lines in general have higher colony-forming efficiencies than cells obtained working directly with biopsy specimens, and assay conditions frequently do not have to be so rigorous, although consistently improved colony formation has been shown with certain human tumour cell lines using the Courtenay procedure (Hill *et al.*, 1982a). However, three methods have been most widely used: (i) plating cells directly onto plastic $\pm$ "feeder" underlayers; (ii) a double agar layer system of 0.3% on a 0.5% base layer $\pm$ "feeders"; (iii) a single agar/agarose concentration of 0.3%–0.18% $\pm$ "feeders". One of the characteristics of malignancy is the ability of cells to form colonies in agar. However, there is increasing evidence that certain tumour cell lines lack this ability. For example, positive colony formation in agar was reported in only 9 of 47 breast cancer cell lines (Engel and Young, 1978) and in only 2 of 5 head and neck tumour cell lines tested (Easty *et al.*, 1981). Certain lines failing to form colonies in semi-solid media or having extremely low efficiencies will form colonies on plastic, suggesting that growth without anchorage is not necessarily a property of malignancy (see e.g. Table 2). A few other lines readily form colonies under either conditions, e.g. LoVo and MCF7 cells (see Table 3).

Table 3 lists cell lines, many currently in use in my laboratory, that have been employed in drug evaluation studies. It can be seen that with most of them colony-forming efficiencies of over 10% can be obtained. These values contrast with figures of 0.1% or less generally obtained with biopsy specimens directly, so again the question of cell selection bias is raised. However, in two

Table 2   Differential colony-forming efficiencies (CFE) in agar or on plastic of some recently established human tumour cell lines. (Rupniak *et al.*, 1982)

Cell line	Tumour type/origin	Growth media	Doubling time (h)	% CFE (in agar)*	% CFE (on plastic)
TR126	s.c.c. tongue	Ham's F12 + 10% FCS	21	0.012	33
TR131	s.c.c. larynx	Ham's F12 + 10% FCS	34	0.001	16
TR138	s.c.c. larynx	Ham's F12 + 10% FCS	22	$0\ (<10^{-4})$	6
TR146	s.c.c. buccal cavity	Ham's F12 + 10% FCS	22	0.019	46

* Using the procedure of Courtenay and Mills (1978).

more recent publications a wider range of colony-forming efficiencies has been quoted, 0.7–53% in 10 melanoma lines (Tveit *et al.*, 1981b), appearing very low amongst 10 lines derived from small cell lung carcinomas (0.03–5.2%), but approaching 30–40% in two adenocarcinoma lines (Gazdar *et al.*, 1980).

It has been proposed that drug sensitivities may be influenced by variations in the following factors: (i) colony-forming efficiencies; (ii) growth media; (iii) passage number; (iv) cell population doubling time; (v) proportion of proliferating versus non-proliferating cells. Evidence to support many of these contentions using human tumour cell lines frequently is not available or is contradictory.

Our experimental data with a neuroblastoma cell line (LAN-1) and a line derived from a colon carcinoma (COLO 205) fail to support the contention that drug sensitivities are influenced by the colony-forming efficiency obtained or the assay method used, *provided that* conditions of drug exposure are identical (Whelan and Hill, 1981; Hill and Whelan, 1983). Indeed variations in conditions of drug exposure can result in a significant drug dose modification factor (Courtenay and Mills, 1981). A variety of media and sera have been employed in drug sensitivity testing (see e.g. Tables 2 and 3), the choice originally being made probably on the basis of availability in each laboratory. Composition of culture medium, however, is known to affect results of certain drug assays. For example, the presence of normal metabolites can significantly modulate cytotoxicity of antimetabolites *in vitro* since thymidine protects from methotrexate and uridine may protect from 5-fluorouracil cytotoxicity (cited by Hakala and Rustum, 1979). Reservations have also been expressed about drug–serum binding which may interfere with the assays, and

Table 3 Characteristics of continuous cell lines used for drug sensitivity evaluations in various types of tumour.

Cell line	Growth media*	Doubling time (h)†	CFE (%)	CF conditions	References
Neuroblastoma					
CHP100	RPMI 1640	29	22	0.18% agarose	Whelan and Hill (1981)
CHP212	RPMI 1640	22	15	0.18% agarose	Hill (unpublished)
LAN-1	Ham's F12 or Waymouths	37	22–50	0.18% agarose	Whelan and Hill (1981)
Prostate					
PC3mA2	RPMI 1640 or Ham's F12	25	15	0.18% agarose	Metcalfe et al. (1983)
DU145	RPMI 1640 or Ham's F12	24	5–20	0.18% agarose	Metcalfe et al. (1983)
HPC36	RPMI 1640 or Ham's F12	28	20	0.18% agarose	Metcalfe et al. (1983)
LNCap	RPMI 1640 or Ham's F12	30	10	0.18% agarose	Metcalfe et al. (1983)
Head and neck					
HN-1	Dulbecco's modified Eagle	38	18	0.18% agarose	Whelan and Hill (1981)
Colon					
COLO 205	RPMI 1640	24	15	0.18% agarose	Whelan and Hill (1981)
COLO 206	RPMI 1640	24	12–20	0.18% agarose	Whelan and Hill (1981)
LoVo	RPMI 1640 or Ham's F12	34	26–50	0.18% agarose	Whelan and Hill (1981)
	Ham's F10 + 20% FCS	29	35–70	on plastic	Drewinko et al. (1979b)
HT29	McCoy's + 20% FCS	n.s.	60	0.27% agarose	Kimball and Brattain (1980)
Breast					
MCF 7	EME + Eagle's salts†	36	5–10	on plastic	Van den Berg et al. (1981)
	IMEM + 5% calf serum †	n.s.	10	0.41% agar	Nawata et al. (1981)

Table 3 (*cont.*)

Cell line	Growth media*	Doubling time (h)†	CFE (%)	CF conditions	References
Lymphoma					
T1	Ham's F10 + 20% FCS	27	40	on plastic	Drewinko et al. (1979a)
CCRF-CEM	RPMI 1640	n.s.	30–60	0.25% agarose	Norman et al. (1978)
KG-1	Alpha + 15% FCS	n.s.	3	0.3% agar	Koeffler et al. (1981)
Raji	McCoy's 5-A	24	29	0.3% agar	Wu et al. (1982)
Bladder					
RT 112	RPMI 1640	24	16	on plastic	Hepburn (unpublished)
T24	RPMI 1640	18	60	on plastic	Hepburn (unpublished)
RT 4	RPMI 1640	47	4	on plastic	Hepburn (unpublished)
Melanoma					
19-4	McCoy's 5A + 20% FCS	25	40	on plastic	Barranco et al. (1972)
26-5	McCoy's 5A + 20% FCS	30	40	on plastic	Barranco et al. (1972)
39-5	McCoy's 5A + 20% FCS	43	40	on plastic	Barranco et al. (1972)
49-5	McCoy's 5A + 20% FCS	48	40	on plastic	Barranco et al. (1972)
EFM	RPMI 1640 + Hepes + 15% FCS	18	53	0.3% agar	Tveit et al. (1981b)
GEM	RPMI 1640 + Hepes + 15% FCS	39	1.1	0.3% agar	Tveit et al. (1981b)
AAM	RPMI 1640 + Hepes + 15% FCS	52	0.7	0.3% agar	Tveit et al. (1981b)

* 10% foetal calf serum (FCS) was included, except where stated otherwise.
† n.s. = not stated; EME = Eagle's minimal essential; IMEM = improved minimal essential.

the variability of different batches of sera is a well recognized problem. In this respect it is of particular interest that serum-free media capable of supporting human tumour cell growth in culture have now been described for growth of small cell lung carcinoma (Carney *et al.*, 1981), malignant urinary bladder epithelia (Messing *et al.*, 1982), and neuroblastoma cells (Bottenstein, 1981).

Properties of cells in culture may change as a function of passage, and this in turn may affect their drug sensitivities. For this reason the use of cells over a restricted number of passages has been recommended, although not frequently adhered to. Evidence supporting this contention, however, is not readily available. Indeed Tveit *et al.* (1981b) reported that, with melanoma lines, permanent cultures showed the same chemosensitivities as earlier subcultures.

Reported doubling times for continuous cell lines range from 15 to 150 hours. There is no apparent relationship between doubling time and colony-forming efficiencies, as shown by the examples in Tables 2 and 3, and by data of Engel and Young (1978), Gazdar *et al.* (1980), and Tveit *et al.* (1981b), who even report positive colony formation with cell lines having doubling times as long as 120 and 149 hours. In a few comparative studies of drug sensitivities, where heterogeneity has been observed (discussed below), this has specifically *not* been related to altered doubling times. Differential responses of proliferating and non-proliferating cells in culture to drug exposure have been investigated in detail by Drewinko *et al.* (1981) (discussed below) but using only one cell line. The influence of variable proportions of proliferating and non-proliferating cells in populations on their overall drug sensitivities therefore remains to be established.

In summary, when proposing the use of continuous human tumour cell lines for drug evaluations, the colony-forming efficiencies should be optimized and media standardized. Disappointingly there are very few reports of attempts to modify and improve colony-forming efficiency by identifying specific conditions for particular tumour types. We have shown that, for many continuous cell lines, colony-forming efficiencies can be increased by reducing the concentration of soft-agar or agarose used (Whelan and Hill, 1981). Benefit also appeared to accrue in all cases tested when August rat red blood cells were incorporated into the assays (Tveit *et al.*, 1981a; Hill *et al.*, 1982a; Hill and Whelan, 1983). The superiority of incubation under conditions of low oxygen tension has been shown in a few studies but only with limited cell types, predominantly from xenografts (Courtenay and Mills, 1978; Tveit *et al.*, 1981a; Gupta and Krishan, 1982). However, there are only conflicting reports of the superiority of agar or agarose, and the value of "feeder" layers has not been firmly established, with certain laboratories favouring their use with all cell types whilst others frequently omit them. So, further studies in this area are needed and should be encouraged.

IV. Results of drug evaluation studies employing clonogenic assays in continuous human tumour cell lines

In general, continuous human tumour cell lines have proved more resistant *in vitro* to most antitumour drugs than animal tumour lines. However, these differences appear quantitative rather than qualitative, and with only a few exceptions comparable patterns of response have been reported.

A. Comparative responses to a range of antitumour drugs using individual cell lines

1. *Dose–response and time–response survival assessments*

Three major studies have established dose–response curves for a large number of antitumour drugs using a single human tumour cell line. Drewinko *et al.* (1979a), using T1 lymphoma cells and 1 hour drug exposures, documented five patterns of cell survival response (see Fig. 1a and Table 4). In a subsequent publication, using LoVo cells (Drewinko *et al.*, 1981), these five divisions were less clear-cut. However, by grouping together types A and C, characterized by exponential curves, and types B and D, characterized by biphasic responses tending to plateau, with the exception of 5-fluorouracil and VP-16-213, the drugs fell into similar categories. (With LoVo cells 5-fluorouracil produced exponential kill, whilst VP-16-213 treatment resulted in a type B survival curve.) Hill and Whelan (1981a), using a neuroblastoma cell line and 24 hour drug exposures, reported that only two types of survival curves were obtained (see Fig. 1b and Table 4). It is of interest that these data correspond exactly with the original Kinetic Classification of Antitumour Agents of Bruce *et al.* (1966) who evaluated responses of normal and malignant stem cells to various antitumour drugs administered *in vivo* over 24 hours to lymphoma-bearing mice.

Wu *et al.* (1982) addressed the question of the influence of drug exposure duration on cell survival using Raji lymphoma cells. Results obtained using 11 anticancer drugs for either 1 hour or continuous drug exposure were compared and three distinct patterns were observed: (a) actinomycin D, adriamycin, bleomycin, mitomycin C, vincristine, and cis-platinum all produced a dose-dependent reduction in colony formation with a 1 hour exposure, which was further augmented by continuous exposure to the drugs; (b) methotrexate, cytosine arabinoside, 5-fluorouracil, and pentamethylmelamine had no suppressive effects on colony formation with a 1 hour exposure, but produced marked cytotoxicity with continuous drug exposure; (c) melphalan had the same degree of colony suppression with both 1 hour and

Table 4   Classification of antitumour agents based on clonogenic cell
survival patterns.

	Drewinko *et al* (1979a)		Hill and Whelan (1981a)
Type A (Simple exponential)	Adriamycin Rubidazone Cis-platinum VP-16-213	*Class II* (Exponential plateau)	ICRF 159 Hydroxyurea Vincristine Vindesine VM-26
Type B (Biphasic exponential)	Bleomycin Peptichemio		VP-16-213
		Class III (Exponential)	Actinomycin D Adriamycin
Type C (Threshold exponential)	Melphalan BCNU CCNU MeCCNU Cis-acid Yoshi 864		Bleomycin Cis-platinum Dibromodulcitol 5-Fluorouracil m-AMSA Melphalan Peptichemio
Type D (Exponential plateau)	Methotrexate Hydroxyurea		
Type E (Ineffective)	Cytosine arabinoside 5-Fluorouracil		

continuous drug exposure. This latter category, however, was considered rather an artifact, resulting from rapid degradation of melphalan to an inactive form. So these data agree with other reports of enhanced cell kill when drug exposure is prolonged beyond 1 hour.

In general these studies are consistent and correspond with earlier studies using animal tumour cell lines. The exceptions which include 5-fluorouracil, VP-16-213, bleomycin, and vindesine may reflect heterogeneity of response (discussed below) and again suggest that a panel of different lines for each tumour type should be examined.

2. *Cell kinetic parameters*
Cell cycle specific events have been established predominantly in non-human cell lines, with the exception of certain HeLa lines (Hill, 1978). Few studies comparing responses in animal and human cell lines have been reported: S-phase specific cell kill has been shown for vincristine and vindesine, using

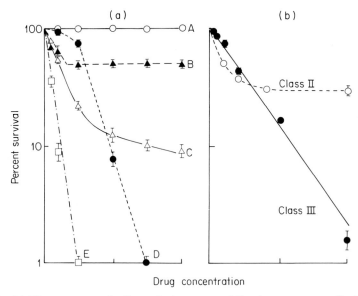

Fig. 1 (a) Five patterns of cell survival response following treatment of a human lymphoma cell line (T1) with antitumour drugs for 1 hour *in vitro*: (A) cis-platinum; (B) bleomycin; (C) CCNU; (D) prednisolone; (E) cytosine arabinoside. (Drewinko *et al.*, 1979a) (b) Two patterns of cell survival response following treatment of a human neuroblastoma cell line (CHP100) with antitumour drugs for 24 hours *in vitro*: Class II, e.g. vincristine; Class III, e.g. cis-platinum. (Hill and Whelan, 1981a)

both NIL8 Syrian hamster ovary cells and CHP100 human neuroblastoma cells (Hill and Whelan, 1981b), whilst cytotoxic and cytokinetic effects of m-AMSA reported in two human tumour lines were similar to those described in Chinese hamster ovary cells (Drewinko *et al.*, 1982). When investigating lethal effects of nitrosoureas as a function of cell position in the cycle at the time of drug administration, it was reported that the pattern of responses differed significantly between the two cell types tested, LoVo and T1 cells (Drewinko *et al.*, 1979b). These authors therefore emphasized the inadequacy of extrapolating results obtained on a given cell line to a generalized statement covering the response of mammalian cells.

In spite of their own reservations, however, Drewinko *et al.* (1981), using LoVo cells, stated that non-proliferating human cells have decreased sensitivity to most antitumour agents. They failed to confirm data from cell lines of rodent origin showing increased efficacy of BCNU, bleomycin, or hydroxyurea on non-proliferating cells. But again there appear differences depending even on the human line studied, which may be related to the definition of "stationary" phase cultures and their cell cycle distribution patterns. Vindesine proved ineffective against stationary phase CHP100 cells over 1 or 24 hour drug exposures (Hill and Whelan, 1981b), but was 20-fold more effective against stationary as opposed to exponentially growing LoVo cells, resulting in at least 2 logs of cell kill following a 1 hour exposure. Such differences may warrant further studies using other cell lines.

B. Comparative drug sensitivity testing using a range of cell lines

Most of these studies have demonstrated significant heterogeneity in drug sensitivities. Indeed, heterogeneity appears to be a widespread phenomenon in both animal and human neoplasms. Its presence has been documented (i) between cells populating an individual tumour, a primary neoplasm and its metastases, and between various metastases (as reviewed by Tsuruo and Fidler, 1981), (ii) between human tumour cells *in vitro* and *in vivo*, and (iii) questionably between normal and malignant cells of the same tissue type. However, many of these studies have only been carried out using animal tumours, and in the few experiments with human tumours rarely have clonogenic assays been employed for establishing drug effects.

The presence of differential sensitivities in subclones derived from a single tumour was first reported by Barranco *et al.* (1972), using four melanoma cell strains and evaluating cytosine arabinoside. Subsequently differential responses to BCNU, but not bleomycin, were also described in the same cell lines (Barranco *et al.*, 1973). Heterogeneity of drug sensitivity has since been identified in subclones from colon carcinomas, to 5-fluorouracil (Kimball and Brattain, 1980) and to 5-fluorouracil, actinomycin D, and methotrexate (Calabresi *et al.*, 1979), and in malignant gliomas when testing BCNU and cis-platinum (Yung *et al.*, 1982).

Studies employing multiple established cell lines have also shown that heterogeneity, in terms of drug responses, is frequently expressed. For example: (i) Tveit *et al.* (1981b) found variable chemosensitivities to six different cytotoxic agents in 9 melanoma lines; (ii) Siegel *et al.* (1980) in two neuroblastoma lines demonstrated significantly varied responses to cyclophosphamide and vincristine; (iii) also using neuroblastoma cells, a 1000-fold difference in response to methotrexate has been documented between five cell lines (Hill, unpublished data); (iv) variable drug responses have been noted by Carney *et al.* (1982) with small cell lung cancer lines.

Differences in *in vivo* and *in vitro* responses to chemotherapeutic agents between cell subclones have been observed by Calabresi and coworkers (1979) using human colon cancers. Tveit *et al.* (1981b) have stressed in their work with melanomas that considerable changes in chemosensitivity may occur when cells are brought from *in vivo* to *in vitro* conditions and vice versa. However, such alterations were not invariable, which may explain the claimed *in vitro–in vivo* correlations of Siegel *et al.* (1980) using two neuroblastoma lines.

Clearly the presence within a tumour of subpopulations of cells with different drug sensitivities has profound implications for designing clinical chemotherapy protocols. Somewhat pessimistically Tsuruo and Fidler (1981) state that, because of differences in drug sensitivities which exist, "it is unlikely that better correlation between *in vitro* sensitivity of tumour cells obtained from a single metastasis and clinical therapy can be achieved". However, the challenge of heterogeneity must be confronted. Models for studying human tumour cell heterogeneity must be developed (as discussed by Baylin, 1982), increased usage of human tumour material must be encouraged, and it is hoped that in this way factors responsible for these differential drug responses amongst heterogeneous tumour cell populations can be determined. In this respect human tumour cell lines appear to have a central role to play since they can be used to screen a large range of cell types. Attempts to study mechanisms associated with these altered responses are remarkable only for their absence. In two studies it was specifically stated that alterations in morphology, growth rate, labelling indices, and chromosome numbers were not involved (Barranco *et al.*, 1973; Yung *et al.*, 1982). Membrane alterations have been implicated, but not documented, and the provocative suggestion that differential mechanisms of cell killing by cytosine arabinoside and BCNU might be responsible for the differential responses observed (Barranco *et al.*, 1973) does not appear to have been followed up.

C. Clinical relevance of laboratory data and attempted laboratory/clinical correlations

In only a few cases have authors suggested, even tentatively, that their data may have clinical application. Drewinko *et al.* (1979a) suggested the following guide lines for clinical investigations on the basis of their classification of antitumour drugs according to patterns of cell survival *in vitro* following 1 hour drug exposures (see Fig. 1a and Table 4): (i) drugs producing type A curves appear potentially effective singly and independent of scheduling; (ii) type B drugs are best used in combinations; (iii) rapid escalation of dosage is favoured for drugs producing type C curves; (iv) judicious scheduling or combination with other agents is recommended with type D drugs; (v) drugs of type E should be administered by continuous intravenous infusion. Reports of clinical studies validating these predictions are still awaited.

Hill and Whelan (1981a) demonstrated that patterns of cell survival after 24 hour drug exposures of human tumour colony-forming cells *in vitro* confirmed the division of drugs as Class II or Class III agents, originally described by Bruce *et al.* (1966) when they proposed their Kinetic Classification of Antitumour Agents (see Fig. 1b and Table 4). This observation may have direct clinical benefit since knowledge of this classification already has proven value in designing safer clinical chemotherapy protocols (Hill, 1978; cited by Price *et al.*, 1981). The administration of drug combinations over approximately 24 hours rather than several days has been shown to reduce toxicity without compromising antitumour effectiveness. When designing such combinations it has been found that toxicity of Class II agents to normal stem cells (e.g. bone marrow) is not dose dependent. Class II drugs therefore may be added to combinations without reducing their dose, provided that the total treatment time is approximately 24 hours. Combinations of Class III drugs will be additively toxic to normal bone marrow, and therefore doses should be reduced proportionately. The use of human tumour cell lines *in vitro* to derive this kinetic classification is of course considerably more convenient than employing the original spleen colony assay procedure, and it can now be used for testing new agents to establish whether they belong to Class II or III. Such information may then be used to predict their safe and effective use as single agents or in drug combinations.

Siegel *et al.* (1980), using two human neuroblastomas, were able to correlate drug sensitivities of the tumours in the patient with those of the cell lines established in culture and in nude mice. They therefore suggested that these lines may provide a relevant model system for evaluating conventional and new chemotherapeutic agents against this disease. Similarly, Hill and Whelan (1981a) used a human neuroblastoma line to screen experimentally for agents specifically effective against this tumour. The preliminary nature of their observations, derived only from a single line, and the inadequacy of pharmacological data available to correlate *in vitro* and *in vivo* tumour drug concentration are stressed. However, tests with 15 drugs allowed their grouping as effective agents, those with some activity, or as ineffective agents. Initial correlations with the clinical activity of the drugs were encouraging since VM26 and adriamycin, used successfully in treating neuroblastomas, were identified as the most effective agents *in vitro*. Studies with other cell lines are now under way. The value of human acute myelogenous leukaemia cell lines as models for the development of new chemotherapeutic schedules and combinations has also been suggested (Koeffler *et al.*, 1981). They compared drug sensitivities of a leukaemic line KG-1 and normal human marrow myeloid clonogenic cells, and found equivalent responses to the drugs tested, including cytosine arabinoside and daunorubicin.

However, most authors would agree that no valid conclusions concerning the sensitivity of a particular tumour type to a specific drug can be reached on the basis of tests carried out on a single or even a few cell lines. For each tumour type a large panel of different cell lines must be examined. Even so, Tveit *et al.* (1981b) suggested that continuous cell lines should be used to study mechanisms of action of chemotherapeutic agents and the development of resistance rather than for direct drug sensitivity evaluations. However, encouragement to pursue the evaluation of drug sensitivities in a range of continuous human tumour cell lines is provided by the recent preliminary report of Carney *et al.* (1982) that such lines derived from small cell lung cancers may be just as useful a screening system for clinical correlations as the original tumour biopsy specimens.

V. Limitations and advantages associated with the use of continuous human tumour cell lines

It is not suggested that continuous human tumour cell lines provide *the* ideal model system for drug sensitivity evaluation; there are many limitations associated with their use, and some examples are listed in Table 5. However, their advantages (see Table 5) can also be stressed and provide a basis for future studies.

VI. Future prospects and conclusions

There is a major requirement for many more human tumour cell lines to be established from a variety of biopsy specimens from all tumour types. This will be aided by improving and optimizing cell culturing techniques and conditions. Such knowledge may also enable improved colony-forming efficiencies to be obtained, so aiding accurate assessments of the influence of drugs on cell survival.

These cell lines may be used for the following studies orientated to antitumour drug evaluations. (i) Elucidation of mechanism(s) of drug action, in particular concentrating on the observed heterogeneity of response to drugs amongst tumour cell populations. (ii) Evaluation of potential improved analogues, comparable to studies using human biopsy specimens to test a range of newer anthracycline derivatives (Salmon *et al.*, 1981). (iii) Establishing dose and time dependent effects on cell survival with antitumour drugs, similar to studies carried out for example with m-AMSA (Drewinko *et al.*, 1982), vindesine (Hill and Whelan, 1981b), and spirogermanium (Hill *et al.*, 1982b). (iv) Determination of valuable drug combinations by identifying synergy or antagonism, and possibly investigations of optimal drug sequences or schedules for use in combination chemotherapy protocols. (v) Identifying mechanisms of drug resistance using not only lines in which resistance is induced *in vitro* experimentally but also those that demonstrate resistance *ab initio*. To date few such studies have involved human tumours, the work on

Table 5 Limitations and advantages associated with the use of continuous human tumour cell lines *in vitro*.

Limitations	Advantages
1. Selected subpopulation of cells—? representative of *in situ* tumour—? retention of tissue specificity	1. Ample supply of material for a large number of assays, which can be carried out rapidly
2. Altered kinetic properties with duration of time in culture	2. Only small quantities of new drug required for testing
3. Contamination with other cell types, e.g. HeLa	3. Detailed study of time and/or dose dependence of cell killing effects of drugs possible
4. Problems of equating drug concentrations used *in vitro* with those achievable clinically, specifically intratumourally	4. Valuable for rapid, inexpensive prescreening of new drugs and potential analogues
5. Proliferation dependence adequately tested but no measure of host toxicities obtainable	5. Valuable source of hormones and growth factors to aid optimization of growth conditions for specific tumour types and clonogenic assay procedures
6. Altered drug metabolism and/or pharmacokinetics *in vitro* and *in vivo*	6. Drug assays may be carried out in serum-free conditions obviating any drug–serum interactions

Vinca alkaloid resistance in CCRF-CEM lymphoblasts (Beck and Cirtain, 1982) proving one of the exceptions. (vi) Clarifying patterns of drug metabolism, which may also be associated with heterogeneity of drug sensitivities and resistance.

It is hoped therefore that both pessimists and optimists concerning the value of cell lines for drug evaluations will be encouraged to pursue these fields of investigation, so providing a more balanced overall approach and some definitive answers.

References

Barranco, S. C., Ho, D. H. W., Drewinko, B., Romsdahl, M. M. and Humphrey, R. M. (1972). Differential sensitivities of human melanoma cells grown *in vitro* to arabinosylcytosine. *Cancer Res.* **32**, 2733–2736.
Barranco, S. C., Drewinko, B. and Humphrey, R. M. (1973). Differential response by

human melanoma cells to 1,3-bis-(2-chloroethyl)-1-nitrosourea and bleomycin. *Mutation Res.* **19**, 277–280.

Baylin, S. B. (1982). Clonal selection and heterogeneity of human solid neoplasms. In *Design of Models for Testing Cancer Therapeutic Agents* (ed. I. J. Fidler and R. J. White), pp. 50–63. Van Nostrand Reinhold, New York.

Beck, W. T. and Cirtain, M. C. (1982). Continued expression of vinca alkaloid resistance by CCRF-CEM cells after treatment with tunicamycin or pronase. *Cancer Res.* **42**, 184–189.

Bottenstein, J. E. (1981). Differentiated properties of neuronal cell lines. In *Functionally Differentiated Cell Lines* (ed. G. Sato), pp. 155–184. Alan R. Liss Inc., New York.

Brodeur G. M., Green, A. A., Hayes, F. A., Williams, K. J., Williams, D. L. and Tsiatis, A. A. (1981). Cytogenetic features of human neuroblastomas and cell lines. *Cancer Res.* **41**, 4678–4686.

Bruce, W. R., Meeker, B. E. and Valeriote, F. A. (1966). Comparison of the sensitivity of normal hematopoietic and transplanted lymphoma colony-forming cells to chemotherapeutic agents administered *in vivo*. *J. Nat. Cancer Inst.* **37**, 233–245.

Calabresi, P., Dexter, D. L. and Heppner, G. H. (1979). Clinical and pharmacological implications of cancer cell differentiation and heterogeneity. *Biochem. Pharmacol.* **28**, 1933–1941.

Carney, D. N., Bunn, Jr, P. A., Gazdar, A. F., Pagan, J. A. and Minna, J. D. (1981). Selective growth in serum-free hormone-supplemented medium of tumour cells obtained by biopsy from patients with small cell carcinoma of the lung. *Proc. Nat. Acad. Sci.* **78**, 3185–3189.

Carney, D. N., Gazdar, A. F. and Minna, J. D. (1982). *In vitro* chemosensitivity of clinical specimens and established cell lines of small cell lung cancer. *Stem Cells* **1**, 296.

Courtenay, V. D. and Mills, J. (1978). An *in vitro* colony assay for human tumours grown in immune-suppressed mice and treated *in vivo* with cytotoxic agents. *Br. J. Cancer* **37**, 261–268.

Courtenay, V. D. and Mills, J. (1981). Factors influencing killing of human tumour cells by melphalan *in vitro*. *Br. J. Cancer* **44**, 306.

Drewinko, B., Roper, P. R. and Barlogie, B. (1979a). Patterns of cell survival following treatment with antitumor agents *in vitro*. *Eur. J. Cancer* **15**, 93–98.

Drewinko, B., Barlogie, B. and Freireich, E. J. (1979b). Response of exponentially growing, stationary-phase, and synchronized cultured human colon carcinoma cells to treatment with nitrosourea derivatives. *Cancer Res.* **39**, 2630–2636.

Drewinko, B., Patchen, M., Yang, L.-Y. and Barlogie, B. (1981). Differential killing efficacy of twenty antitumor drugs on proliferating and nonproliferating human tumor cells. *Cancer Res.* **41**, 2328–2333.

Drewinko, B., Yang, L.-Y. and Barlogie, B. (1982). Lethal activity and kinetic response of cultured human cells to 4′-(9-acridinylamino)methanesulfon-*m*-anisidide. *Cancer Res.* **42**, 107–111.

Easty, D. M., Easty, G. C., Carter, R. L., Monaghan, P. and Butler, L. J. (1981). Ten human carcinoma cell lines derived from squamous carcinomas of the head and neck. *Br. J. Cancer* **43**, 772–785.

Engel, L. W. and Young, N. A. (1978). Human breast carcinoma cells in continuous culture: a review. *Cancer Res.* **38**, 4327–4339.

Fogh, J., Wright, W. C. and Loveless, J. D. (1977a). Absence of HeLa cell contamination in 169 cell lines derived from human tumors. *J. Nat. Cancer Inst.* **58**, 209–214.

Fogh, J., Fogh, J. M. and Orfeo, T. (1977b). One hundred and twenty-seven cultured human tumor cell lines producing tumors in nude mice. *J. Nat. Cancer Inst.* **59**, 221–225.

Gazdar, A. F., Carney, D. N., Russell, E. K., Sims, H. L., Baylin, S. B., Bunn, Jr, P. A., Guccion, J. G. and Minna, J. D. (1980). Establishment of continuous, clonable cultures of small-cell carcinoma of the lung which have amine precursor uptake and decarboxylation cell properties. *Cancer Res.* **40**, 3502–3507.

Gupta, V. and Krishan, A. (1982). Effect of oxygen concentration on the growth and drug sensitivity of human melanoma cells in soft-agar clonogenic assay. *Cancer Res.* **42**, 1005–1007.

Hakala, M. T. and Rustum, Y. M. (1979). The potential value of *in vitro* screening. In *Methods in Cancer Research*, Vol. XVI (ed. V. T. DeVita, Jr, and H. Bush), pp. 247–287. Academic Press, New York.

Hamburger, A. W. and Salmon, S. E. (1977). Primary bioassay of human tumour stem cells. *Science* **197**, 461–463.

Hepburn, P. and Masters, J. R. W. (1983). The biological characteristics of continuous cell lines derived from human bladder. In *The Pathology of Bladder Cancer* (ed. G. T. Bryan and S. M. Cohen). CRC Press (in press).

Hill, B. T. (1978). Cancer chemotherapy: the relevance of certain concepts of cell cycle kinetics. *Biochim. Biophys. Acta* **516**, 389–417.

Hill, B. T. and Whelan, R. D. H. (1981a). Assessments of the sensitivities of cultured human neuroblastoma cells to anti-tumour drugs. *Pediatr. Res* **15**, 1117–1122.

Hill, B. T. and Whelan, R. D. H. (1981b). Comparative cell killing and kinetic effects of vincristine or vindesine in mammalian cell lines. *J. Nat. Cancer Inst.* **67**, 437–443.

Hill, B. T. and Whelan, R. D. H. (1983). Attempts to optimise colony-forming efficiencies using three different survival assays and a range of continuous human tumour cell lines. *Cell Biol. Int. Rep.* (in press).

Hill, B. T., Rupniak, H. T., Whelan, R. D. H. and Metcalfe, S. A. (1982a). Improved colony formation with human tumours using the Courtenay clonogenic assay. *Stem Cells* **1**, 322.

Hill, B. T., Whatley, S. A., Bellamy, A. S., Jenkins, L. Y. and Whelan, R. D. H. (1982b). Cytotoxic effects and biological activity of 2-aza-8-germanspiro[4,5]decane-2-propanamine-8,8-diethyl-*N*,*N*-dimethyl dichloride (NSC 192965; spirogermanium) *in vitro. Cancer Res.* **42**, 2852–2856.

Kimball, P. M. and Brattain, M. G. (1980). Isolation of a cellular subpopulation from a human colonic carcinoma cell line. *Cancer Res.* **40**, 1574–1579.

Koeffler, H. P., Yen, J. and Lowe, L. (1981). An *in vitro* model for acute myelogenous leukemia chemotherapy. *Cancer* **48**, 1958–1963.

Leibovitz, A., Stinson, J. C., McCombs, III, W. B., McCoy, C. E., Mazur, K. C. and Mabry, N. D. (1976). Classification of human colorectal adenocarcinoma cell lines. *Cancer Res.* **36**, 4562–4569.

Messing, E. M., Fahey, J. L., deKernion, J. B., Bhuta, S. M. and Bubbers, J. E. (1982). Serum-free medium for the *in vitro* growth of normal and malignant urinary bladder epithelial cells. *Cancer Res.* **42**, 2392–2397.

Metcalfe, S. A., Whelan, R. D. H., Masters, J. R. W. and Hill, B. T. (1983). *In vitro* responses of human prostate tumor cell lines to a range of antitumor agents. *Int. J. Cancer* (in press).

Nawata, H., Bronzert, D. and Lippman, M. E. (1981). Isolation and characterization of a tamoxifen-resistant cell line derived from MCF-7 human breast cancer cells. *J. Biol. Chem.* **256**, 5016–5021.

Norman, M. R., Harmon, J. M. and Thompson, E. B. (1978). Use of a human lymphoid cell line to evaluate interactions between prednisolone and other chemotherapeutic agents. *Cancer Res.* **38**, 4273–4278.

Pettengill, O. S., Sorenson, G. D., Wurster-Hill, D. H., Curphey, T. J., Noll, W. W., Cate, C. C. and Maurer, L. H. (1980). Isolation and growth characteristics of continuous cell lines from small-cell carcinoma of the lung. *Cancer* **45**, 906–918.

Price, L. A., Hill, B. T. and Ghilchik, M. W. (eds) (1981). *Safer Cancer Chemotherapy*, pp. 1–120. Baillière Tindall, London.

Reid, L. M., Minato, N. and Rojkind, M. (1980). Human prostatic cells in culture and in conditioned animals. In *Male Accessory Sex Glands* (ed. E. Spring-Mills and E. S. E. Hafez), pp. 617–640. Elsevier/North-Holland Biomedical Press.

Roper, P. and Drewinko, B. (1976). Comparison of *in vitro* methods to determine drug induced cell lethality. *Cancer Res.* **36**, 2182–2188.

Rupniak, H. T., Lane, E. B., Trejdosiewicz, L. K., Steele, J. G., Laskiewicz, B., Shaw, H. J. and Hill, B. T. (1982). Preliminary characterization of some recently established human cell lines derived from squamous cell carcinomas of the head and neck. Proc. 1st Eur. Congr. on Cell Biology. Abstract No. 22.

Salmon, S. E., Liu, R. M. and Casazza, A. M. (1981). Evaluation of new anthracycline analogs with the human tumor stem cell assay. *Cancer Chemother. Pharmacol.* **6**, 103–110.

Siegel, M. M., Chung, H. S., Rucker, N., Siegel, S. E., Seeger, R. C., Isaacs, Jr, H. and Benedict, W. F. (1980). *In vitro* and *in vivo* preclinical chemotherapy studies of human neuroblastoma. *Cancer Treat. Rep.* **64**, 975–979.

Sinkovics, J. G., Gyorkey, F., Kusyk, C. and Siciliano, M. J. (1978). Growth of human tumor cells in established culture. *Methods Cancer Res.* **14**, 243–323.

Smith, H. S. and Dollbaum, Ch. M. (1981). Growth of human tumors in culture. In *Tissue Growth Factors* (ed. R. Baserga), pp. 451–490. Springer Verlag.

Tsuruo, T. and Fidler, I. J. (1981). Differences in drug sensitivity among tumor cells from parental tumors, selected variants, and spontaneous metastases. *Cancer Res.* **41**, 3058–3064.

Tveit, K. M., Fodstad, O. and Pihl, A. (1981a). Cultivation of human melanomas in soft agar: factors influencing plating efficiency and chemosensitivity. *Int. J. Cancer* **28**, 329–334.

Tveit, K. M., Fodstad, O. and Pihl, A. (1981b). The usefulness of human tumor cell lines in the study of chemosensitivity: a study of malignant melanomas. *Int. J. Cancer* **28**, 403–408.

Van Den Berg, H. W., Clarke, R. and Murphy, R. F. (1981). Failure of 5-fluorouracil and methotrexate to destroy the reproductive integrity of a human breast cancer cell line (MCF-7) growing *in vitro*. *Eur. J. Cancer Clin. Oncol.* **17**, 1275–1281.

Whelan, D. H. and Hill, B. T. (1981). The influence of agarose concentration on the cloning efficiency of a series of established human cell lines. *Cell Biol. Int. Rep.* **5**, 1137–1142.

Wu, P.-C., Ozols, R. F., Hatanaka, M. and Boone, C. W. (1982). Anticancer drugs: effect on the cloning of Raji lymphoma cells in soft agar. *J. Nat. Cancer Inst.* **68**, 115–121.

Yung, W.-K. A., Shapiro, J. R. and Shapiro, W. R. (1982). Heterogeneous chemosensitivities of subpopulations of human glioma cells in culture. *Cancer Res.* **42**, 992–998.

13. Growth of Tumour Cells as Multicellular Spheroids and Antitumour Drug Evaluation

T. NEDERMAN

I. Introduction

Several factors may modify the effectiveness of chemotherapy of solid tumours. These include problems with drug penetration due to poor vascularization, proliferation gradients, which have varying effects depending on the cell-cycle specificity of the drug, and differences in the microenvironment (i.e. pH and pO_2) as a function of the distance from supporting blood vessels. Most of these factors are to some degree simulated *in vitro* by multicellular spheroids (Fig. 1a).

The tumour-like properties of spheroids have been described in detail by Sutherland and Durand (1976). Briefly, spheroids consist of aggregated cells in a spherical configuration (Fig. 1b). Peripheral cells proliferate intensively and contribute to spheroid growth. Deeper lying cells probably suffer from a poor supply of nutrients and inadequate clearance of catabolic products. Proliferation decreases as a function of depth (Carlsson, 1977; Haji-Karim and Carlsson, 1978; Wibe *et al.*, 1981) and, if spheroids are big enough (0.4–0.8 mm, depending on the cell line), massive, necrotic regions will develop in the central parts. A wide variety of research applications of cellular spheroids has been demonstrated: these applications were reviewed by Sutherland *et al.* (1981).

II. Culture of spheroids

A. Spinner flask technique

The spinner flask technique has been used extensively for cultivating rodent cell spheroids (Sutherland *et al.*, 1971; Sutherland and Durand, 1976). A

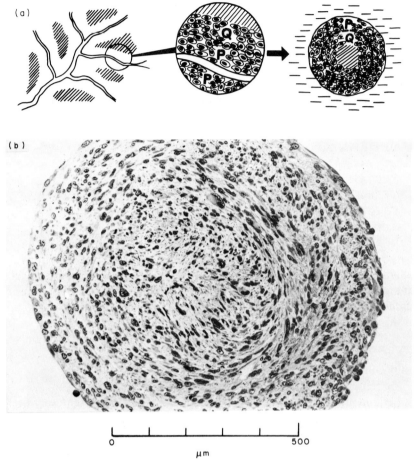

Fig. 1 (a) Schematic drawing of tumour vascularization on the left, with a branching vessel leading through the tumour mass. Necrotic areas are indicated as hatched areas. The nodular structure, with proliferative cells (P) close to vessels or capillaries and non-proliferative cells (Q) near the necrotic areas, is shown in the middle. The corresponding structure in a cultured cellular spheroid is shown on the right. (Carlsson, 1982) (b) Section of a human glioma (U-118 MG) spheroid. The spheroid was embedded in methacrylate, sectioned (2 μm), and stained with haematoxylin and eosin.

single-cell suspension is put into a spinner flask containing culture medium. Small cell-aggregates form during initial hours of culture, and subsequent spheroid growth is due mainly to proliferation. This technique seems to be especially useful when large amounts of equal-sized spheroids are needed.

B. Liquid overlay technique

This technique has been used for cultivating human tumour spheroids. The culture is initiated by seeding trypsinized cells from monolayers or suspension cultured cells into dishes with non-adhesive surfaces. The non-adhesive surface may be a thin layer of agarose on the bottom of a culture dish or bacterial culture dishes, although when using the latter some loose cell attachment may occur. If cells of the studied line have the capacity to grow as spheroids, spherical aggregates can be observed in the dishes a few days after initiation of culture. At this stage single cells and irregular aggregates have been removed. The liquid overlay technique has been described by Yuhas *et al.* (1977) and Haji-Karim and Carlsson (1978). A combination of the spinner flask technique and the liquid overlay technique has been presented by Sano *et al.* (1982).

One advantage of the liquid overlay technique is that it is easy to handle for small scale production and provides an easy method of screening the capacity of new cell types to form and grow as spheroids. From the reports of Sutherland *et al.* (1981) and Carlsson (1982) it is evident that tumour cells have a special capacity to form growing spheroids. About 50% of human tumour cells tested have shown this capacity.

III. Different end points for toxicity testing

There are three different methods for analysing disturbances induced by agents such as drugs, hyperthermia, or radiation, which are outlined schematically in Fig. 2. These involve measuring (i) changes in growth of the intact spheroid, i.e. rate of volume increase, which is a rather insensitive method since all spheroids sooner or later reach a plateau phase, (ii) changes in the capacity of cells to attach to an adhesive surface and to form a growing monolayer, and (iii) changes in clonogenicity of the individual cells of the spheroids, if the spheroids can be disintegrated. These methods may be supplemented by cell kinetics analysis using, for example, pulse labelling with ^{3}H-thymidine to measure the number of S-phase cells in the populations.

A. Volume growth

After exposure to drugs, spheroids are individually transferred to agarose-coated wells in plastic tissue-culture multidishes (one spheroid per well). Growth of individual spheroids is examined by inverted microscopy. Two diameters, *a* and *b*, at right-angles are measured repeatedly. The spheroid volume is calculated from the relation $V = (4/3) \times \pi \times (a \times b)^{3/2}$. Volume

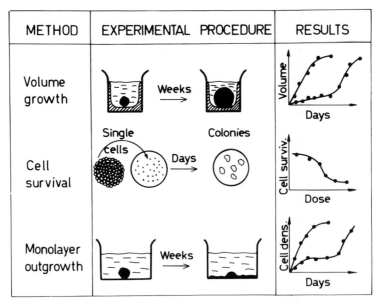

METHOD	EXPERIMENTAL PROCEDURE	RESULTS
Volume growth	Weeks →	Volume / Days
Cell survival	Single cells → Days → Colonies	Cell surviv. / Dose
Monolayer outgrowth	Weeks →	Cell dens. / Days

Fig. 2 Three different methods of analysing disturbances induced by drugs or other cytotoxic agents. Experimental procedures and the type of results obtained are outlined. For further details see text.

growth curves can be constructed and, for example, growth inhibition caused by drug treatment can be evaluated (Yuhas *et al.*, 1978; Twentyman, 1980a).

Volume growth analysis permits the spheroid structure to be left intact after treatment. A special feature of this method is that surviving cells in the central region may not be able to contribute to growth, owing to their unfavourable position in the spheroid, and it seems likely that this is also the situation in a tumour nodule *in vivo*.

B. Survival of individual cells

This method requires that spheroids are disaggregated into single-cell suspensions after drug treatment, usually by trypsinization, combined with shaking or some other, gentle, mechanical influence (Sutherland and Durand, 1976). Enzymes other than trypsin also have been used (Sano *et al.*, 1982). Single cells obtained are then seeded into culture dishes, as in conventional cloning (Sutherland and Durand, 1976), and survival curves can be constructed as a function of drug dose.

By this method all clonogenic cells can be studied, including those in the centre of spheroids, which would otherwise have been lysed owing to their unfavourable position. If sequential trypsinization is performed (Freyer and Sutherland, 1980; Wibe, 1980), successive "shells" of the spheroid can be removed and differences in drug action as a function of depth in the spheroid may be analysed. However, caution is required when proteolytic enzymes are used to dissociate spheroids, since they may in some cases produce loss of cells (Sutherland *et al.*, 1981). Another disadvantage of the method is that the spheroid structure is destroyed, yielding growth conditions more similar to monolayer cultures than to tumour nodules.

Most analyses of this type are made with rodent cell lines. Human spheroids may be difficult to disaggregate. For example, Carlsson (1982) has reported on three different human tumour cell lines (two glioma and one osteosarcoma) which resisted enzymatic treatment with trypsin, collagenase, hyaluronidase, protease, DNAase, and RNAase in different combinations. In addition, this method may be inapplicable because most human cells have a low cloning efficiency.

C. Outgrowth as a monolayer

The spheroids are, after exposure to drugs, transferred to conventional culture dishes (multidishes with one spheroid per well). Spheroids attach and, within a few days, cells migrate out and form small, monolayer cultures around the spheroids. Monolayers continue to grow by proliferation. After cytotoxic treatment both migration and proliferation may be inhibited. Outgrowth from spheroids can be observed for several weeks. The number of outgrowing cells from drug-treated and control spheroids can be compared by inverted microscopy or by trypsinization of the monolayer and counting. From these data, growth curves can be constructed, and outgrowth delays caused by different treatments can be compared. Alternatively reduction in the number of outgrowing cells, after an appropriate time of outgrowth, can be used as an endpoint.

The method can be simplified to measure only survival after treatment. It may be said that a spheroid has survived when it has retained the ability to give rise to a growing monolayer. A satisfactory criterion for survival has been found to be outgrowth of more than 1000 cells within 5 weeks. Measurement of monolayer outgrowth from spheroids as a method of determining chemo- and radio-sensitivity of human tumour spheroids has been described and discussed in detail by Carlsson and Nederman (1982). This method is relatively easy and allows large-scale experiments to be performed. Another advantage is that recovery after several weeks can be detected. For example, growth delays as long as 20–25 days have been detected with human tumour spheroids after exposure to 5-fluorouracil or vinblastine (unpublished observations).

One disadvantage of this method may be that cells that migrate out of the spheroid obtain growth conditions that are more similar to those of normal, monolayer-cultured cells than to those of tumour nodules. However, as with the "volume growth" method, surviving cells in the central region may not be able to contribute to outgrowth (at least not until after several days) owing to their unfavourable position in the spheroids. Another feature of this method is that changes in the migration capacity also may influence results.

D. Comparisons of the use of different endpoints

Cytotoxicity of eight drugs following a 1 hour exposure to EMT6 mouse mammary tumour spheroids was studied using both volume growth delay and cell survival as endpoints (Twentyman, 1980a). For nitrogen mustard, melphalan, BCNU, CCNU, and cis-platinum, a considerable recovery in cell survival was observed if trypsinization was delayed for 24 hours instead of being performed immediately after drug exposure. A reasonably good correlation between growth delay and cell survival (measured at 24 h) was observed for these five drugs. However, for adriamycin, actinomycin D, and 5-fluorouracil, no increase in clonogenic cell survival was observed after a 24 hours delay in assay, and with these agents a poor correlation between the two endpoints used was obtained. It appears therefore that, for many drugs, surviving fractions measured immediately after exposure to drugs do not reflect the degree of damage which determines the regrowth of intact spheroids. Survival of clonogenic cells measured 24 hours after drug treatment seems, at least for some drugs, to be a more realistic endpoint.

Yuhas et al. (1978) used the outgrowth method to measure the killing of spheroids exposed to nitrogen mustard and cyclophosphamide (100% killing being equal to lack of monolayer outgrowth for all spheroids in the group). The surviving spheroids were, in addition, analysed by the "volume growth" method. It was found that the primary effect of nitrogen mustard was to produce a dose-dependent increase in the "lag" period before normal, volume growth rate was resumed. No killing at all was achieved until the growth delay was as long as about 14 days (dose of $HN2 = 1 \mu g \, ml^{-1}$ for 1 h). The killing was then less than 10%. However, when spheroids were exposed to cyclophosphamide (in the peritoneal cavities of mice), the surviving spheroids showed considerably shorter growth delays. For example, when 8% of the spheroids were killed (50 mg kg^{-1} i.v. in the mice and 4 h exposure in vivo before the spheroids were harvested for in vitro analysis), surviving spheroids showed a growth delay of only 3 days.

Radiation sensitization by the drug misonidazole has been determined using both "cell survival" and "outgrowth" methods (Sutherland, 1980). Enhancement of the effect of 1750 rad by exposure to 15 mM misonidazole for

3 hours can be compared. When determined by the cloning of trypsinized cells, the surviving fraction was found to be decreased from 10% to 1% by the addition of misonidazole. The amount of surviving spheroids determined by the outgrowth assay was, however, found to decrease from more than 90% to about 60% by the same treatment. Thus the enhancement ratio is greater when measured on single cells than when measured on whole spheroids. This may indicate that many of the additional cells killed by the combination treatment were located in such unfavourable positions that they could not contribute to spheroid outgrowth. This hypothesis seems reasonable, since hypoxic cells known to be sensitized by misonidazole are located about 200 μm inside the V79 spheroids used in this study.

IV. Applications of studies with spheroids

Studies of the actions of many different cytotoxic drugs on cellular spheroids have been made. Table 1 gives a brief summary of some of these studies.

Some problems regarding chemotherapy can be considered as being of particular interest when spheroids are used as a model system. For example,

Table 1   Drugs studied by the use of cellular spheroids

Drug	Cells	References
Alkylating agents		
BCNU	Mouse mammary tumours (EMT 6)	Twentyman (1980a,b, 1982)
BCNU	Rat brain tumour (9L)	Deen *et al.* (1980)
CCNU	EMT 6	Twentyman (1980a, 1982)
Cyclophosphamide	Mouse mammary tumour (MCa-11)	Yuhas *et al.* (1978)
Melphalan	EMT 6	Twentyman (1980a, 1982)
Nitrogen mustard	EMT 6	Twentyman (1980a,b, 1982)
Nitrogen mustard	MCa-11	Yuhas *et al.* (1978)
Antimetabolites		
5-Fluorouracil	EMT 6	Twentyman (1980a)
5-Fluorouracil	Human glioma (U-118 MG)	Nederman *et al.* (1981)
Methotrexate	Human osteosarcoma	West *et al.* (1980)
2-Deoxy-D-glucose	Chinese hamster, embryonic lung (V79)	Sridhar *et al.* (1979)
5-Thio-D-glucose	V79	Sridhar *et al.* (1979)

Table 1 (*cont.*)

Drug	Cells	References
Antibiotics		
Actinomycin D	EMT 6	Twentyman (1980a)
Adriamycin	EMT 6	Sutherland *et al.* (1979, 1980)
		Twentyman (1980a,b, 1982)
Adriamycin	V79	Durand (1976, 1981)
		Olive (1981)
		Durand and Brown (1982)
Plant alkaloids		
Vinblastine	U-118 MG	Nederman *et al.* (1981)
Vincristine	Human cervix	Wibe (1980)
	carcinoma	Wibe and Oftebro (1981)
	(NHIK 3025)	
Radiosensitizers (nitroimidazoles)		
Metronidazole (Flagyl)	V79	Sutherland (1974, 1980)
		Sridhar *et al.* (1976)
		Olive (1981)
Misonidazole	EMT 6	Sutherland and Macfarlane (1978)
		Sutherland *et al.* (1980)
		Twentyman (1980b, 1982)
Misonidazole	V79	Sridhar *et al.* (1976)
		Sutherland and Macfarlane (1978)
		Sutherland (1980)
		Durand and Brown (1982)
Ro-05-8863	EMT 6	Sutherland and Macfarlane (1978)
		Sutherland *et al.* (1980)
Ro-07-0207	EMT 6	Sutherland and Macfarlane (1978)
Ro-07-0741	EMT 6	Sutherland and Macfarlane (1978)
Ro-11-3696	EMT 6	Sutherland and Macfarlane (1978)
SR 2508	EMT 6	Sutherland *et al.* (1980)
Miscellaneous		
AF-2 (a nitrofuran)	V79	Olive (1981)
m-AMSA	V79	Wilson *et al.* (1981)
Cis-platinum	EMT 6	Twentyman (1980a)
Nifuroxine	V79	Olive (1981)
NY 3170 (a metaphase		
inhibitor)	NHIK 3025	Wibe and Oftebro (1981)

the drug penetration barriers which may exist in poorly vascularized regions of tumours can, in part, be simulated by spheroids (Nederman *et al.*, 1981). Since cells in different parts of spheroids have different microenvironments and different growth conditions regarding cell cycle distribution, oxygen tension, nutrition supply, etc., the phenomenon of preferential toxicity towards cells growing under different conditions can also be studied.

A. Drug penetration studies

To reach cells in the deeper regions of spheroids, drugs must penetrate through several layers of cells without the aid of capillaries. This may mimic the situation when chemotherapy is applied in the clinic.

It has been suggested that drug penetration barriers exist to, for example, adriamycin, vinblastine, methotrexate, and m-AMSA. Spheroids of EMT 6 mammary tumour cells have been found to be markedly more resistant to adriamycin than monolayer cells in exponential or plateau growth phases (Sutherland *et al.*, 1979).

Measurements of the natural fluorescence of adriamycin indicated the existence of a significant penetration barrier. However, measurements of the drug sensitivity of the inner spheroid cells as a function of absorbed drug concentration indicated that other factors also were involved in the drug resistance of these cells. Durand (1981) used flow cytometry to determine intracellular adriamycin content in V79 spheroids. A limited penetration was demonstrated, but also in this case equal toxicity required greater intracellular fluorescence (and thus more adriamycin) for spheroid cells than for mono-layer cells.

Low drug concentration in deep lying, spheroid cells may be due to limited penetration but may also be due to their altered metabolic state. To judge whether real penetration barriers exist or not, the soluble fraction of the drug also has to be studied. A histological method of preserving the distribution of water-soluble substances has been developed (Nederman *et al.*, 1981). For example, by this technique 5-fluorouracil was shown to be isotropically distributed inside human glioma spheroids after a 15 min exposure. After a corresponding exposure to vinblastine, however, the main part of the drug was present in the outer cell layers and only small amounts seemed to have reached the central parts (Fig. 3). Recent studies also indicated that spheroids were more resistant to vinblastine than to 5-fluorouracil (unpublished observations).

The action of vincristine, a drug closely related to vinblastine, was studied by Wibe (1980) and Wibe and Oftebro (1981). Spheroids were remarkably more resistant to the lethal effects of the drug (24 h exposure) than exponentially growing, monolayer cultures of the same cell line (NHIK 3025, originating from a human cervix carcinoma). Sequential trypsinization showed that the surviving fraction increased only slightly as a function of distance from the spheroid surface. The relative concentration of intracellular, bound drug was studied by autoradiography. It was shown that considerable

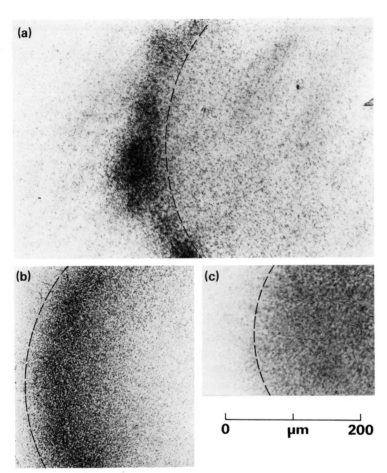

Fig. 3 Contact autoradiograms with grain distributions which show the penetration pattern of (a) ^{125}I-albumin, (b) ^{3}H-vinblastine, and (c) ^{3}H-5-fluorouracil after (b and c) 15 min or (a) 20 min exposure to the substance. After exposure to the test substances the spheroids were quickly frozen, freeze-dried, vapour-fixed, wax-embedded, sectioned, and dry-mounted. Autoradiograms were prepared by exposure of a dry thin layer of photoemulsion to the spheroid sections. These procedures did not significantly disturb the distribution of the water-soluble substances tested (Nederman *et al.*, 1981). The broken lines indicate spheroid peripheries. Three quite different penetration patterns were observed. Most of the ^{125}I-albumin was confined to the periphery while ^{3}H-vinblastine had a limited penetration and ^{3}H-5-fluorouracil seemed to be isotropically distributed inside the spheroid.

amounts of the drug reached cells located up to 160 μm inside the spheroid after 2 hours of exposure (60–70% of peripheral value). This indicated that resistance to vincristine was not mainly an effect of penetration barriers.

Methotrexate has been used in the clinical management of human osteosarcoma, and its binding to the intracellular target (dihydrofolate reductase) was studied in human osteosarcoma spheroids (West *et al.*, 1980) by standard histological and autoradiographic methods. It was found that, at a diameter of 250 μm, drug penetration was limited to the outer two to three cellular layers of the spheroidal mass, and there was no evidence of the presence of methotrexate in the centre. These results may explain the limited effectiveness of methotrexate in certain adjuvant trials for osteosarcoma.

Deep lying cells in V79 (Chinese hamster) spheroids have been found to be more resistant to m-AMSA treatment than monolayer cells or spheroid cells disaggregated prior to exposure to drugs (Wilson *et al.*, 1981). Resistance appeared to be partly a result of the non-cycling or slowly cycling state of most of these cells, but may also have been partly due to drug penetration limitations.

B. Studies of preferential toxicities

Cells in different parts of spheroids have quite different growth conditions. Peripheral cells have a good supply of nutrients and proliferate at a high rate. Deeper lying cells are mainly resting, probably owing to the poor supply of oxygen and other nutrient factors, and this may also be related to accumulation of catabolic products and decreased pH. Such gradients are believed to exist in solid tumours *in vivo*. It is obvious that cells under different conditions in terms of cell cycle distribution, oxygen tension, pH, etc. may differ in their susceptibilities to drugs.

Preferential toxicity towards different cell populations within spheroids can, for example, be studied using sequential trypsinization, as mentioned above. An alternative method has been described by Olive (1981). Thioguanine-resistant cells were introduced into spinner flasks containing spheroids; the mutant cells attached to the surface of the spheroids. The composite spheroids thus formed consisted of external (cycling, oxic), thioguanine-resistant and internal (non-cycling, hypoxic), thioguanine-sensitive cells. Differential effects of drugs on external and internal cells of composite spheroids could be assayed by plating cells trypsinized from spheroids into both standard medium and medium containing thioguanine. The latter allowed growth of only the external, thioguanine-resistant cells. By using this technique on V79 spheroids it was shown that adriamycin acts mainly on external cells while AF-2, a nitrofuran, acts mainly on internal, hypoxic cells.

The cytotoxic action of several nitroimidazoles has been evaluated.

Metronidazole was shown to kill preferentially internal, non-cycling cells in V79 spheroids (Sutherland, 1974). The same phenomenon was shown for both metronidazole and misonidazole (Sridhar et al., 1976). Cytotoxicity seemed to be related to the hypoxic environment of the killed cells. The cytotoxic effects of misonidazole and two other nitroimidazoles (Ro-05-9963 and SR 2508) to mouse mammary tumour spheroids have been shown to be predictive of the relative effectiveness of the drugs in treating the corresponding tumours in vivo (Sutherland et al., 1980). However, the rate and extent of the cytotoxicity were greater in vivo especially at low drug concentrations.

The internal cells, sensitive to nitroimidazoles, may be resistant to other forms of therapy, including radiation (oxygen effect) and other drugs (e.g. penetration barriers). Therefore experiments have been performed to determine the potential usefulness of this preferential cytotoxicity. As previously discussed, adriamycin has been found to kill preferentially peripheral cells in spheroids, mainly owing to penetration barriers (Sutherland et al., 1979; Durand, 1981). When misonidazole and adriamycin were combined, the preferential toxicity of each agent was demonstrated in V79 spheroids (Durand and Brown, 1982). Additionally, prolonged exposure to misonidazole increased cell susceptibility to adriamycin. Sutherland et al. (1980) also showed that the addition of adriamycin immediately after a 24 hour exposure to misonidazole resulted in an apparently supra-additive response in mouse mammary tumour spheroids (EMT 6). However, using another subline of the same cell line, Twentyman (1980b) showed no enhanced sensitivity to nitrogen mustard, adriamycin, or BCNU of cells surviving 21 hours of misonidazole treatment.

Most studies of the action of drugs have indicated that cells cultured as spheroids were more resistant to chemotherapy than the corresponding monolayer cells. However, the glucose antimetabolites 2-deoxy-D-glucose and 5-thio-D-glucose were shown to be more toxic to spheroid cells than to monolayer cells (Sridhar et al., 1979). These drugs are selectively toxic to hypoxic cells grown as monolayer cultures. When V79 spheroids were exposed to these drugs, the cell killing observed was much more than could be predicted on the basis of the hypoxic fraction known to be present in these spheroids. It was suggested that the crowded, tumour-like environment in some way made the cells vulnerable to the cytotoxic action of glucose analogues and other glycolytic inhibitors.

V. Discussion

A solid tumour in vivo is a complex system of cells. Tumours may have gradients in oxygen, glucose, and other nutrients. The poorly vascularized regions may also contain increased concentrations of catabolic products. Regions with chronically hypoxic cells may develop when the tumour mass grows. The pH in the central parts of the tumour mass will probably decrease and other microenvironmental changes may also occur. Proliferation gradients will develop, and large local variations in growth rates will exist.

This complex system is very difficult to model *in vitro*. However, multicellular tumour spheroids seem to offer many of the characteristics of *in vivo* tumours which are unavailable in monolayer or suspension cultures (e.g. Sutherland and Durand, 1976; Yuhas *et al.*, 1977; Haji-Karim and Carlsson, 1978; Wibe *et al.*, 1981). Cellular spheroids provide a system that is easy to handle, with a complexity intermediate between "solid" tumours and conventional, monolayer cultures. This system allows studies of different therapy modalities and problems associated with metabolic and proliferative gradients, pH and pO_2 gradients, drug penetration barriers, and possibly also the development of drug resistance.

In combination with knowledge of the spatial and temporal distribution of the drug in the body and its toxicity to normal tissue, spheroids seem to provide a relevant model system for development of new chemotherapeutic principles. An obvious limitation is that cells in the spheroids may not be representative of tumours *in vivo*, owing to selection of certain cells when cultures are established. In addition, diversity of spheroids originating from the same cell line has been shown to exist (Durand, 1980). This indicates the necessity of adequate characterization of the spheroid system and the methods used. However, these limitations are essentially the same for all *in vitro* systems.

Chemotherapy studies with cellular spheroids may have many clinical implications. For example, the necessity of taking the drug penetration problem into account has been clearly pointed out. Other studies have shown potential advantages in the combination of different treatments (Sutherland and Macfarlane, 1978; Durand and Brown, 1982). The development of drug resistance has in a few cases been shown to be similar in the spheroid system to that in the corresponding animal tumour system (Sutherland *et al.*, 1981; Yuhas, 1982). The spheroid system is likely to be useful in the development of new chemotherapy modalities.

Acknowledgements

I am grateful to Dr Jörgen Carlsson and to Prof. Börje Larsson for the helpful discussion I had with them and for their valuable criticism of the manuscript. The work was financially supported by the Swedish Cancer Society, the Max Planck Gesellschaft, Munich, and the Swedish National Defence Research Institute.

References

Carlsson, J. (1977). A proliferation gradient in three-dimensional colonics of cultured human glioma cells. *Int. J. Cancer* **20**, 129–136.

Carlsson, J. (1982). Personal communication.

Carlsson, J. and Nederman, T. (1982). A method to measure the radio- and chemosensitivity of human spheroids. In *Oxygen Transport to Tissue*, IV (ed. J. Matzka), pp. 399–417. Plenum, New York (in press).

Deen, D. F., Hoshio, T., Williams, M. E., Muraoka, I., Knebel, K. D. and Barker, M. (1980). Development of a 9L rat brain tumour cell multicellular spheroid system and its response to 1,3-bis(2-chloroethyl)-1-nitrosourea and radiation. *J. Nat. Cancer Inst.* **64**, 1373–1382.

Durand, R. E. (1976). Adriamycin: a possible indirect radiosensitizer of hypoxic tumour cells. *Radiology* **119**, 217–222.

Durand, R. E. (1980). Variable radiobiological responses of spheroids. *Radiat. Res.* **81**, 85–99.

Durand, R. E. (1981). Flow cytometry studies of intracellular adriamycin in multicell spheroids *in vitro*. *Cancer Res.* **41**, 3495–3498.

Durand, R. E. and Brown, S. M. (1982). Combination adriamycin/misonidazole toxicity in V79 spheroids. *Int. J. Radiat. Oncol. Biol. Phys.* **8**, 603–605.

Freyer, J. P. and Sutherland, R. M. (1980). Selective dissociation and characterization of cells from different regions of multicell tumour spheroids. *Cancer Res.* **40**, 3956–3965.

Haji-Karim, M. and Carlsson, J. (1978). Proliferation and viability in cellular spheroids of human origin. *Cancer Res.* **38**, 1457–1464.

Nederman, T., Carlsson, J. and Malmqvist, M. (1981). Penetration of substances into tumour tissue: a methodological study on cellular spheroids. *In Vitro* **17**, 290–298.

Olive, P. L. (1981). Different sensitivity to cytotoxic agents of internal and external cells of spheroids composed of thioguanine-resistant and sensitive cells. *Br. J. Cancer* **43**, 85–92.

Sano, Y., Deen, D. F. and Hoshino, T. (1982). Factors that influence initiation and growth of 9L rat brain gliosarcoma multicellular spheroids. *Cancer Res.* **42**, 1223–1226.

Sridhar, R., Koch, C. and Sutherland, R. (1976). Cytotoxicity of two nitroimidazole radiosensitizers in an *in vitro* tumour model. *Int. J. Radiat. Oncol. Biol. Phys.* **1**, 1149–1157.

Sridhar, R., Stroude, E. C. and Inch, W. R. (1979). Cytotoxicity of glucose analogues, in V79 multicell spheroids. *In Vitro* **15**, 685–690.

Sutherland, R. M. (1974). Selective chemotherapy of noncycling cells in an *in vitro* tumour model. *Cancer Res.* **34**, 3501–3503.

Sutherland, R. M. (1980). The multicellular spheroid system as a tumour model for studies of radiation sensitizers. *Pharmacol. Ther.* **8**, 105–123.

Sutherland, R. M. and Durand, R. E. (1976). Radiation response of multicell spheroids: an *in vitro* tumour model. *Curr. Top. Radiat. Res.* **11**, 87–139.

Sutherland, R. and Macfarlane, W. (1978). Cytotoxicity of radiosensitizers in multicell spheroids: combination treatment with hyperthermia. *Br. J. Cancer* **37** (Suppl. III), 168–171.

Sutherland, R. M., McCredie, J. A. and Inch, W. R. (1971). Growth of multicell spheroids in tissue culture as a model of nodular carcinomas. *J. Nat. Cancer Inst.* **46**, 113–120.

Sutherland, R. M., Eddy, H. A., Bareham, B., Reich, K. and Vanantwerp, D. (1979). Resistance to adriamycin in multicellular spheroids. *Int. J. Radiat. Oncol. Biol. Phys.* **5,** 1225–1230.

Sutherland, R. M., Bareham, B. J. and Reich, K. A. (1980). Cytotoxicity of hypoxic cell sensitizers in multicell spheroids. *Cancer Clin. Trials* **3,** 73–83.

Sutherland, R. M., Carlsson, J., Durand, R. and Yuhas, J. (1981). Spheroids in cancer research. *Cancer Res.* **41,** 2980–2984.

Twentyman, P. R. (1980a). Response to chemotherapy of EMT 6 spheroids, as measured by growth delay and cell survival. *Br. J. Cancer* **42,** 297–304.

Twentyman, P. R. (1980b). The response of EMT 6 tumour spheroids to combined treatment with misonidazole and either nitrogen mustard, adriamycin or BCNU. *Cancer Clin. Trials* **3,** 253–256.

Twentyman, P. R. (1982). *In vitro* pre-incubation with misonidazole under hypoxic conditions: effect on drug response of EMT 6 spheroids. *Int. J. Radiat. Oncol. Biol. Phys.* **8,** 607–609.

West, G. W., Weichselbaum, R. and Little, J. B. (1980). Limited penetration of methotrexate into human osteosarcoma spheroids as a proposed model for solid tumour resistance to adjuvant chemotherapy. *Cancer Res.* **40,** 3665–3668.

Wibe, E. (1980). Resistance to vincristine of human cells grown as multicellular spheroids. *Br. J. Cancer* **42,** 937–941.

Wibe, E. and Oftebro, R. (1981). A study of factors related to the action of 1-propargyl-5-chloropyrimidin-2-one (NY 3170) and vincristine in human multicellular spheroids. *Eur. J. Cancer Clin. Oncol.* **17,** 1053–1059.

Wibe, E., Lindmo, T. and Kaalhus, O. (1981). Cell kinetic characteristics in different parts of multicellular spheroids of human origin. *Cell Tissue Kinet.* **14,** 639–651.

Wilson, W. R., Whitmore, G. F. and Hill, R. P. (1981). Activity of 4'-(9-acridinyl-amino-methanesulfon-*m*-aniside against Chinese hamster cells in multicellular spheroids. *Cancer Res.* **41,** 2817–2822.

Yuhas, J. M. (1982). Personal communication.

Yuhas, J. M., Li, A. P., Martinez, A. O. and Ladman, A. J. (1977). A simplified method for production and growth of multicellular tumour spheroids. *Cancer Res.* **37,** 3639–3643.

Yuhas, J. M., Tarleton, A. E. and Harman, J. G. (1978). *In vitro* analysis of the response of multicellular tumour spheroids exposed to chemotherapeutic agents *in vitro* or *in vivo*. *Cancer Res.* **38,** 3595–3598.

14. An Overview of the Role of Organ Culture for Human Tumour Biopsies

J. R. W. MASTERS

I. Introduction

The aim of this chapter is to provide an introduction to organ culture of human malignant tumours and to summarize its use in studies of hormone and chemotherapeutic drug sensitivities. Organ culture is the maintenance or growth of tissue *in vitro* to allow differentiation and preservation of architecture and/or function (Schaeffer, 1979). Because the purpose of the technique is to retain the integrity of three-dimensional cellular interrelationships, it might be expected to yield data more accurately reflecting drug sensitivity *in vivo* than other tissue culture systems. Whilst this concept may be correct, a major limitation is the objective and reproducible measurement of *in vitro* sensitivity of heterogeneous tumour explants. Most studies use subjective or non-specific measurements, and as yet there are no simple quantitative means by which to distinguish the response of tumour cells, and particularly those neoplastic cells capable of indefinite proliferation, from the rest of the cellular constituents in this system. Despite this limitation, many studies on maintenance of human malignant tumours in organ culture have been described, and assessments of sensitivity to hormones, chemotherapeutic drugs, X-irradiation, and hyperthermia have been made. Organ culture provides an experimental approach for studying effects of drugs and hormones on tissue maintained *in vitro* in a manner more akin to that encountered physiologically than any other tissue culture system, but it requires further study to evaluate its potential for predicting *in vivo* response to chemotherapy.

II. Methodology

The concept of organ culture was developed by Fell more than 50 years ago, and applied to the maintenance of embryonic tissue on plasma-embryo extract clots (Fell and Robison, 1929). Subsequent technical innovations include use of agar supports (Spratt, 1947), co-culture with chick embryonic tissues (Wolff, 1970), and porous matrices (Leighton, 1951). The most popular method is to position thin slices of tissue at a liquid–gas interface on some form of support such as a stainless steel grid (Trowell, 1959). The methodology has been reviewed by Easty (1970) and the applications by Hodges (1981).

The technique has been applied to most types of human "solid" malignant tumour (see Table 1). Despite the abundance of such studies, standard and defined culture conditions for each tumour type have not been established. In contrast to embryonic, normal and benign tumour tissues, in many studies malignant tumours are maintained in a viable state for short periods, often less than 1 week. Nevertheless, malignant tumours can be maintained in organ culture for many years in the presence of complex and undefined nutrients, such as chick embryonic mesonephros (Wolff, 1970). Development of defined media for the purpose of long-term culture should make the technique more widely applicable.

While the basic methodology is simple and applicable to most tumours, many factors need to be considered (see review by Hodges, 1981). These include medium, substrate, pH, gaseous atmosphere, temperature, osmolarity, and particularly tissue handling. Each of these factors can influence viability of the tissue.

III. Hormone sensitivity

Most prostate cancers and approximately one-third of tumours of the breast and endometrium will respond to some form of endocrine manipulation. Numerous attempts to distinguish hormone-sensitive tumours have been made, but no reliable system for predicting clinical response has been achieved using organ culture. Three factors in particular have made it difficult to determine the potential value of organ culture for this purpose. First, because the quantity of tumour tissue is often limited, in order to make experimental samples representative, only a single or limited range of hormone concentrations is tested. Secondly, most assessments of sensitivity require the cultures to be terminated, and therefore sequential changes are not investigated. Thirdly, it has not been possible to retain complete viability in all tumours, the more anaplastic tumours being most difficult to maintain. Criteria for viability in organ culture explants are usually morphological, but if biochemical characteristics are not also retained then specific hormonal effects are unlikely to be observed. A finding relevant to all studies on hormone-sensitive tumours in organ culture has been made by Satyaswaroop and Mortel (1982).

Table 1 Survey of organ culture studies of human malignant tumours, listed according to site of origin and showing features investigated, maximum culture period, and number of tumours examined. This is not a comprehensive list and in general includes only the most recent publication from each group of workers

Number of tumours studied	Maximum culture period (days)	Features investigated	Reference
Bladder			
47	7	Morphology/prognosis	Abaza *et al.* (1978)
8	28	Scanning E.M.	Hodges (1978)
Brain (Glioma)			
13	14	Morphology	Holmstrom (1975)
5	137	Morphology	Rubinstein *et al.* (1973)
15	14	Invasiveness	Sorour *et al.* (1975)
Breast			
10	4	Hormone sensitivity	Aspegren (1976)
34	3	Hormone sensitivity	Beeby *et al.* (1975)
16	1	Hormone sensitivity	Chayen *et al.* (1970)
9	2	Glycoprotein synthesis	Dermer and Sherwin (1975)
44	1	Drug sensitivity	Dickson and Suzanger (1976)
17	3	Steroid metabolism	Duncan *et al.* (1981)
30	3	Osteolysis	Easty *et al.* (1976)
130	1	Hormone sensitivity	Flax *et al.* (1973)
17	5	Hormone sensitivity	Finkelstein *et al.* (1975)
5	5	Steroid metabolism	Geier *et al.* (1975)
22	2	Hormone sensitivity	Gorlich *et al.* (1981)
94	14	Hormone sensitivity	Heuson *et al.* (1975)
19	3	Lactalbumin production	Kleinberg (1975)
67	8	Tumour immunology	Kiricuta *et al.* (1978)
8	3	Hormone sensitivity	Lagios (1974)
18	7	Hormone sensitivity	Masters *et al.* (1980)
20	4	Tumour immunology	Nissen and Tanneberger (1976)
15	4	Hormone sensitivity	Sellwood and Castro (1974)
31	2	Hormone sensitivity	Stoll (1970)
10	3	Glycoprotein synthesis	Tokes and Dermer (1977)
16	11	Hormone sensitivity	Wellings and Jentoft (1972)
26	2	Hormone sensitivity	Welsch *et al.* (1976)
19	3	Steroid metabolism	Willcox and Thomas (1972)
10	10	Lactalbumin production	Wilson *et al.* (1980)
Genital tract (female)			
Cervix			
60	20	Herpes virus infection	Mandeville *et al.* (1979)
32	7	Morphology/cell kinetics	Siracky *et al.* (1974)
Endometrium			
46	1	Tumour antigens	Brockas and Wiernik (1976)
30	7	Hormone sensitivity	Hustin (1975)
15	4	Hormone sensitivity	Jacobelli *et al.* (1978)
10	3	Hormone sensitivity	Kohorn and Tchao (1968)
15	9	Hormone sensitivity	Matoska (1970)

Table 1 (*cont.*)

Number of tumours studied	Maximum culture period (days)	Features investigated	Reference
47	7	Hormone sensitivity	Nordquist (1970)
9	2	Hormone sensitivity	Satyaswaroop and Mortel (1982)
20	7	Morphology/cell kinetics	Siracky *et al.* (1974)
Ovary			
27	3	Fibrinolysis activation	Svanberg and Astedt (1976)
Gastrointestinal tract			
Colorectal			
20	14	Tumour marker production	Breborowicz *et al.* (1975)
26	21	Tumour invasiveness	Kalus (1972)
11	1	Glycoprotein synthesis	O'Gorman and Lamont (1978)
26	28	Poliovirus infection	Tsypkin *et al.* (1976)
Stomach			
1	> 5 yrs	X-Radiation sensitivity	Dendy (1968)
17	4	Tumour immunology	Nissen and Tanneberger (1976)
1	> 5 yrs	Drug sensitivity	Simpson (1969)
26	18	Poliovirus infection	Tsypkin *et al.* (1976)
Lung			
13	2	Metabolic activity	Cohen *et al.* (1981)
1	8	Protein synthesis	McCully (1968)
Nephroblastoma			
15	22	Differentiation	Rousseau-Merck *et al.* (1977)
Neuroblastoma			
7	19 wks	Morphology/E.M.	Lyser (1976)
Prostate			
12	2	Steroid metabolism	Bard and Lasnitzki (1977)
6	2	Steroid metabolism	Ghanadian *et al.* (1981)
3	1	Steroid metabolism	Kadohama *et al.* (1977)
12	6	Hormone sensitivity	Lasnitzki (1979)
3	4	Hormone sensitivity	McMahon *et al.* (1972)
5	3	Glycoprotein synthesis	Tokes and Dermer (1977)
More than one tumour type			
62	6	Morphology	Archer (1968)
30	17	Morphology	Cooper and Goldring (1964)
140	4	Collagenolytic activity	Dresden *et al.* (1972)
84	2	Histochemistry/E.M.	Hecker and Deutschmann (1976)
105	21	Morphology	Kalus *et al.* (1968)
241	14	Drug sensitivity	Lazarus *et al.* (1966)
30	13	Morphology	Leighton *et al.* (1969)
29	12	Morphology	Matoska and Stricker (1967)
91	11	Morphology	Roller *et al.* (1966)
27	19	Morphology	Rovin (1962)
147	2	Drug sensitivity	Tanneberger and Mohr (1973)
17	5	Drug sensitivity	Tchao *et al.* (1968)
	> 5 yrs	Morphology	Wolff (1970)

Progesterone receptor activity (PR) and stimulation of oestradiol dehydrogenase activity (E_2DH) by medroxyprogesterone acetate (MA) were measured in organ cultures of normal proliferative and neoplastic endometrium. While PR activity was retained and stimulation of E_2DH activity by MA observed in normal endometrium, in carcinomas the PR activity was lost within 24 hours and E_2DH activity was not stimulated by MA. Partial or complete loss of receptor activity in organ culture may explain the failure in many studies to observe specific hormonal effects.

Apart from the many factors that need to be considered in determinations of *in vitro* drug sensitivities, three additional points need to be examined in measurements of hormonal sensitivity. First, endocrine therapy results in either permanent changes in circulating hormone levels following surgery or continuous administration of synthetic or natural hormones for as long as the tumour remains under control. Thus it may be necessary to expose tissue to hormones throughout the culture period, and take account of the metabolism and stability of the hormone under *in vitro* conditions. Secondly, an implicit assumption in many *in vitro* studies is that the hormone exerts a direct effect on tumour cell growth. Alterations in circulating levels of one hormone will result in changes in hormonal balance, and in some instances tumour growth may be controlled by these secondary phenomena. The direct influence of one hormone *in vitro* therefore may not reflect the pattern *in vivo*. Thirdly, it is difficult to monitor endogenous levels of hormones within explanted tissue, and these may be sufficient to obscure effects of hormone addition to the culture medium. Furthermore, sera contain hormones and should be avoided if possible, although serum "stripped" of its hormone content may provide a suitable alternative.

Data relating to hormonal sensitivity of human malignant tumours in organ culture are summarized in Table 2. Frequently results are contradictory and it is not valid to draw general conclusions regarding particular hormones or tumours for the following reasons.

1. A wide range of exposure periods and hormone concentrations have been used, often far in excess of those encountered physiologically.
2. Many different sera, media, and culture periods have been tested.
3. It is not possible to compare directly the various non-specific or subjective methods of assessment of *in vitro* hormone sensitivity.

IV. Chemotherapeutic drug sensitivity

Many of the comments made in the preceding section in relation to assessment of hormone sensitivity in organ culture apply equally to chemotherapeutic

Table 2 Survey of organ culture studies on the hormone sensitivity of human malignant tumours, giving brief details of hormone concentrations, methods used to assess *in vitro* sensitivity, and the effects observed

Hormone concentrations (μg ml^{-1})	Methods of assessment	Hormonal effects	Reference
Breast			
T, 0.5–50; Prog, 0.8–80; E, 0.02–20 (with 20% HS)	Histology; ^{3}H-TdR and ^{3}H-U autoradiography and incorporation	Variable, perhaps non-specific	Aspegren (1976)
E, 0.03–3; T, 0.03–3.0; OP, 0.01–1; Tamoxifen, 3 (with 10 μg ml^{-1} I)	Histochemistry/ biochemistry of PSD activity; ^{3}H-TdR and ^{3}H-U incorporation	No significant effects	Beeby *et al.* (1975)
E, T, drostanolone	Morphology; histochemistry	7/16 tumours sensitive to E	Chayen *et al.* (1970)
T, 20; E, 1 (with 20% male CS)	Morphology, ^{3}H-TdR, ^{3}H-U, and ^{14}C-amino acid incorporation	Stimulation and inhibition observed	Finkelstein *et al.* (1975)
E, 0.1–1	Histochemistry of LDH, E$_2$DH, and LAD activity; electron microscopy	Decrease in activity or no effect in 21/22 tumours	Gorlich *et al.* (1981)
E, 0.01 ng–10 μg ml^{-1}; OP, 5; I, 10; HC, 1	Morphology	E improved survival of "scirrhous" tumours, but could be replaced by pretreatment with collagenase	Heuson *et al.* (1975)
OP, 0.1; MA, 0.1 (with I and HC and 20% female HS)	α-Lactalbumin production	Stimulation in 2/19 tumours	Kleinberg (1975)
E, 0.5; T, 0.5; OP, 22–220 mIU ml^{-1}	Morphology; mitotic index; electron microscopy	Higher mitotic index in some cases	Lagios (1974)
E, 0.272 and 2.72; T, 0.288 and 2.88; OP, 22 and 220 mIU ml^{-1}	Histochemistry of PSD activity	No reproducible effects	Masters *et al.* (1977)
E, 0.0272 ng–27.2 μg ml^{-1}	Morphology; ^{125}I-Udr uptake	Stimulation and inhibition observed	Masters *et al.* (1980)
E, 0.272 and 2.72; T, 0.288 and 2.88; OP, 22 and 220 mIU ml^{-1}	Histochemistry of PSD activity	Enhancement by E (11%), T (11%), OP (15%), OP and E (10%), OP and T (6%) of 130 tumours	Flax *et al.* (1973) Salih *et al.* (1972a,b)
T, 10; E, 10; HC, 10; stilboestrol, 10 (with 12% CS and 6 μg ml^{-1} I)	Morphology	No influence on survival	Sellwood and Castro (1974)
Diethylstilboestrol and ethynyloestradiol 50 ng–1 mg ml^{-1}; MA, 0.05–5 (with 10% CS and 20 μg ml^{-1} I)	Histochemistry of acid phosphatase; biochemistry	No significant effects	Stoll (1970)
I, 1–5 (0.3 U ml^{-1}); D-aldosterone, 1; E, 0.1–10; OP, 2–4	Morphology	No effect on survival except toxicity by high E concentration	Wellings and Jentoft (1972)
OP (33 IU mg^{-1}), 10; bovine I (22.5 IU mg^{-1}), 5; HC, 1	^{3}H-TdR incorporation; morphology	Stimulation by I, and in 3/20 tumours by OP	Welsch *et al.* (1976)
OP, 0.5–50	α-Lactalbumin production; morphology	No effect	Wilson *et al.* (1980)

Table 2 (*cont.*)

Hormone concentrations ($\mu g\ ml^{1}$)	Methods of assessment	Hormonal effects	Reference
Endometrium			
E, 5–20; Prog, 5–100; GH, 2 U ml^{-1}; HCG, 100 U ml^{-1} various progestogens and oestrogens 5–100 (with 10% HS and 0.1 IU ml^{-1} I)	Morphology; ^{3}H-TdR autoradiography	Viability enhanced by pregnenolone, unaffected by peptide hormones, reduced by progesterone	Hustin (1975)
Progesterone and various progestogens, 0.8%–8.0 (with 30% FCS and 5 U ml^{-1} I)	Morphology; ^{3}H-TdR incorporation	No significant effects on ^{3}H-TdR incorporation	Jacobelli *et al.* (1978)
Prog, 10–50; E, 1; T, 10; I, 10 (with 10% CS ± patient's serum)	Morphology	Viability enhanced by 10 μg ml^{-1} and reduced by 50 μg ml^{-1} Prog	Kohorn and Tchao (1968)
Prog, 25–50 (with 25% autologous serum, yeast extract, chick ovovitelline membrane)	Morphology; ^{3}H-TdR autoradiography	Viability enhanced in 1, but decreased in 6/14 tumours	Matoska (1970)
E, 20; Prog, 10–100 (with 20% adult HS and 10% CEE)	Morphology	High Prog concentrations impaired survival	Nordquist (1970)
MA, 0.5 (with 10% FCS, 10 μg ml^{-1} I, 2.5 ng ml^{-1} E)	PR and E$_2$DH activity	Loss of PR activity and no stimulation by MA	Satyaswaroop and Mortel (1982)
Prostate			
T, 0.136 and 1.36; Estracyt, 0.1 and 10	5α-Reductase activity; morphology	Range of effect	Kadohama *et al.* (1977)
T, E, DHT, 3α and 3β androstanediol, androstenedione, 3 each (with 10% CS)	Morphology; ^{3}H-TdR and ^{3}H-U autoradiography	DNA synthesis rate reduced by all hormones; RNA synthesis stimulated by androgens, depressed by E; similar effects in tumour and stromal cells	Lasnitzki (1979)
T, 3; stilboestrol, 4 (with 10% FCS and 25 μg ml^{-1} I)	Morphology; mitotic index	T increased mitotic index in 1, and stimulated differentiation in 2/3 tumours	McMahon *et al.* (1972)
Kidney			
MA, testosterone propionate, HC, stilboestrol, 1–5 each	Morphology	Range of effect	Tchao *et al.* (1968)

Normal ranges of hormone concentrations vary slightly between laboratories. As an approximate guide, plasma levels of 17β-oestradiol are <68 pg ml^{-1} in males and post menopausal females and 20–400 pg ml^{-1} in premenopausal menstruating females; testosterone, 2.6–6.9 ng ml^{-1} in adult males and 0.14–0.72 ng ml^{-1} in adult females; progesterone, <0.9 ng ml^{-1} in males and postmenopausal females and 0.9–29.9 ng ml^{-1} in premenopausal menstruating females; prolactin, <0.36 mIU ml^{-1} in adult males and females.

Abbreviations used: CEE, chick embryo extract; CS, calf serum; DHT, dihydrotestosterone; E, 17β-oestradiol; E$_2$DH, oestradiol dehydrogenase; FCS, foetal calf serum; GH, growth hormone; HC, hydrocortisone; HCG, human chorionic gonadotrophin; HS, human serum; ^{3}H-TdR, ^{3}H-thymidine; ^{3}H-U, ^{3}H-uridine; I, insulin; ^{125}I-Udr, ^{125}I-iodo-2'-deoxyuridine; LAD, lipoamide dehydrogenase; LDH, lactate dehydrogenase; MA, medroxyprogesterone acetate; OP, ovine prolactin; Prog, progesterone; PR, progesterone receptor; PSD, pentose shunt dehydrogenase; T, testosterone.

drugs. In common with all such *in vitro* assessments, numerous factors require careful consideration, including:

1. Drug concentration and half-life.
2. Drug metabolism, particularly of compounds in which the active metabolite is produced at a site distant from the tumour (e.g. cyclophosphamide in liver).
3. Exposure and recovery periods.
4. Effect of culture conditions, particularly in relation to maintenance of the tissue and drug activity.
5. Method of assessing *in vitro* sensitivity.

In addition, studies using organ culture should take account of tumour heterogeneity and the presence of normal tissue.

A few thorough studies on the practicalities of using this approach have been published (see Table 3). A comparison of assay systems by Lazarus *et al.* (1966) indicated that three-quarters of the tumours tested could be grown in the chick mesonephros system devised by Wolff (1970). It was concluded that this system was too complex for use as a routine assay, and that the presence of chick tissue made assessment of sensitivity difficult. Nevertheless it is clear from the study of Dendy (1968) that this methodology, when applied to a tumour capable of continuous long-term growth in organ culture, provides an exceptional means for studying serial changes in replicate samples. Dickson and Suzangar (1976) attempted to counter some of the criticisms applied to *in vitro* measurements of chemosensitivity. Using a simplified methodology, the incidence of sensitivity to a range of anticancer agents in melanoma, breast, stomach, colon, and lung cancer was determined. The only group who have related *in vitro* data to clinical response in a large series of cases used methodology described by Tanneberger and Mohr (1973). No correlation was observed in adjuvant therapy trials of ovarian and lung cancer (Nissen *et al.*, 1978), but more encouraging results were obtained in a breast cancer adjuvant therapy trial (Peek *et al.*, 1981).

V. Hormone and chemotherapeutic drug metabolism

Response to endocrine therapy and chemotherapy may be related in part to the metabolism of the agents used, and measurement of metabolites in organ culture may be relevant clinically. Studies using organ culture have shown that there are differences in metabolism of hormones and anticancer agents by normal and neoplastic tissue (for references see Table 1). Normal lung tissue predominantly forms sulphate ester conjugates with 1-naphthol, whereas squamous cell carcinomas from the same patients form mainly glucuronic

Table 3 Survey of organ culture studies on effects of chemotherapeutic drugs on human malignant tumours, giving brief details of drug concentrations, period of exposure, and methods of assessing *in vitro* sensitivity

Chemotherapeutic drug concentrations (μg ml^{-1})	Exposure (days)	Method of assessing *in vitro* sensitivity	Reference
MTX, 4; 5FU, 26; CP, 70; TT, 6; PAM, 2.5; VB, 2.5; ACT D, 0.2 In presence of 15% pooled AB serum $\pm$ hyperthermia (4 h at 42°C)	1	O_2 consumption and CO_2 production; incorporation of ^{3}H-thymidine and ^{14}C-uridine into nucleic acids and ^{14}C-leucine into protein; morphology	Dickson and Suzangar (1976)
DG, 0.5; DA, 0.5; MTX, 2.5 and 5.0; 5-FUDR, 2.5 and 5.0; 6MP, 2.5 and 5.0 (In presence of various substrates and additions, enveloped by chick mesonephros and vitelline membrane)	7	Morphology	Lazarus *et al.* (1966)
Melphalan, 67–336 (In presence of chick embryo extracts and surrounded by chick vitelline membrane)	7	Histology	Simpson (1969)
TR, 0.01 and 0.1; Methyl-GAG, 6 and 60; sarcolysin, 0.4 and 4.0; VB, 0.2 and 2.0; VC, 0.08 and 0.8; 5FU, 20 and 200; MTX, 0.6 and 60 (In presence of 20% CS)	2	Incorporation of ^{3}H-thymidine	Tanneberger and Mohr (1973)
Thiotepa, MTX, melphalan, mannitol-myleran, 1–10 (Culture additions not stated)	3 5	Incorporation of ^{3}H-thymidine into DNA; autoradiography of ^{3}H-thymidine uptake; morphology	Tchao *et al.* (1968)
MTX and melphalan 2.5 and 25	2	Incorporation of ^{32}P-phosphate into nucleic acids; morphology	Yarnell *et al.* (1964)

In order to compare *in vitro* dose levels with those achieved clinically, a tabular summary of pharmacokinetic parameters has been produced by Alberts and Chen (1980).

Abbreviations used: Act D, actinomycin D; CP, cyclophosphamide; CS, calf serum; DA, 2′-deoxyadenosine; DG, 2′-deoxyguanosine; 5FU, 5-fluorouracil; 5-FUDR, 2′-deoxy-5-fluorouridine; Methyl-GAG, Methyl-bis-(guanylhydrazone); 6MP, 6-mercaptopurine; MTX, methotrexate; PAM, L-phenylalanine mustard; TR, trenimon; TT, triethylene thiophosphoramide; VB, vinblastine; VC, vincristine.

acid conjugates with this substrate (Cohen *et al.*, 1981). Identification of such biochemical differences could be used in the design of agents with greater selective toxicity for neoplastic cells. Bearing in mind the advantages of the organ culture technique for maintaining the structure and function of tissue *in vitro*, it is surprising that the vast majority of such biochemical studies are carried out using homogenates (in which the cellular integrity is destroyed) or short-term incubations of tissue slices in buffered salt solutions (in which viability is limited). This is an area in which organ culture should be exploited.

VI. Methods of assessment

Application of organ culture to drug sensitivity testing has been limited by the lack of a simple objective method for measuring *in vitro* sensitivity. Not only must tumour heterogeneity be taken into account, but measurements should differentiate, ideally, between the response of the neoplastic and other cell types. Many different methods have been used (see Tables 2 and 3). Histological and histochemical examinations are useful, and in part essential to examine viability, but subjective assessments are unsatisfactory unless clear-cut and rigid criteria can be applied. Autoradiography provides an alternative and quantitative approach, but it is laborious and time-consuming. Biochemical measurements of incorporation of radioactively labelled precursors have been used in many studies, but they may not differentiate response of the tumour cells. In addition, differences in the effects of drugs on individual biochemical pathways, and uncertainty concerning the relationship between changes in rates of DNA, RNA, or protein synthesis and subsequent viability, raise doubts as to the validity of this approach. Similar reservations may be made concerning other biochemical and physiological measurements, such as respiration rate. More reliable data might be obtained by measuring individual biochemical markers related to the mechanism of action of each chemotherapeutic drug (e.g. dihydrofolate reductase activity following treatment with methotrexate). Changes in the rate of tumour marker production, such as α-lactalbumin in breast cancer (Kleinberg, 1975; Wilson *et al.*, 1980), may be useful both *in vitro* and *in vivo*, but not all tumours produce measurable quantities of such substances. However, the advent of tissue-specific monoclonal antibodies could provide an answer to this problem. Measurement of antigen production in culture medium may permit serial, quantitative and tumour-specific assessments of *in vitro* sensitivity to be made.

VII. Perspective

A technique that maintains structural and functional integrity *in vitro* has obvious advantages. Tumours can be maintained in organ culture for many years, and the next step is to replace the complex media and substrates used by defined media. Each tumour cell type probably will require different culture conditions, and it must be shown that characteristics such as clonogenicity, steroid receptor activity, and specific antigen production are retained. Once these objectives are achieved, it should be possible to use organ culture more effectively to investigate *in vitro* sensitivity to hormones and chemotherapeutic drugs.

Acknowledgements

I wish to thank Dr G. M. Cohen, Dr Gisele M. Hodges, and Dr G. D. Wilson for their helpful comments.

References

Abaza, N. A., Leighton, J. and Zajac, B. A. (1978). Clinical bladder cancer in sponge matrix tissue culture. *Cancer* **42,** 1364–1374.

Alberts, D. S. and Chen, H.-S. G. (1980). Tabular summary of pharmacokinetic parameters relevant to in vitro drug assay. In *Cloning of Human Tumor Stem Cells* (ed. S. E. Salmon), pp. 351–359. Alan R. Liss, New York.

Archer, F. L. (1968). Normal and neoplastic human tissue in organ culture. *Arch. Path.* **85,** 62–71.

Aspegren, K. (1976). Hormone effects on human mammary cancer in organ cultures. *Am. J. Surg.* **131,** 575–580.

Bard, D. R. and Lasnitzki, I. (1977). The influence of oestradiol on the metabolism of androgens by human prostatic tissue. *J. Endocr.* **74,** 1–9.

Beeby, D. I., Easty, G. C., Gazet, J. C., Grigor, K. and Neville, A. M. (1975). An assessment of the effects of hormones on short term organ cultures of human breast carcinomata. *Br. J. Cancer* **31,** 317–328.

Breborowicz, J., Easty, G. C., Birbeck, M., Robertson, D., Nery, R. and Neville, A. M. (1975). The monolayer and organ culture of human colorectal carcinomata and the associated "normal" colonic mucosa and their production of carcinoembryonic antigens. *Br. J. Cancer* **31,** 559–569.

Brockas, A. J. and Wiernik, G. (1976). Isolation of labelled glycoproteins from organ cultured carcinoma of the cervix. In *Human Tumours in Short Term Culture* (ed. P. P. Dendy), pp. 270–276. Academic Press, London.

Chayen, J., Altmann, F. P., Bitensky, L. and Daly, J. R. (1970). Response of human breast-cancer tissue to steroid hormones in vitro. *Lancet* **i,** 868–870.

Cohen, G. M., Gibby, E. M. and Mehta, R. (1981). Routes of conjugation in normal and cancerous tissue from human lung. *Nature* **291,** 662–664.

Cooper, P. and Goldring, I. P. (1964). Organ culture studies of human normal tissues and tumors. *Acta Unio Contra Cancrum* **20,** 1288–1291.

Dendy, P. P. (1968). The effects of X-rays on a human tumour growing in organo-typic culture. *Eur. J. Cancer* **4,** 163–172.

Dermer, G. B. and Sherwin, R. P. (1975). Autoradiographic localization of glycoprotein in human breast cancer cells maintained in organ culture after incubation with (^{3}H)fucose or (^{3}H)glucosamine. *Cancer Res.* **35,** 63–67.

Dickson, J. A. and Suzangar, M. (1976). The in-vitro response of human tumours to cytotoxic drugs and hyperthermia (42°) and its relevance to clinical oncology. In *Organ Culture in Biomedical Research* (ed. M. Balls and M. Monnickendam), pp. 417–461. Cambridge University Press.

Dresden, M. H., Heilman, S. A. and Schmidt, J. D. (1972). Collagenolytic enzymes in human neoplasms. *Cancer Res.* **32,** 993–996.

Duncan, J. N., Davis, J. C., Wade, A. P. and Walker, S. (1981). Short term organ culture of human breast tumour tissue and its application in studies of steroid metabolism. *Eur. J. Cancer Clin. Oncol.* **17,** 1133–1142.

Easty, G. C. (1970). Organ culture methods. *Methods Cancer Res.* **5,** 1–43.

Easty, G. C., Powles, T., Easty, D. M., Dowsett, M. and Neville, A. (1976). The detection of osteolytic substances produced by human breast tumours. In *Organ Culture in Biomedical Research* (ed. M. Balls and M. Monnickendam), pp. 367–377. Cambridge University Press.

Fell, H. B. and Robison, R. (1929). The growth, development and phosphatase activity of embryonic avian femora and limb buds cultivated in vitro. *Biol. J.* **23**, 767–785.

Finkelstein, M., Geier, A., Horn, H., Levij, I. S. and Ever-Hadani, P. (1975). Effect of testosterone and estradiol-17β on synthesis of DNA, RNA and protein in human breast in organ culture. *Int. J. Cancer* **15**, 78–90.

Flax, H., Salih, H., Newton, K. A. and Hobbs, J. R. (1973). Are some women's breast cancers androgen dependent? *Lancet* **i**, 1204–1207.

Geier, A., Horn, H., Levij, I. S., Lichtshtein, E. and Finkelstein, M. (1975). The metabolism of ^{3}H-estradiol-17β in human breast cancer in organ culture. *Eur. J. Cancer* **11**, 127–130.

Ghanadian, R., Masters, J. R. W. and Smith, C. B. (1981). Altered androgen metabolism in carcinoma of the prostate. *Eur. Urol.* **7**, 169–170.

Gorlich, M., Hecker, D. and Heise, E. (1981). Comparison of estradiol receptor investigations and histochemical investigations on enzymes in human mammary cancers. *J. Nat. Cancer Inst.* **67**, 521–527.

Hecker, D. and Deutschmann, A. (1976). Histochemical and ultrastructural investigations on organ culture of malignant tumors. *Acta Histochem.* **55**, 8–13.

Heuson, J.-C., Pasteels, J.-L., Legros, N., Heuson-Stiennon, J. and Leclercq, G. (1975). Estradiol-dependent collagenolytic enzyme activity in long-term organ culture of human breast cancer. *Cancer Res.* **35**, 2039–2048.

Hodges, G. M. (1978). Normal and neoplastic urothelium of human bladder in vivo and in vitro: an assessment of SEM studies. *Scanning Electron Microscopy* **2**, 983–990.

Hodges, G. M. (1981). Growth differentiation and function of tumours in organ culture. In *Regulation of Growth in Neoplasia* (ed. G. V. Sherbet), pp. 52–130. Karger, Basel.

Holmstrom, T. (1975). Human brain tumor cells in matrix culture. In *Human Tumor Cells in Vitro* (ed. J. Fogh), pp. 161–174. Plenum Press, New York.

Hustin, J. (1975). Effect of protein hormones and steroids on tissue cultures of endometrial carcinoma. *Br. J. Obstet. Gynaecol.* **82**, 493–500.

Jacobelli, S., Sica, G., Ranelletti, F. and Barile, G. (1978). An assessment of the effects of steroid hormones and antiestrogens on short-term organ culture of human endometrial carcinoma. *Eur. J. Cancer* **14**, 931–938.

Kadohama, N., Kirdani, R. Y., Murphy, G. P. and Sandberg, A. A. (1977). 5α-Reductase as a target enzyme for anti-prostatic drugs in organ culture. *Oncology* **34**, 123–128.

Kalus, M. (1972). Carcinoma and adenomatous polyps of the colon and rectum in biopsy and organ tissue culture. *Cancer* **30**, 972–982.

Kalus, M., Ghidoni, J. J. and O'Neal, R. M. (1968). The growth of tumors in matrix cultures. *Cancer* **22**, 507–516.

Kiricuta, I., Todorutiu, C., Mulea, R. and Risca, R. (1978). Axillary lymph-node and breast carcinoma interrelations in organ culture. *Cancer* **42**, 2710–2715.

Kleinberg, D. L. (1975). Human α-lactalbumin: measurement in serum and in breast cancer organ cultures by radioimmunoassay. *Science* **190**, 276–278.

Kohorn, E. I. and Tchao, R. (1968). The effect of hormones on endometrial carcinoma in organ culture. *J. Obstet. Gynaec. Br. Cwlth.* **75**, 1262–1267.

Lagios, M. D. (1974). Hormonally enhanced proliferation of human breast cancer in organ culture. *Oncology* **29**, 22–33.

Lasnitzki, I. (1979). Metabolism and action of steroid hormones on human benign prostatic hyperplasia and prostatic carcinoma grown in organ culture. *J. Steroid Biochem.* **11**, 625–630.

Lazarus, H., Tegeler, W., Mazzone, H. M., Leroy, J. G., Boone, B. A. and Foley, G. E. (1966). Determination of sensitivity of individual biopsy specimens to potential inhibitory agents: evaluation of some explant culture methods as assay systems. *Cancer Chemother. Rep.* **50**, 543–555.

Leighton, J. (1951). A sponge matrix method for tissue culture: formation of organised aggregates of cells in vitro. *J. Nat. Cancer Inst.* **12**, 545–562.

Leighton, J., Justh, G. and Mark, R. (1969). The use of three-dimensional matrix tissue culture for bioassay of cancer: a progress report. *Recent Results Cancer Res.* **17**, 147–167.

Lyser, K. M. (1976). Organ culture of human nervous system tumors. *In Vitro* **12**, 48–56.

Mandeville, R., Holloway, A., Lauchlan, S. C. and Simard, R. (1979). Replication of *Herpes simplex* virus type 2 in normal dysplastic and neoplastic human cervical epithelia. *Eur. J. Cancer* **15**, 351–361.

Masters, J. R. W., Sangster, K. and Smith, I. I. (1977). Hormonal sensitivity of human breast tumors in vitro: pentose-shunt activity. *Cancer* **39**, 1978–1980.

Masters, J. R. W., Krishnaswamy, A., Rigby, C. C. and O'Donoghue, E. P. N. (1980). Quantitative organ culture: an approach to prediction of tumour response. *Br. J. Cancer* **41**, Suppl. IV, 199–202.

Matoska, J. (1970). Effect of progesterone on endometrial cancer in the organ culture. *Neoplasma* **17**, 525–533.

Matoska, J. and Stricker, F. (1967). Following human tumours in primary organ culture. *Neoplasma* **14**, 507–519.

McCully, K. S. (1968). Protein synthesizing activity of human neoplastic and normal thyroid tissue in chick embryo mesonephros organ culture. *Int. J. Cancer* **3**, 142–149.

McMahon, M. J., Butler, A. V. J. and Thomas, G. H. (1972). Morphological responses of prostatic carcinoma to testosterone in organ culture. *Br. J. Cancer* **26**, 388–394.

Nissen, E. and Tanneberger, S. (1976). Mixed organ culture as a tool for considering cellular tumor-host relationships in tumor patients. *Arch. Geschwulstforsch.* **46**, 281–293.

Nissen, E., Tanneberger, S., Projan, A., Morack, G. and Peek, U. (1978). Recent results of in vitro drug prediction in human tumour chemotherapy. *Arch. Geschwulstforsch.* **48**, 667–672.

Nordquist, S. (1970). Survival and hormonal responsiveness of endometrial carcinoma in organ culture. *Acta Obstet. Gynec. Scand.* **49**, 275–283.

O'Gorman, T. A. and Lamont, J. T. (1978). Glycoprotein synthesis and secretion in human colon cancers and normal colonic mucosa. *Cancer Res.* **38**, 2784–2789.

Peek, U., Tanneberger, S., Heise, E., Gorlich, M., Nissen, E., Marx, G., Projan, A., Winkler, R., Kunde, D. and Bodek, B. (1981). High risk breast cancer: long-term surgical adjuvant therapy based on predictive tests—preliminary report. *Arch. Geschwulstforsch.* **51**, 139–151.

Roller, M.-R., Owen, S. P. and Heidelberger, C. (1966). Studies on the organ culture of human tumors. *Cancer Res.* **26**, 626–637.

Rousseau-Merck, M. F., Lombard, M. N., Nezelof, C. and Mouly, H. (1977).

Limitation of the potentialities of nephroblastoma differentiation in vitro. *Eur. J. Cancer* **13**, 163–170.

Rovin, S. (1962). The influence of carbon dioxide on the cultivation of human neoplastic explants in vitro. *Cancer Res.* **22**, 384–387.

Rubinstein, L. J., Herman, M. M. and Foley, V. L. (1973). In vitro characteristics of human glioblastomas maintained in organ culture systems. *Am. J. Path.* **71**, 61–80.

Salih, H., Flax, H. and Hobbs, J. R. (1972a). In-vitro oestrogen sensitivity of breast-cancer tissue as a possible screening method for hormonal treatment. *Lancet* **i**, 1198–1202.

Salih, H., Flax, H., Brander, W. and Hobbs, J. R. (1972b). Prolactin dependence of human breast cancers. *Lancet* **ii**, 1103–1105.

Satyaswaroop, P. G. and Mortel, R. (1982). Failure of progestins to induce estradiol dehydrogenase activity in endometrial carcinoma, in vitro *Cancer Res.* **42**, 1322–1325.

Schaeffer, W. I. (1979). Proposed usage of animal tissue culture terms. *In Vitro* **15**, 649–653.

Sellwood, R. A. and Castro, J. E. (1974). The effect of hormones on organ cultures of human mammary carcinoma. *J. Path.* **113**, 223–225.

Simpson, P. (1969). La sensibilité différentielle d'une tumeur humaine et des tissus somatiques et germinaux des gonades embryonnaires en culture organotypique in vitro. *Eur. J. Cancer* **5**, 331–337.

Siracky, J., Matoska, J. and Siracka, E. (1974). Morphology and autoradiography studies of gynaecological tumours in organ culture. *Neoplasma* **21**, 307–312.

Sorour, O., Raafat, M., El-Bolkainy, N. and Rifaat, M. (1975). Infiltrative potentiality of brain tumors in organ culture. *J. Neurosurg.* **43**, 742–749.

Spratt, N. T. (1947). A simple method for explanting and cultivating early embryos in vitro. *Science* **106**, 452.

Stoll, B. A. (1970). Investigation of organ culture as an aid to the hormonal management of breast cancer. *Cancer* **25**, 1228–1233.

Svanberg, L. and Astedt, B. (1976). Release of fibrinolytic activators from human ovarian tumours in organ culture. *Ann. Chirurg. Gynaecol.* **65**, 405–407.

Tanneberger, S. and Mohr, A. (1973). Biological characterization of human tumours by means of organ culture and individualized cytostatic cancer treatment. *Arch. Geschwulstforsch.* **42**, 307–315.

Tchao, R., Easty, G. C., Ambrose, E. J., Raven, R. W. and Bloom, H. J. G. (1968). Effect of chemotherapeutic agents and hormones on organ cultures of human tumours. *Eur. J. Cancer* **4**, 39–44.

Tokes, Z. A. and Dermer, G. B. (1977). Glycoprotein synthesis as a function of epithelial cell arrangement: biosynthesis and release of glycoproteins by human breast and prostate cells in organ culture. *J. Supramol. Struct.* **7**, 515–530.

Trowell, O. A. (1959). The culture of mature organs in a synthetic medium. *Exp. Cell Res.* **16**, 118–147.

Tsypkin, L. B., Voroshilova, M. K., Goryunova, A. G., Lavrova, I. K. and Koroleva, G. A. (1976). The morphology of tumors of the human gastrointestinal tract in short-term organ culture and the reaction of these tumors to infection with poliovirus. *Cancer* **38**, 1796–1806.

Wellings, S. R. and Jentoft, V. L. (1972). Organ cultures of normal, dysplasic, hyperplasic, and neoplasic human mammary tissues. *J. Nat. Cancer Inst.* **49**, 329–338.

Welsch, C. W., Iturri, G. C. and Brennan, M. J. (1976). DNA synthesis of human, mouse and rat mammary carcinomas in vitro. *Cancer* **38,** 1272–1281.

Willcox, P. A. and Thomas, G. H. (1972). Oestrogen metabolism in cultured human breast tumours. *Br. J. Cancer* **26,** 453–460.

Wilson, G. D., Woods, K. L., Walker, R. A. and Howell, A. (1980). Effect of prolactin on lactalbumin production by normal and malignant human breast tissue in organ culture. *Cancer Res.* **40,** 486–489.

Wolff, E. (1970). Organ chimeras and organ culture of malignant tumors. In *Organ Culture* (ed. D. Thomas), pp. 459–496. Academic Press, New York.

Yarnell, M., Ambrose, E. J., Shepley, K. and Tchao, R. (1964). Drug assays on organ cultures of biopsies from human tumours. *Br. Med. J.* **2,** 490–491.

15. The Xenograft as an Intermediate Model System

J. A. HOUGHTON and P. J. HOUGHTON

I. Introduction

The principle of effective chemotherapy, established by Ehrlich, depends upon the agent causing selective toxicity to an invading organism. Such selective toxicity is a consequence of metabolic differences between target and host cells, and appears pertinent to bacterial, viral, and cancer chemotherapy. It is apparent, however, that cancer is a diverse group of diseases, each one individual with regard to its natural history, metabolic characteristics, and responses to chemotherapy. Furthermore, within a disease type there exists both intertumour (interpatient) and intratumour variability. Thus, when one considers model systems that may have application for new agent evaluation, or for developing therapies using cytotoxic agents of known utility, certain demands can be made of the model. These include (a) that selectivity of drug action can be assessed, (b) that metabolic characteristics of the model parallel that of a particular cancer type, and (c) that the model reflects at least some of the intertumour variability observed in the clinical disease.

Because of the individual metabolic characteristics of each type of cancer, it may well be that truly selective agents can be found only by using each type of human cancer as its own test system. A logical development of this concept, which fulfils the demands placed upon the model, is to grow human cancers in laboratory animals. Although this is not a new concept, the practical application has been realized only in the past decade.

II. Xenografts as models

Human tumours transplanted into immune-deficient (athymic nude) or immune-deprived mice essentially retain the histological and morphological characteristics of the original human tumour, although there are exceptions.

The stroma, which is derived from the host (Giovanella and Fogh, 1978), is generally decreased (Povlsen, 1976; Shimosato et al., 1979). Other changes may be indicative of host selection pressures. Tokita et al. (1980) found that the parabasal type cells of the Yumoto cervical carcinoma became dominant after 8 serial transfers in nude mice. Shimosato et al. (1979) reported distinct changes in hepatoblastomas transplanted into nude mice, and a Wilms tumour was subsequently classified as a rhabdomyosarcoma in the mouse. The fact that first passage transplants may differ from the patient tumour may be explained by variation within the original tumour rather than a process of cell selection in mure. The fact that changes occur with subsequent transfer becomes more disturbing, and is indicative of selection pressure within the host. Several workers have observed xenografts to be more differentiated after serial passage (Shimosato et al., 1976; Tokita et al., 1980), but again there are exceptions. Breast carcinomas passaged in immune-deprived mice in most cases retained histological features of the original patient specimen. However, in some of the first-generation transplants, and increasingly with further passage, there was a tendency for tumour to become less differentiated with fewer ducts or acini, increased mitoses, nuclear pleomorphism and atypia (Bailey et al., 1981). The prominent desmoplastic response and elastosis typical of many breast carcinomas were also lost upon transplantation. That human tumours retain many of their original features growing as xenografts in mice may be fortuitous, since animal cancers often change dramatically when passaged serially in syngeneic hosts (Greene and Harvey, 1968).

III. Histochemical, hormone, and antigen production

Houghton and Taylor (1978a) observed maintenance of epithelial mucin, and carcinoembryonic antigen (CEA) was maintained in colon adenocarcinoma xenografts. Kim et al. (1976) found that CEA concentrations (units g^{-1} wet weight) decreased with serial transfer in athymic nude mice, but these values may be related to tumour size and degree of necrosis at the time of sampling. In general, xenografts retain their ability to produce peptide hormones. Thus, choriocarcinomas produce human chorionic gonadotrophin (Hayashi et al., 1978); adenocorticotropin and β-melanocyte-stimulating hormone were produced by a small cell carcinoma of lung (Shimosato et al., 1976).

Hormone dependency of BR-10 breast tumour was also demonstrated in nude mice. Epithelial membrane antigen was maintained during serial passage in breast tumour xenografts (Bailey et al., 1981), whereas expression of CEA decreased. Other changes have been noted also. Giovanella et al. (1978) failed to detect osteoid in an osteosarcoma xenograft, and melanin was absent in xenografts derived from poorly melanotic xenografts, although other bio-chemical criteria (e.g. tyrosinase) were maintained.

Chromosomal evolution has been observed during serial passage (Reeves and Houghton, 1978), but whether the xenograft or primary transplant reflects the cell clones present in the patient's tumour remains an important but unanswered question.

IV. Cell proliferation kinetics

Cell cycle kinetics of xenografts derived from several different tumour types are summarized in Table 1. Cell cycle phase durations in colorectal xenografts are consistent with the limited data obtained in patients, but growth rate of xenografts is greater than that reported for human cancers in man. Sharkey *et al.* (1980) reported that the mitotic index increased after xenotransplantation, and found a greater increase for sarcomas compared with tumours of epithelial origin. For many tumours transplanted into immune-deficient mice, growth rates increase for the first several serial passages (Pickard *et al.*, 1975; Houghton and Taylor, 1978b). This appears to be due to a decreasing cell loss factor rather than a change in phase duration or growth fraction (see Table 1). This may indicate an adaptive change, or a process of selection, and requires further examination.

V. Sensitivity to known agents

For the xenograft model to be of value it must either reflect the known clinical sensitivity of the human disease or, more specifically, it should demonstrate sensitivity similar to that of the original donor tumour. It is unfortunate that many studies of the former type have used adenocarcinomata of the digestive tract (stomach, colon, rectum), which are relatively unresponsive to chemo-therapy. Experimental design is such that agents of known clinical efficacy are evaluated against a series of xenografts of the same histological type, to determine whether the spectrum of clinical sensitivity is reflected in the model. In order to carry out such a study many xenograft lines must be used, and consequently these experiments are both time-consuming and expensive. Table 2 summarizes results obtained using colorectal adenocarcinoma xenografts, where an agent has been examined against a reasonable number of tumour lines. 5-Fluorouracil, the nitrosoureas, and cyclophosphamide show activity in this screen, and have also demonstrated efficacy against large bowel cancer. Correlations of this type are of critical importance if the xenograft models are to be of value in detecting new effective agents. However, it must be

Table 1 Cell cycle kinetics of xenografts from different tumour types

Xenograft	LI (%)	MI (%)	G_1	S	G_2	T_c	T_{pot}	GF (%)	CLF (%)
Colorectal									
1. P76/3*	27	1.7	3.8	13.9	5.2	24.8	42	50	—
2. P116/4	11	0.85	8.4	13.2	6.6	30.9	87	—	—
3. Hx23/1	9	0.54	14.5	10.1	7.3	34.4	99	29	—
4. Hx18/1	25	1.1	7.0	14.8	3.7	28	50	46	—
5. Hx18/2	19	1.0	7.6	11.9	4.6	26.1	52	44	—
6. Hx18/3	20	1.3	14.7	11.8	4.9	34.8	50	—	—
7. HxGC$_3$/3	20	2.3	8.7	9.0	3.8	23.6	38	65	86
8. HxGC$_3$/10	18	2.3	9.4	8.0	3.9	23.4	37	69	76
9. HxHC$_1$/10	16	1.8	12.0	11.8	7.3	34.2	60	52	64
10. Hx13/6	22	1.07	13.1	17	2.5	35	—	47	80
11. Hx18/2	19	1.0	7.6	11.9	4.6	26.1	—	46	66
Lung									
12. Hx29/7	26	2.2	10.9	12.4	5.2	30.3	—	61	81
13. TO-1/9	16	1.9	10	8	7	25	39	55	84
14. LU-9/11	20	2.5	13	14	6	33	71	38	79
15. LU-24/8	15	1.9	1	13	12	26	109	18	62
Rhabdomyosarcoma									
16. HxRD/3	20	1.3	19.5	22.2	4.8	50.7	88	57	65
17. HxLL/3	15	0.72	23	24.2	3.7	55.8	123	37	67

T_{pot} = potential doubling time; GF = growth fraction; CLF = cell loss factor.

* Denotes passage number.

(1–6) Pickard _et al._, 1975. (1, 8) Houghton and Taylor, 1978b. (9, 16, 17) Houghton and Houghton, unpublished results. (10–12) Kopper and Steel, 1975. (13–15) Shimosato _et al._, 1979.

stated also that a response according to the criteria used would not meet the clinical criterion of a 50% decrease in the product of the tumour diameters. Table 3 shows results obtained using rhabdomyosarcoma xenografts derived from untreated children. This model identifies agents active against this disease, and appears capable of discriminating between vincristine and vinblastine.

Where sufficient data exist, xenografts of a particular cancer type appear to identify agents of known clinical activity against that disease. Criteria for regarding a drug as active are rather less demanding in experimental studies

Table 2 Response of colorectal xenografts to chemotherapy.

Agent	Tumours	Responses	% Responses
5-Fluorouracil	35	13	37
Methyl CCNU	22	7	32
BCNU	7	3	42
Cyclophosphamide	15	5	31
Doxorubicin	7	0	0
Actinomycin D	13	0	0
Cis-platinum	10	0	0
Melphalan	9	1	11
Methotrexate	8	1	12

A response is defined as (i) volume of treated tumours (mean) $\leqslant 40\%$ that of control mean volume, or (ii) a growth delay $\geqslant 2$ tumour volume doubling times.

Data are from: Kubota et al. (1978); Fodstad (1979); Giulani et al. (1981a); Ovejera et al. (1978); Fujita et al. (1980); Nowak et al. (1978); Catane et al. (1979); Kopper and Steel (1975); Giulani and Kaplan (1980); Osieka et al. (1977); Houghton and Houghton (1978).

Table 3 Responses of rhabdomyosarcoma xenografts to single agents.

Agent	Tumours	Responses
Vincristine	4	4
Vinblastine	3	0
Vindesine	3	3
Actinomycin D	4	1
Doxorubicin	4	3
Cyclophosphamide	4	3
DTIC	4	3
Mitomycin C	4	2
Cis-dichlorodiammineplatinum	4	1

From Houghton et al. (1982) and unpublished data.

compared with the clinical situation, which may lead to the identification of false positives. One observation common to almost every study is that xenografts, established from individual patients with the same type of malignancy, show marked variation in response to chemotherapeutic agents.

Consequently a single xenograft line is not capable of reliably identifying agents of value in the treatment of the disease. Hence the National Cancer Institute screening programme using human tumour xenografts has failed to identify clinically active agents. For example, the mammary carcinoma MX-1 used in this screen is not responsive to doxorubicin (Goldin *et al.*, 1981), unlike other mammary carcinoma xenografts (Giulani *et al.*, 1981b). Ideally the model should reflect clinical heterogeneity, and be representative of histological subtypes. The number of tumour lines required will depend upon the heterogeneity of responses within that cancer type. Goldin *et al.* (1981) have suggested that it may be advisable to employ a battery of human tumours of the same histologic type, i.e. a series of colon tumours. This would reduce the incidence of false positive or false negative results.

An alternative approach has been to compare responses of the human tumour in the mouse and in the donor patient. Such studies are fraught with difficulties and, although positive correlations have been claimed, usually the number of observations has been few. The exception is a study by Shorthouse and colleagues (1980) in which responses of lung carcinomas were compared with their respective xenografts. The results strongly suggest that xenografts retain the chemosensitivity of the parent tumour.

VI. Methods

Human tumour xenografts may be grown in a variety of laboratory animals using several preparative procedures. Only those models suitable for chemotherapy studies will be considered.

A. Congenitally athymic nude mouse

Since the initial report by Rygaard and Povlsen (1969) that human epidermoid cancers could be grown in the athymic nude mouse mutant, numerous reports concerning growth of other tumour types have appeared. The nude (nu/nu) gene has been established in many mouse strains, although the BALB/c backcross is used most frequently (for a detailed review of nude mouse variants see Hansen, 1978). Without a thymus gland, approximately 1% of spleen and lymph node cells are positive for antigen using indirect immunofluorescence, and these T-cell precursors can be activated to recognize allo-antigens (Ramseier, 1975). In addition, nude mice may have a normal or augmented humoral immunity and, approximately 3 weeks after birth, levels of natural killer cells increase. Even with these limitations the athymic nude mouse has proved suitable for growing human tumours as xenografts, and the presence of residual T-cell and normal humoural immunity offers the possibility to suppress the mouse further in order to enhance tumour growth.

1. *Antilymphocyte or antithymocyte serum*

Antilymphocyte (ALS) or antithymocyte (ATS) serum is prepared by the method of Levey and Medawar (1966). Injections of active serum commence 1 day prior to tumour implantation and continue thereafter as 0.25 ml doses intraperitoneally three times each week (Ohsugi *et al.*, 1980).

2. *X-irradiation*

At 1 day before tumour transplantation, nude mice are X-irradiated at 320 rad min^{-1} to a total of 500 rads. Although the original technique utilized a 6 MeV machine, presumably other radiation sources would be suitable. This technique was found to enhance the transplantability of human malignant lymphoblasts, and was superior to ALS manipulation. Ziegler *et al.* (1982) have reported enhanced growth of MOLT-4 human T-cell leukaemia in BALB/c nude female mice irradiated three times with 200 rad over a 3 week period.

3. *Maternal thymectomy*

Epstein *et al.* (1976) found that the progeny of maternally thymectomized NIH Swiss nude mice had a higher percentage of tumour-bearing animals compared with progeny of normal mothers when injected with human lymphoma cells intracranially. The latent period for tumour development was also shorter.

4. *Pretreatment with immunosuppressive agents*

Injection of cyclophosphamide (300 mg kg^{-1}) 4 days before implantation subcutaneously of human retinoblastoma resulted in the growth of 3 out of 4 specimens, whereas none of 13 attempts in untreated Swiss nude mice was successful (Gallie *et al.*, 1977). Cyclophosphamide decreased the white cell count from 10 000 to 400 mm^{-3}.

Under conventional housing conditions nude mice have a relatively short lifespan of between 4 and 5 months. Two viruses are responsible for most deaths, namely murine hepatitis virus and Sendai virus. Evaluations of cytotoxic therapy in infected mice must be regarded with caution. Giovanella and Stehlin (1973) have described conditions under which nude mice may be kept healthy and have a normal lifespan of 1.5–2 years. Essentially, mice are maintained under strictly pathogen-free conditions; cages, water, and food are sterilized. All manipulations and surgical procedures are conducted under a laminar flow hood by personnel gowned and masked in sterile attire. To reduce further the possibility of infection, a solution containing antibiotics is added to the drinking water from birth to 3 months of age. Pinworm infestation may be controlled by periodically adding piperazine hexahydrate to drinking water (Giulani *et al.*, 1981a). Control of such parasitic infections may prove critical in xenograft studies (see later).

B. Immune-deprived mouse

1. *Thymectomized irradiated bone marrow reconstituted mice ($T^- B^+$)*

The most successful mouse strain has been the CBA, which is thymectomized at 4 weeks of age and given 900 rad whole body irradiation 3 weeks later, and an injection of syngeneic bone marrow within a few hours. The appropriate conditions may vary with the CBA strain used. In our experience CBA/lac (Laboratory Animal Centre, Carshalton, Surrey) and the CBA/CaJ (Jackson Laboratory, Maine) are similar although in the former 900 rads and in the latter 850 rads are used. Both CBA/J and BDF$_1$ mice are inferior hosts compared with CBA/CaJ. The number of cells required to rescue from radiation-induced aplasia varies. We have used routinely 2.5×10^6 nucleated cells per mouse derived from syngeneic thymectomized donors; other have rescued using as few as 5×10^5 cells.

2. *Thymectomized cytosine arabinoside irradiated mouse*

This model is based upon an observation by Millar (1976) that a low dose of cytosine arabinoside (ara-C) protected mice from a subsequent potentially lethal dose of ^{60}Co radiation. Steel *et al.* (1978) reported that CBA/lac mice given ara-C (200 mg kg^{-1}) 48 hours prior to 900 rads were better immune-deprived than were nude mice or CBA/lac prepared in the conventional manner. This preparation is technically less tedious than rescue with bone marrow.

The immune-deprived status may deteriorate with time, hence tumour should be transplanted within 4 weeks of irradiation. In our experience the bone marrow reconstituted mouse will support progressive growth of primary human explants for periods in excess of 12 months.

Essentially such immune-deprived mice may be housed under conventional conditions, although in a room separate from other animals. The major disadvantage of this type of preparation is that there is at least some permanent damage from the irradiation. This may be manifest as a greater variation in toxicity during chemotherapy trials, and necessitates some reduction in drug dose compared with that giving equivalent toxicity in normal CBA mice. Immune-deprived mice and the athymic nude mouse support the growth of similar spectra of human tumours.

C. Immune-suppressed mouse

Although there are some data indicating that T-cell mediated immunity may be depressed for a considerable time after administration of a short course of ATS, immunity may recover with time. We have classified such animals as immune-suppressed rather than as immune-deprived.

The most extensive studies have been reported by Cobb and Mitchley (1974a) and Mitchley *et al.* (1977). In these experiments mice were thymecto-mized at 4 weeks of age and then treated with ATS during weeks 6–9. Mice were injected with 0.5 cm^3 subcutaneously in the interscapular region three times weekly and tumour was implanted 2 weeks after the last injection. Alternatively ATS treatment may be started 1 day prior to tumour inoculation, and continued throughout growth. Tibbetts *et al.* (1977) reported that mice immunosuppressed by repeated injections of ATS for longer than 1 month tend to become unhealthy, and tumour growth rate slows after about 30 days.

The major problems associated with ATS or ALS are production of sufficient quantities for routine use, and standardization of batches. In addition, prolonged administration may induce formation of anti-ATS antibodies that would reduce the immune-suppressive activity of ATS, as well as leading to immune complex formation.

The study by Mitchley *et al.* (1977) is of considerable interest, since hexamethylmelamine cured a human lung tumour xenograft grown in ATS treated mice but failed to eradicate the tumour in immune-deprived mice. These results suggest caution in the use of mice prepared with ATS alone to evaluate chemotherapeutic efficacy.

D. Athymic nude rat

The athymic Rowett nude rat (rnu/rnu) has recently become available, and several studies suggest that in many respects it is biologically and immunologi-cally similar to the nude mouse. Successful transplantations of human tumours and athymic mouse xenografts have been reported (see Davis *et al.*, 1981). The role of the athymic nude rat remains to be defined but, despite its immunoincompetence, it appears to tolerate conventional housing conditions with no increase in morbidity or mortality compared with animals housed in isolators.

E. Immune-privileged sites

Implantations of human tumours to immune-privileged sites, such as the anterior chamber of the eye, the brain, subrenal capsule, or cheek-pouch of the hamster, have been successful but allow limited growth of the xenograft, render progressive growth measurements difficult, and are not necessarily useful models for chemotherapy studies. However, such sites may prove valuable for establishing certain tumour types that otherwise fail to grow in alternative more practical sites, or where therapy specific for that site is being investigated, e.g. uveal melanoma, retinoblastoma, or brain tumours.

Gallie *et al.* (1977) reported growth of retinoblastoma in the anterior chamber of the eye in Swiss nude mice, but failed to detect growth in several other species. Epstein and colleagues (1976) successfully transplanted human lymphomas to the brains of Swiss nudes and BALB/c nudes ($1–5 \times 10^5$ cells in 0.03 ml), and reported that these failed to grow in nude mice with isologous neonatal thymus grafts. The hamster cheek-pouch presents a useful site for transplantation. With ATS as an adjunct, such animals are equally as receptive as thymectomized irradiated bone marrow reconstituted CBA mice (Cobb and Mitchley, 1974b). However, relatively few chemotherapy studies utilizing this model have been reported.

VII. Response to chemotherapy

In certain respects studies in which xenografts have been used to evaluate agents are reminiscent of early clinical trials. There is little standardization, with respect to time of initiation of therapy, scheduling, dosage levels, and assessment of response. Thus, an attempt to interrelate studies from different groups is often futile. This point is not trivial. Few researchers have either the time or financial support to evaluate routinely agents against sufficient xenografts of a particular cancer type in order to state, with statistical conviction, that the agent, or combination, justifies clinical evaluation against that disease. If results of a clinical trial based upon three or four patients are unacceptable, why should we accept as meaningful results based upon three or four xenograft lines? One possible solution would be to form collaborative groups, essentially analogous to clinical cooperatives. An alternative, and probably more realistic, proposal is to accept a uniform approach to the time of treatment and assessment of response.

A. Site of implantation

Most frequently fragments (3–5 mm cubes) or cell suspensions (5×10^6 cells) are inoculated subcutaneously in the inguinal region. All surgical procedures should be carried out using aseptic procedures. The use of bilateral implants allows fewer animals to be used in order to achieve the same degree of statistical certainty (Warenius *et al.*, 1980). Implantation of a further two tumour fragments in the axillary region allows growth of four ·discrete tumours per animal, but does not allow sufficient time to evaluate therapy where tumours fuse together. The subcutaneous site offers the advantage that tumours may be readily detected by palpation, and margins can be determined. Inoculation of tumour cells into the gastrocnemius muscle of a hind limb is less satisfactory in these respects and also, with increasing tumour mass, vascular occlusion and accumulated oedema may influence the response to therapy.

B. Time of treatment

Few xenografts, even after serial transplantation, grow consistently in 100% of recipient animals. Thus, tumours should be well established and palpable at the initiation of therapy. In our experiments mice are treated when the mean tumour diameter is 6–8 mm. The time taken to grow to this size varies within a group of mice and is also a tumour-specific phenomenon; however, in immune-deprived mice the growth rate is at least partially host-determined (Houghton and Taylor, 1978b). Thus, in our studies mice are randomized into treatment groups when tumours are the appropriate size, and this necessitates treating groups of mice at different times. The "late growing" xenografts have a similar spectrum of growth rates to those that attain 6–8 mm more rapidly, so variation may represent differences in viability of the original tumour fragment implanted, and hence primarily in lag phase. When xenografts have achieved a diameter of 6–8 mm spontaneous regressions are observed only rarely.

C. Assessing responses

Xenografts tend to grow as localized, well circumscribed masses, and do not readily metastasize. Hence the lifespan of a tumour-bearing animal is not necessarily related to tumour burden. For this reason, assessment of antitumour activity by use of indices such as increased lifespan is not possible.

Mice bearing well established palpable tumours are randomized into groups of seven or more. Where necessary the hair over the tumour is clipped, and the tumour measured using two perpendicular diameters. Measurements are made at 7 day intervals, or more frequently if the rate of tumour growth is rapid. To calculate tumour volume it is necessary to make certain generalizations. If the shape is ellipsoid, volume = 0.5[length × (width)^2]. For tumours approximating to a sphere, volume = $\pi d^3/6$, where d is the mean diameter. Essentially similar results may be obtained irrespective of the formula used.

1. *Inhibition-of-growth method*

Growth curves for groups of treated or control tumours are constructed by plotting volume against time using semilogarithmic graph paper. At a given time after cessation of treatment the ratio of volumes for treated and control tumours can be calculated, and degree of inhibition of growth deduced.

$$\text{Inhibition of growth} = [(1 - T/C) \times 100]\%$$

where T is the mean volume of treated tumours and C that of controls. Alternatively tumours may be excised and weight substituted for volume (see Fig. 1). From the hypothetical curves in Fig. 1 it is clear that the T/C ratio constantly changes with time until the growth rate of treated tumours returns to that of untreated tumours. Giulani and his associates (1981a) have expressed activity as an optimal inhibition, i.e. the greatest difference between treated and control groups, irrespective of time. In our hypothetical study drug A has an optimal T/C (80% inhibition) at day 7, but subsequent regrowth leads to only a marginal growth delay. For drug B optimal inhibition occurs at day 21 (80%) but is obviously more effective at inhibiting tumour growth. Consequently the time for assessment should, within an experiment (and between experiments), remain invariant. For solid tumours the criterion for an agent to be considered active is a 60% growth inhibition. The method is suitable for detecting activity *per se* but does not allow accurate ranking of efficacy between active agents.

2. *Growth-delay method*

From our hypothetical growth curves (Fig. 1) it is apparent that growth inhibition becomes constant at such time that treated tumours regrow at the rate measured in control tumours of similar volume. The growth pattern of xenografts, particularly more rapidly growing types, follows a Gompertz function (Spang-Thomsen *et al.*, 1980), but there is a considerable period that approximates closely to exponential growth. It is important that chemotherapy evaluation be made during this period before growth approaches the horizontal asymptote. Growth delay is assessed when treated tumours return to the control growth rate. In our studies growth delay is assessed when treated tumours reach four times their volume at treatment. Steel and his colleagues (Shorthouse *et al.*, 1980) assess growth delay at twice the treatment volume, although tumours at this point may not have reached the control rate of growth. Mean growth delay (GD) may be calculated thus:

$$\text{GD} = \frac{\Sigma(T_y - T_0)}{n} - \frac{\Sigma(C_y - C_0)}{n}$$

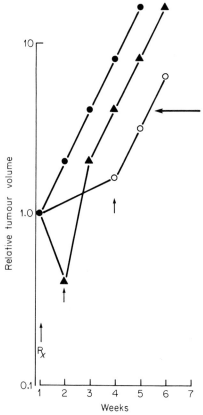

Fig. 1 Hypothetical growth curves for groups of xenografts receiving different therapy. The optimal T/C is shown (↑), and assessment of growth inhibition is made when treated tumours attain 4 times their volume at the time of treatment (↑R_x); ● untreated, ▲ drug A, ○ drug B. Relative tumour volume $= (V_x - V_0)/V_0$ where V_x is the volume at day x and V_0 is the volume on the day of treatment.

where T_y and C_y are the days at which individual tumours reached four times their volume from the day of treatment (T_0, C_0) for treated and control tumours respectively, and n is the number of tumours per group. Growth delay may be normalized for tumour lines with different growth rates by expressing the delay in terms of tumour-volume doublings. Thus the average time taken for untreated tumours to double in volume (T_d) is calculated and the growth delay expressed in terms of doublings saved (GD/T_d). Making certain assumptions (e.g. that the repopulation rate is similar to the growth rate for untreated tumours of equivalent size, and that repopulation is exponential), we may derive an approximate surviving or repopulation fraction (P):

$$P = (0.5)^{t/c}$$

where t is the growth delay (days) and $c = T_d$ (Houghton and Houghton, 1979). Hence, for a growth delay of 100 days and a $T_d = 10$ days, $P = 0.5^{10}$ or about 0.001. This type of quantitation is useful where long-term regressions or "cures" are obtained. From the P values obtained at various subcurative doses, the slope of the dose–response curve can be calculated and some idea of probable cell survival at "curative" dose levels may be determined.

Schabel *et al.* (1980) have suggested that assessment of antitumour activity in the laboratory should utilize some of the criteria used in clinical assessment. Such a system for evaluating single agents is currently in use in our laboratory and is presented in Table 4. This system, although it accounts for only some of the possible tumour responses, incorporates both laboratory and clinical criteria for antitumour activity, and allows for a greater degree of sensitivity in ranking agents.

Table 4   System for the evaluation of antitumour agents

Tumour response	Representation
No growth inhibition	−
Transient response, inhibition $< Td_2$*	±
Growth inhibition $\geqslant Td_2$	+
Growth inhibition $\geqslant 2 \times Td_2$	+ +
Growth inhibition $\geqslant 3 \times Td_2$	+ + +
Growth inhibition $\geqslant 3\ Td_2 +$ volume regression $\geqslant 50\%$	+ + + +
Complete regression with regrowth	+ + + + +
Complete regression with no regrowth	+ + + + + +

* $Td_2 =$ mean time for tumour volume to double.

In our studies an agent is evaluated at the LD_{10} level of dosage in seven mice bearing bilateral tumours. If the drug shows significant activity (+ +), a dose–response relationship is established using 75, 50, and 25% of the LD_{10} dose. Establishing a dose–response relationship is important, and is essential where this agent is subsequently used in combination chemotherapy.

D. Alternative measurement of response

1. *In vitro clonogenic assay*
Steel and his associates have attempted to evaluate tumour response using *in*

vitro clonogenic assays. In these experiments tumour-bearing mice are treated with an agent, and the tumours are subsequently excised and cells disaggregated. The ability to form colonies in semisolid medium *in vitro* or in diffusion chambers implanted in the peritoneum of mice (Smith, 1979) has been compared between treated and untreated tumour xenografts. Varied results have been obtained with these assays, and further work is required to relate adequately clonogenic survival to tumour response *in situ*. Such assays offer the advantage that response may be determined in the absence of host factors although they introduce other potential artifacts. Taetle *et al.* (1981) reported that the cloning efficiency varied between different untreated xenografts of the same tumour line, which suggests that considerable caution should be exercised using this technical approach. Thomas (1979) has adapted a lung colony assay developed using the B16 melanoma of mouse origin to a human melanoma xenograft. Results of this assay are consistent with *in vitro* clonogenic assays, but it is of note that relatively few human tumours form lung colonies subsequent to intravenous inoculation of cell suspensions.

2. *Histological changes*
Several studies have attempted to evaluate tumour response to treatment using histological criteria. While this approach may give interesting data regarding sensitivities of different cell types, Hayashi *et al.* (1978) noted haemorrhage, necrosis, and cystic degeneration in both treated and control tumours.

3. *Short-term assays*
Because growth inhibition studies take a relatively long time to complete, alternative methods have been evaluated. One of these is the short-term growth of human tumours implanted beneath the kidney capsule in athymic or normal mice (Bogden *et al.*, 1978). Animals are treated 1 day after implantation, and growth or regression of the tumour fragment is assessed on day 6. This system may select more "false positives" (Goldin *et al.*, 1981) but may prove to be a practical pre-screen for further evaluation of agents in other xenograft models. We have previously described a method by which growth inhibition could be related to changes in [6-^{3}H]thymidine incorporation into DNA (Houghton *et al.*, 1977) of colorectal adenocarcinoma xenografts. The application of such an assay to other tumour types may be of interest.

VIII. Tumour heterogeneity

A single donor tumour, cut into fragments and transplanted into 10 or 20 mice, will give rise to xenografts with a spectrum of growth rates. This variation is observed not only in immune-deprived mice but also in athymic mice, and in some instances it makes the effect of therapy difficult to evaluate. Using immune-deprived mice Kopper *et al.* (1980) confirmed our initial observation that growth of xenografts was partially host-determined, and extended this observation to responses of tumours subsequent to therapy. In this study within a treatment group complete regressions were achieved in some mice while tumours in other similarly treated hosts progressed. It is thus pertinent to question whether this situation arises in syngeneic tumour models, or is this unique to xenografts? Indeed, such variable regression rates among similarly staged advanced syngeneic or transplantable solid tumours in mice, under identical drug treatment, are observed with representatives of the major clinically useful anticancer agents. Schabel *et al.* (1980) suggested that such variation may indicate variable drug pharmacodynamics and metabolism among presumed identical inbred or syngeneic host mice. Thus, although we must be aware that we are using an allogeneic system, variable responses may be due to factors other than host immunity.

IX. Characterization

It is essential that tumours arising subsequent to transplantation of human neoplastic tissue are characterized in order to establish that the tumour is indeed human. Subsequent to implantation of colorectal adenocarcinomas from different patients, we observed the growth of a mammary carcinoma and a fibrosarcoma, both of mouse origin. Both grew at the site of xenotransplantation, although each may have been radiation-induced during the immune-deprivation procedure. Of greater concern are reports concerning induction of lymphomas in athymic nude mice following chronic stimulation with antigens (pinworms or xenografts; Baird *et al.*, 1982), or the possible transformation of host stroma within human xenografts growing in these mice (Beattie *et al.*, 1982; Goldenburg and Pavia, 1982). Greene and Harvey (1967) also reported induction of lymphomas in hamsters bearing heterografts. It is essential therefore to characterize xenografts routinely after primary transplantation and after serial passage in order to detect potential overgrowth with murine cells. Routine procedures should include histological examination of tissue at the time of transplantation, karyotype analysis and/or lactate dehydrogenase (LDH) isoenzyme analysis. Karyotype analysis is time-consuming and requires considerable expertise. Separation of human and mouse isoenzymes of LDH is readily accomplished by electrophoresis, and where necessary the ratio of mouse to human isoenzymes can be quantitated by scanning densitometry. The overgrowth of human adenocarcinoma T362 by murine sarcoma is detailed in Fig. 2. Kaplan and his group routinely assay LDH isoenzymes and serially transplant only tumours with less than 20% mouse

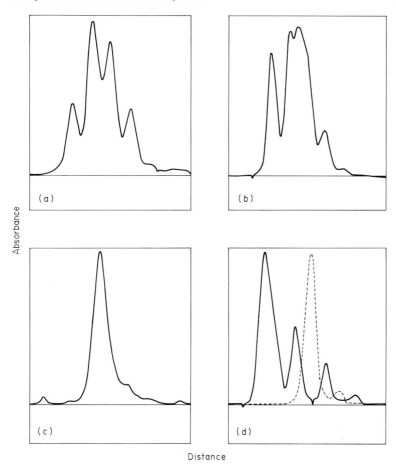

Fig. 2   Changes in lactate dehydrogenase isoenzyme profiles during overgrowth of T362 human adenocarcinoma xenograft by murine sarcoma. (a) Isozyme profile of T362 homogenate from passage 10; 100% human by analysis. (b) Isozyme profile of T362 homogenate from passage 11; 50% mouse isozyme by analysis. (c) Isozyme profile of T362 homogenate from passage 12; 100% mouse isozyme by analysis. (d) Isozyme profile of human liver (solid line) and mouse connective tissue (dotted line) for comparison. (Beattie *et al.*, 1982)

LDH (Giulani *et al.*, 1981a). An alternative may be to examine the ratio of fast (mouse) to slow (human, caucasian) glucose-6-dehydrogenase isoenzymes.

X.   Limitations

It is unlikely that the human tumour xenograft model will be valuable in selecting therapy for individual patients, although xenografts in mice have been shown in some studies to respond similarly to their donor tumours in man (Fujita *et al.*, 1980; Shorthouse *et al.*, 1980). The time necessary to establish xenografts precludes this use. Short-term methods such as the subrenal capsule assay may have value in these situations although convincing data have still to be presented.

The value of the xenograft screen lies in the possible detection of agents that may have application to a particular cancer type. Consequently, in the laboratory one is looking for an agent that is active against a high proportion of xenografts derived from a single cancer type. By definition this demands that each agent be evaluated against five to ten tumour lines representative of a particular disease. The use of such a screen utilizing types of neoplasm most frequently found in man (lung, colon, breast) obviously presents a formidable problem.

In addition to the logistical limitations, xenograft models are expensive in comparison with conventional murine tumour systems. Breeding and maintenance of athymic mice essentially demands aseptic procedures in order to minimize morbidity of experimental animals. The alternative immune-deprived CBA mouse is considerably less expensive, and may be maintained under conventional housing conditions for periods in excess of 18 months.

XI. Conclusions and future directions

Virtually all types of human cancer may be propagated in immune-deficient deprived or suppressed hosts. These include neoplasms such as lymphomas, leukaemias, and adenocarcinomas of the breast, although these types continue to present problems. Contrary to a previous report (Steel, 1978) the transplantability of sarcomata is high both in athymic nude mice (Giovanella *et al.*, 1978) and in immune-deprived mice (Houghton *et al.*, 1982). Xenografts of human tumours retain histological and functional integrity, differing from the original in having a reduced stromal component and generally having localized encapsulated growth. There is increasing evidence that xenografts of many tumour types metastasize, but as yet no reproducible model has been reported that would allow lifespan to be used as an endpoint in chemotherapy studies. Development of such models would be an advantage.

The role of xenografts is not limited to screening. These models offer a unique opportunity to examine activity of agents that selectively perturb biochemical and cell kinetic parameters within tumours and which may be exploited subsequently. The models may be used to examine and optimize kinetic or biochemical scheduling, to examine determinants of drug sensitivity, and to examine the emergence or selection of drug-resistant populations of human tumour cells *in situ* (Houghton *et al.*, 1981). The xenograft model may have specific applications to less frequently diagnosed cancers, which include many paediatric neoplasms, where large-scale randomized clinical evaluation is not possible. The future role of xenografts in developmental therapeutics is a valuable one if they are used to their full potential.

Acknowledgements

Work reported from this laboratory was supported by American Cancer Society grants CH-156A and CH-172, by National Cancer Institute grants CA-23099 and CA-21677, and by the American, Lebanese, Syrian Associated Charities.

References

Bailey, M. J., Ormerod, M. G., Imrie, S. F., Humphreys, J., Roberts, J. D. B., Gazet J.-C. and Neville, A. M. (1981). Comparative functional histopathology of human breast carcinoma xenografts. *Br. J. Cancer* **43**, 125.

Baird, S. M., Beattie, G. M., Lannom, R. A., Lipsick, J. S., Jensen, F. C. and Kaplan, N. O. (1982). Induction of lymphoma in antigenically simulated athymic mice. *Cancer Res.* **42**, 198.

Beattie, G. M., Knowles, A. F., Jensen, F. C., Baird, S. M. and Kaplan, N. O. (1982). Induction of sarcomas in athymic mice. *Proc. Nat. Acad. Sci.* **79**, 3033.

Bogden, A. E., Kelton, D. E., Cobb, W. R., Gulkin, T. A. and Johnson, R. K. (1978). Effect of serial passage in nude athymic mice on the growth characteristics and chemotherapy responsiveness of 13762 and R3230 AC mammary tumor xenografts. *Cancer Res.* **38**, 59.

Catane, R., Von Hoff, D. D., Glaubiger, D. L. and Muggia, F. M. (1979). Azaserine, DON, and azotomycin: three diazo analogs of L-glutamine with clinical antitumor activity. *Cancer Treat. Rep.* **63**, 1033.

Cobb, L. M. and Mitchley, B. C. V. (1974a). Development of a method for assessing the antitumor activity of chemotherapeutic agents using human tumor xenografts. *Cancer Chem. Rep.* (Part 1) **58**, 645.

Cobb, L. M. and Mitchley, B. C. V. (1974b). The growth of human tumours in immune deprived mice. *Eur. J. Cancer* **10**, 473.

Davis, G., Duke, D., Grant, A. G., Kelly, S. A. and Hermon-Taylor, J. (1981). Growth of human digestive tumour xenografts in athymic nude rats. *Br. J. Cancer* **43**, 53.

Epstein, A. L., Herman, M. M., Kim, H., Dorfman, R. F. and Kaplan, H. S. (1976). Biology of the human malignant lymphomas. III. Intracranial heterotransplantation in the nude, athymic mouse. *Cancer* **37**, 2158.

Fodstad, Ø. (1979). Human gastrointestinal cancer grown in nude mice used to test new chemotherapeutic agents. In *Frontiers in Gastrointestinal Research*, Vol. 5, p. 71. Karger, Basel.

Fujita, M., Hayata, S. and Taguchi, T. (1980). Relationship of chemotherapy on human cancer xenografts in nude mice to clinical response in donor patient. *J. Surg. Oncol.* **15**, 211.

Gallie, B. L., Albert, D. M., Wang, J. J. Y., Buyukmihci, N. and Puliafito, C. A. (1977). Heterotransplantation of retinoblastoma into the athymic "nude" mouse. *Invest. Ophthalmol. Visual Sci.* **16**, 256.

Giovanella, B. C. and Stehlin, J. S. (1973). Heterotransplantation of human malignant tumors in "nude" thymusless mice. I. Breeding and maintenance of "nude" mice. *J. Nat. Cancer Inst.* **51**, 615.

Giovanella, B. C. and Fogh, J. (1978). Present and future trends in investigations with the nude mouse as a recipient of human tumor transplants. In *The Nude Mouse in Experimental and Clinical Research* (ed. J. Fogh and B. C. Giovanella), p. 281. Academic Press, New York.

Giovanella, B. C., Stehlin, J. S., Williams, L. J., Lee, S. S. and Shepard, R. C. (1978). Heterotransplantation of human cancers into nude mice. *Cancer* **42**, 2269.

Giulani, F. C. and Kaplan, N. O. (1980). New doxorubicin analogs active against doxorubicin-resistant colon tumor xenografts in the nude mouse. *Cancer Res.* **40**, 4682.

Giulani, F. C., Zirvi, K. A., Kaplan, N. O. and Goldin, A. (1981a). Chemotherapy of human colorectal tumor xenografts in athymic mice with clinically active drugs: 5-fluorouracil and 1,3-bis-(2-chloroethyl)-1-nitrosourea (BCNU): comparison with doxorubicin derivatives, 4'-deoxydoxorubicin and 4'-O-methyldoxorubicin. *Int. J. Cancer* **27**, 5.

Giulani, F. C., Zirvi, K. A. and Kaplan, N. O. (1981b). Therapeutic response of human tumor xenografts in athymic mice to doxorubicin. *Cancer Res.* **41**, 325.

Goldenberg, D. M. and Pavia, R. A. (1982). In vivo horizontal oncogenesis by a human tumor in nude mice. *Proc. Nat. Acad. Sci.* **79**, 2389.

Goldin, A., Venditti, J. M., MacDonald, J. S., Muggia, F. M., Henney, J. E. and DeVita, V. (1981). Current results of the screening program at the Division of Cancer Treatment, National Cancer Institute. *Eur. J. Cancer* **17**, 129.

Greene, H. S. N. and Harvey, E. K. (1967). The induction of lymphomas in hamsters by heterologous tumor transplants. *Am. J. Pathol.* **51**, 447.

Greene, H. S. N. and Harvey, E. K. (1968). Metaplasia and progressive growth of heterologous tumor transplants in the subcutaneous space of mice. *Am. J. Pathol.* **53**, 293.

Hansen, C. T. (1978). The nude gene in animal models for oncologic research. In *Proceedings of the Symposium on the Use of Athymic (Nude) Mice in Cancer Research* (ed. D. P. Houchens and A. A. Ovejera), p. 11. Gustav Fischer, New York.

Hayashi, H., Kameya, T., Shimosato, Y. and Mukojima, T. (1978). Chemotherapy of human choriocarcinoma transplanted to nude mice. *Am. J. Obstet. Gynecol.* **131**, 548.

Houghton, P. J. and Houghton, J. A. (1978). Evaluation of single-agent therapy in human colorectal tumor xenografts. *Br. J. Cancer* **37**, 833.

Houghton, J. A. and Houghton, P. J. (1979). Evaluation of cytotoxic agents in human colonic tumor xenografts and mouse gastrointestinal tissues using a ^{3}H-thymidine incorporation assay. *Eur. J. Cancer* **15**, 763–769.

Houghton, J. A. and Taylor, D. M. (1978a). Maintenance of biological and biochemical characteristics of human colorectal tumours during serial passage in immune-deprived mice. *Br. J. Cancer* **37**, 199.

Houghton, J. A. and Taylor, D. M. (1978b). Growth characteristics of human colorectal tumours during serial passage in immune-deprived mice. *Br. J. Cancer* **37**, 213.

Houghton, P. J., Houghton, J. A. and Taylor, D. M. (1977). Effects of cytotoxic agents on TdR incorporation and growth delay in human colonic tumour xenografts. *Br. J. Cancer* **36**, 206.

Houghton, J. A., Houghton, P. J., Brodeur, G. M. and Green, A. A. (1981). Development of resistance to vincristine in a childhood rhabdomyosarcoma growing in immune-deprived mice. *Int. J. Cancer* **28**, 409.

Houghton, J. A., Houghton, P. J. and Green, A. A. (1982). Chemotherapy of childhood rhabdomyosarcomas growing as xenografts in immune-deprived mice. *Cancer Res.* **42**, 535.

Kim, D. K., Kakita, A., Cubilla, A., Fleisher, M. and Fortner, J. G. (1976). Unique features of serially transplanted human pancreatic cancer in nude mice. *Surg. Forum* **27**, 142.

Kopper, L. and Steel, G. G. (1975). The therapeutic response of three human tumor lines maintained in immune-suppressed mice. *Cancer Res.* **35**, 2704.

Kopper, L., Lapis, K. and Hegedus, C. S. (1980). Chemotherapeutic sensitivity of human colorectal tumor xenografts. *Oncology* **37**, 42.

Kubota, T., Shimosato, Y., and Nagai, K. (1978). Experimental chemotherapy of carcinoma of the human stomach and colon serially transplanted in nude mice. *Gann* **69**, 299.

Levey, R. H. and Medawar, P. B. (1966). Some experiments on the action of antilymphoid antisera. *Ann. New York Acad. Sci.* **129**, 164.

Millar, J. L. (1976). Protective effect of cyclophosphamide or cytosine arabinoside pretreatment on animals given a lethal dose of gamma irradiation. *Exp. Haematol.* **4**, Suppl. 68.

Mitchley, B. C. V., Clarke, S. A., Connors, T. A., Carter, S. M. and Neville, A. M. (1977). Chemotherapy of human tumors in T-lymphocyte-deficient mice. *Cancer Treat. Rep.* **61**, 451.

Nowak, K., Peckham, M. J. and Steel, G. G. (1978). Variation in response of xenografts of colorectal carcinoma to chemotherapy. *Br. J. Cancer* **37**, 576.

Ohsugi, Y., Gershwin, M. E., Owens, R. B. and Nelson-Rees, W. A. (1980). Tumorigenicity of human malignant lymphoblasts: comparative study with unmanipulated nude mice, antilymphocyte serum-treated nude mice and X-irradiated nude mice. *J. Nat. Cancer Inst.* **65**, 715.

Osieka, R., Houchens, D. P., Goldin, A. and Johnson, R. K. (1977). Chemotherapy of human colon cancer xenografts in athymic nude mice. *Cancer* **40**, 2640.

Ovejera, A. A., Houchens, D. P. and Barker, A. D. (1978). Chemotherapy of human tumor xenografts in genetically athymic mice. *Ann. Clin. Lab. Sci.* **8**, 50.

Pickard, R. G., Cobb, L. M. and Steel, G. G. (1975). The growth kinetics of xenografts of human colorectal tumours in immune-deprived mice. *Br. J. Cancer* **31**, 36.

Povlsen, C. O. (1976). Heterotransplantation of human malignant melanomas to the mouse mutant nude. *Acta Path. Microbiol. Scand.* **84**, 9.

Ramseier, H. (1975). Specific activation of T-lymphocytes from nude mice. *Immunogenetics* **1**, 507.

Reeves, B. R. and Houghton, J. A. (1978). Serial cytogenetic studies of human colonic tumour xenografts. *Br. J. Cancer* **37**, 612.

Rygaard, J. and Povlsen, C. O. (1969). Heterotransplantation of a human malignant tumour to "nude" mice. *Acta Path. Microbiol. Scand.* **77**, 758.

Schabel, F. M., Skipper, H. E., Trader, M. W., Laster, W. R., Corbett, T. H. and Griswold, D. P. (1980). Concepts for controlling drug-resistant tumor cells. In

Breast Cancer: Experimental and Clinical Aspects (ed. H. T. Mouridsen and T. Palshoff), *Eur. J. Cancer* Suppl. 1, 199.

Sharkey, F. E., Bains-Grebner, M. and Kimak, M. (1980). Increased mitotic activity in human tumors transplanted to nude mice. *Proc. Am. Assoc. Cancer Res.* **21,** 272.

Shimosato, Y., Kameya, T., Nagai, K., Hirohashi, S., Koide, T., Hayashi, H. and Nomura, T. (1976). Transplantation of human tumors in nude mice. *J. Nat. Cancer Inst.* **56,** 1251.

Shimosato, Y., Kameya, T. and Hirohashi, S. (1979). Growth, morphology, and function of xenotransplanted human tumors. In *Pathology Annual 14* (ed. S. C. Sommers and P. P. Rosen), p. 215. Appleton-Century-Crofts, New York.

Shorthouse, A. J., Peckham, M. J., Smyth, J. F. and Steel, G. G. (1980). The therapeutic response of bronchial carcinoma xenografts: a direct patient-xenograft comparison. *Br. J. Cancer* **41** (Suppl IV), 142.

Smith, I. E. (1979). Chemosensitivity studies on human tumour cells from a pancreatic carcinoma xenograft. *J. Roy. Soc. Med.* **72,** 260.

Spang-Thomsen, M., Nielsen, A. and Visfeldt, J. (1980). Growth curves of three human malignant tumors transplanted to nude mice. *Exp. Cell Biol.* **48,** 138–154.

Steel, G. G. (1978). The growth and therapeutic response of human tumours in immune deficient mice. *Bull. Cancer* (Paris) **65,** 465.

Steel, G. G., Courtenay, V. D. and Rostom, A. Y. (1978). Improved immune-suppression techniques for the xenografting of human tumours. *Br. J. Cancer* **37,** 224.

Taetle, R., Koessler, A. K. and Howell, S. B. (1981). In vitro growth and drug sensitivity of tumor colony-forming units from human tumor xenografts. *Cancer Res.* **41,** 1856.

Thomas, J. M. (1979). A lung colony clonogenic cell assay for human malignant melanoma in immune-suppressed mice and its use to determine chemosensitivity, radiosensitivity, and the relationship between tumor size and response to therapy. *Br. J. Surg.* **66,** 696.

Tibbetts, L. M., Chu, M. Y., Hager, J. C., Dexter, D. L. and Calabresi, P. (1977). Chemotherapy of cell-line-derived human colon carcinomas in mice immunosuppressed with antithymocyte serum. *Cancer* **40,** 2651.

Tokita, H., Tanaka, N., Sekimoto, K., Veno, T., Okamoto, K. and Fujimura, S. (1980). Experimental model for combination chemotherapy with metronidazole using human uterine cervical carcinomas transplanted into nude mice. *Cancer Res.* **40,** 4287.

Warenius, H. M., Freedman, L. A. and Bleehen, N. M. (1980). The response of a human tumour xenograft to chemotherapy: intrinsic variation between tumours and its significance in planning experiments. *Br. J. Cancer* **41** (Suppl. IV), 128.

Ziegler, H. W., Frizzera, G. and Bach, F. H. (1982). Successful transplantation of a human leukemia cell line into nude mice: conditions optimizing graft acceptance. *J. Nat. Cancer Inst.* **68,** 15.

16. Use of Xenografts for Drug Sensitivity Testing *in vitro*

K. M. TVEIT

I. Introduction

Human tumour xenografts transplanted into immunodeficient animals or to certain organs of immunocompetent animals have been increasingly used for *in vivo* studies of tumour biology and various aspects of cancer treatment. The usefulness of the xenograft model to investigate effects of established antitumour agents and of new drugs and analogues on human cancer has been discussed in Chapter 15.

Different endpoints for assaying effects of chemotherapy have been employed after treatment *in vivo*. The two most commonly used are (i) tumour volume measurements and calculation of the number of doubling times saved by the treatment, the growth delay (Nowak *et al.*, 1978), and (ii) *in vitro* assay of the number of residual clonogenic cells (Courtenay and Mills, 1978).

Human tumour xenografts can also be used for *in vitro* studies of drug sensitivities of tumour cells. By using xenografts serially heterotransplanted into immune-deprived animals as a bank of easily available tumour tissue, repeated studies of tumour cells from the same patient can be performed, and thus the reproducibility of an *in vitro* assay can be examined. Moreover, the relationship between *in vitro* sensitivity and *in vivo* response can be established in detail. In Fig. 1 survival curves for five different xenografted melanomas treated *in vitro* with CCNU and vinblastine are shown. Clearly, different tumours of the same histological type show different sensitivities *in vitro*. In this chapter, *in vitro* data obtained using human tumour xenografts will be discussed.

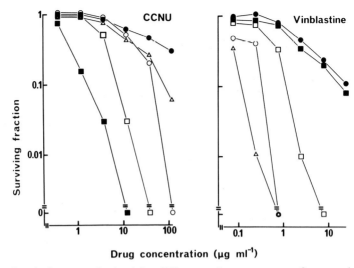

Fig. 1 Survival curves obtained for different melanoma xenografts treated *in vitro* with CCNU and vinblastine. The residual ability to form colonies in soft agar was assayed according to the method of Courtenay and Mills (1978).

II. Comparisons of the sensitivity of human tumour xenografts and the parent tumours to antitumour agents

A. Response to xenografts *in vivo*

It is generally considered that human tumour xenografts retain the chemosensitivity of the parent tumour. Evidence for this is largely indirect: tumours of a certain histological type show approximately the same pattern of response to different agents as experienced in the clinic (reviewed by Steel and Peckham, 1980). However, only a few reports of direct individual comparisons of the response of patients' tumours and of the corresponding xenografts have appeared. Thus, Giovanella *et al.* (1977) found good correlations in four cases of breast carcinoma. Similar findings were made by Nowak *et al.* (1978) in colonic carcinoma. Shorthouse *et al.* (1980) have presented convincing evidence for the chemotherapeutic validity of response data obtained on xenografts. In 14 patients with bronchial carcinomas of different histological types, 16 direct patient/xenograft comparisons were made and positive correlations were observed in all cases. A positive correlation was also found by Fodstad *et al.* (1980) with malignant melanomas.

B. *In vitro* assay of xenografts and parent tumours

Human melanomas were established as serially heterotransplanted xenografts in athymic nude mice (Fodstad *et al.*, 1980). *In vitro* sensitivity to DTIC, CCNU, vinblastine, procarbazine, abrin, and ricin was assessed on cell suspensions prepared directly from the patients' tumours and from established xenografts at different passages. In all cases the colony-forming assay, described by Courtenay and Mills (1978), was used after incubation with drugs at various concentrations for 1 hour. The residual number of colony-forming cells was determined after 2 weeks' incubation, and dose–response curves were established. Representative curves obtained in two cases after treatment with CCNU and abrin are shown in Fig. 2. In the case of K.A. the sensitivity of the different xenografts was about the same as that of the patient's tumour. However, with K.F. the xenografts were more sensitive to the drugs than the patient's original tumour.

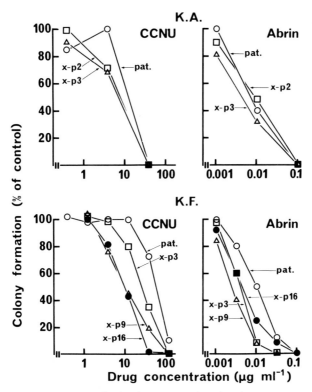

Fig. 2 Dose–response curves obtained on two patients' melanoma metastases (K.A. and K.F.) treated *in vitro* with CCNU and abrin, and of the established xenografts, at different passages.

In order to compare data obtained for different tumours and drugs, *in vitro* sensitivity was quantitated in terms of "expected growth delay" (EGD) by means of the calibration curves obtained on melanoma xenografts (Tveit *et al.*, 1980; explained in more detail below). Direct xenograft/patient comparisons were performed for 8 different melanomas; sensitivities found are shown in Table 1. In most cases changes in sensitivity were small and insignificant. However, in some cases changes were more pronounced in the direction of either increased or decreased sensitivity. A change in expected growth delay greater than or equal to 1.0 was observed in 4 out of the 41 patient/xenograft

Table 1 Plating efficiency and drug sensitivity *in vitro* of patients' melanomas (pat.) and the established xenografts (x) in athymic mice

Tumour sample		Plating efficiency (%)	Sensitivity (expected growth delay) to					
			DTIC	CCNU	vinblas- tine	procarb- azine	abrin	ricin
R.V.	pat.	0.1	1.9	2.2	1.3	2.0	2.0	1.0
	x-P5	0.2	2.0	2.2	1.5	2.0	1.6	1.2
	x-P9	0.8	1.9	2.4	1.4	2.0	1.6	1.4
K.F.	pat.	2.0	0.5	0	0	0	1.6	0.6
	x-P3	1.0	0.5	0.5	0	0.5	1.9	1.1
	x-P9	1.6	0.8	1.0	0.1	NT	2.1	1.1
	x-P15	3.5	1.0	1.0*	0.1	0.5	1.9	0.8
K.A.	pat.	0.1	0.3	0.3	0.3	0	2.0	0.6
	x-P2	1.6	0.8	0.8	1.2	0	1.6	0.4
	x-P3	2.1	0.8	0.8	1.3*	0	2.2	0.7
N.R.	pat.	0.2	1.8	0.6	1.1	NT	3.0	NT
	x-P7	0.6	2.6	1.1	1.2	NT	3.5	NT
G.N.	pat.	0.9	2.0	0.4	1.4	0	3.0	1.6
	x-P12	1.1	1.6	0.4	1.2	0	1.2*	0.5*
G.E.2	pat.	0.2	0.5	0	1.2	2.0	2.0	1.5
	x-P8	0.2	0.7	0.3	1.0	2.0	1.5	1.5
	x-P12	0.4	NT	0	1.0	NT	1.5	NT
	x-P15	0.4	1.0	0.4	1.5	NT	NT	1.5
L.Ø.	pat.	1.0	1.1	2.1	1.4	NT	NT	NT
	x-P2	6.1	1.4	2.2	1.3	0	3.0	2.0
S.L.	pat.	2.2	1.5	0.8	1.7	NT	1.5	0.5
	x-P2†	2.9	0.8	0.7	1.5	NT	1.8	0.9
	x-P6†	1.5	1.2	0.8	1.6	NT	2.0	1.0

NT = not tested.
* Change in expected growth delay ⩾ 1.0.
† Passaged *in vitro* before implantation in mice.

comparisons. When xenografts at different passages were examined, only insignificant differences were observed.

Altogether, both *in vivo* data and *in vitro* data show that human tumour xenografts, with a few exceptions, retain the chemosensitivity of the original patients' tumours. Also, sensitivity of xenografted tumours seems in general to be retained upon serial transplantation.

III. The value of tumour xenografts in *in vitro* chemosensitivity assays

A. Establishment of optimal conditions for *in vitro* testing

Important information regarding conditions used in the *in vitro* assay can be obtained using tumour xenografts. Thus, the effect of different disaggregation methods on cell yield, viability, ability to grow, and chemosensitivity can be studied in detail. In such experiments we found that different enzymatic procedures gave the same sensitivity as a mechanical procedure, indicating that chemosensitivity data obtained after use of different disaggregation methods can be compared (Tveit *et al.*, 1981b).

The influence of tumour size on *in vitro* growth and sensitivity to antitumour agents also can easily be studied using xenografts of different sizes (Tveit *et al.*, 1981b). In Fig. 3 the relation between plating efficiency (PE; number of colonies formed as a percentage of the number of viable cells plated) and tumour size is shown for two cases of melanoma xenografts. The fraction of clonogenic cells was apparently higher in small tumours than in

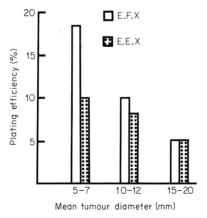

Fig. 3 Plating efficiency of two xenografted melanomas at different tumour sizes.

large tumours. However, chemosensitivity of the clonogenic cells was similar even in these xenografts of different sizes.

One of the major problems associated with colony-forming assays is that many tumours give insufficient colony growth. An important task is therefore to improve culture conditions so that more tumours grow with higher plating efficiencies. Effects of different culture conditions including various stimulating factors can easily be examined using human tumour cells derived from xenografts. Courtenay and Mills (1978) showed in a pancreatic carcinoma xenograft that red blood cells and a low oxygen concentration stimulate colony formation. In melanoma xenografts we found that the same two factors considerably improved colony growth (Tveit *et al.*, 1981b), a finding confirmed when the investigations were extended to biopsy material from patients (Tveit *et al.*, 1981a,b, 1982). The influence of different culture conditions on colony formation using a melanoma xenograft is shown in Fig. 4.

Different culture conditions may also influence the sensitivity of tumour cells to antitumour agents, as was shown in xenografted melanomas when the chemosensitivities obtained using two different colony-forming assays were compared (Tveit *et al.*, 1981a). Recently Gupta and Krishan (1982) found that drug sensitivity of tumour cells from a human melanoma xenograft was dependent on the oxygen concentration in the atmosphere during the incubation.

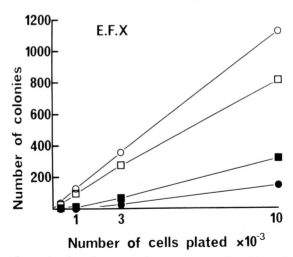

Fig. 4 Colony formation from human melanoma xenografts cultivated under various conditions employing rat red blood cells (RBC) and oxygen concentration. ○ RBC added, 5% O_2; □ RBC added, 20% O_2; ■ RBC omitted, 5% O_2; ● RBC omitted, 20% O_2.

B. *In vitro/in vivo* correlation using tumour xenografts

Human tumour xenografts are extremely useful in establishing the overall validity of an *in vitro* chemosensitivity assay. Data obtained with such tumours are probably more relevant to the clinic than those obtained with murine tumours. Using these xenografts, relationships can be established between the chemosensitivity of the cells responsible for tumour growth *in situ* and the sensitivity of the cells assayed *in vitro* (either the total cells disaggregated or only the clonogenic cells). More important, *in vitro/in vivo* correlations can be established in a quantitative way, since *in vivo* sensitivity can be evaluated in terms of growth delay or by assessing the number of residual clonogenic cells *in vitro*.

In a study of human pancreatic carcinoma xenografted into immune-suppressed mice, Bateman *et al.* (1979) found good correlations between the ranking order of different drugs *in vivo* and *in vitro*. In xenografted human melanomas Bateman *et al.* (1980) observed different sensitivities to different drugs *in vitro* in accordance with clinical experience. They also found a positive correlation between the *in vitro* and *in vivo* sensitivities to melphalan, methyl-CCNU, and adriamycin. In three human tumour xenografts (colon, breast, and lung carcinomas) Rice *et al.* (1980) also obtained a positive correlation between *in vitro* and *in vivo* sensitivities.

In an investigation of xenografted melanomas with different growth rates and chemosensitivities *in vivo* we found positive correlations between *in vitro* sensitivity (defined by $1/ID_{50}$ values) and the *in vivo* response (judged by growth delay) to DTIC, CCNU, vinblastine, procarbazine, abrin, and ricin (Tveit *et al.*, 1980). The correlation coefficients ranged from 0.866 up to 0.985. In Fig. 5 dose–response curves obtained *in vitro* for five different melanoma xenografts exposed to ricin, abrin, and DTIC are shown. Also, the correlations with the *in vivo* responses to the same drugs are included. The correlation curves serve as a calibration of the *in vitro* assay, and can be used to convert the *in vitro* sensitivity of other melanomas into the same *in vivo* unit, viz. the expected growth delay.

So far *in vitro* sensitivity data obtained using xenografts are limited. However, for the drugs and tumours studied, a close relationship has been found between *in vitro* sensitivity of the cells assayed and *in vivo* response in xenografts. Probably similar relationships exist for other tumour types and drugs, but this has to be examined further. Positive correlations established for xenografts can be used as a calibration of *in vitro* tests of patients' tumour specimens, as discussed later in Chapter 25.

C. *In vitro* screening of new drugs

The currently employed procedures for evaluation of the effectiveness of new

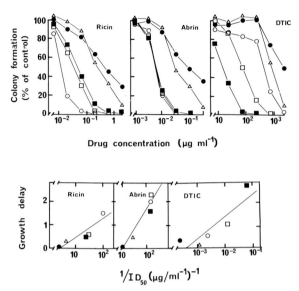

Fig. 5 Dose–response curves obtained on five xenografted melanomas treated *in vitro* with ricin, abrin, or DTIC. In the same melanomas correlations are shown between *in vitro* sensitivity ($1/ID_{50}$) and *in vivo* response (growth delay) of the melanomas after treatment with the same agents. (Data from Tveit *et al.*, 1980)

agents in the treatment of human cancer have substantial shortcomings. *In vivo* tests of potential anticancer drugs on human tumour xenografts have obvious advantages over previous methods. It has become clear that a panel of tumours of the same histological type has to be tested (Fodstad *et al.*, 1980), and such investigations are necessarily expensive and time-consuming. However, important information can also be obtained *in vitro* by testing the sensitivity of fresh tumour samples from patients or tumour xenografts. Tumour lines of different histological types that give sufficient colony growth *in vitro* can be kept as xenografts *in vivo* and used for *in vitro* screening at moderate cost (Tveit *et al.*, 1980; Taetle *et al.*, 1981). Different drugs or analogues can be tested reproducibly on previously untreated tumour tissue. Moreover, human tumour xenografts can be used to calibrate an *in vitro* sensitivity assay of the effectiveness of a new drug. Thus the antitumour activity of the toxic plant proteins abrin and ricin was examined against human melanoma cells. Five melanoma xenografts with known *in vivo* sensitivity (Fodstad *et al.*, 1980) were tested *in vitro* and positive correlations with *in vivo* growth delay were obtained (Fig. 5; Tveit *et al.*, 1980). The correlation curves established were then used to quantitate the effectiveness of abrin and ricin and also of other drugs on a large number of previously untreated patients' melanomas *in vitro* (Tveit *et al.*, 1982). The proportion of tumours with expected growth delay $\geqslant 2.0$ to different agents is given in Table 2. Using this approach, human melanomas were found to be more sensitive to abrin than to the conventional drugs used in the treatment of this tumour type.

Table 2 Sensitivity of untreated melanomas to two experimental drugs and to currently used cancerostatic agents

Cytotoxic agent	Proportion of patients in which expected growth delay $\geqslant 2.0$	
Abrin	29/50	58.0%
Ricin	6/50	12.0%
DTIC	19/72	26.4%
Vinblastine	9/66	13.6%
CCNU	9/67	13.4%
Procarbazine	3/33	9.1%

IV. Conclusions

Human tumour xenografts are useful not only for *in vivo* chemosensitivity experiments but also for *in vitro* studies. Conditions used in sensitivity assays *in vitro* of patients' tumours can certainly be improved, and such work is greatly facilitated by the use of tumour xenografts. It would be a great advantage for the future use of *in vitro* chemosensitivity tests if the usefulness of all available methods were validated using tumour xenografts, to establish whether a close relationship exists between a quantitatively measured *in vivo* response and *in vitro* sensitivity for all drugs and tumour types. *In vitro* studies of the chemosensitivity of patients' tumours would be more reliable if such correlations were established.

Acknowledgement

This work was supported by The Norwegian Cancer Society.

References

Bateman, A. E., Peckham, M. J. and Steel, G. G. (1979). Assays of drug sensitivity for cells from human tumours: *in vitro* and *in vivo* tests on a xenografted tumour. *Br. J. Cancer* **40,** 81–88.

Bateman, A. E., Selby, P. J., Steel, G. G. and Towse, G. D. W. (1980). *In vitro* chemosensitivity tests on xenografted human melanomas. *Br. J. Cancer* **41,** 189–198.

Courtenay, V. D. and Mills, J. (1978). An *in vitro* colony assay for human tumours grown in immune-suppressed mice and treated *in vivo* with cytotoxic agents. *Br. J. Cancer* **37,** 261–268.

Fodstad, Ø., Aass, N. and Pihl, A. (1980). Response to chemotherapy of human, malignant melanoma xenografts in athymic, nude mice. *Int. J. Cancer* **25,** 453–458.

Giovanella, B. C., Stehlin, J. S. and Shepard, R. C. (1977). Experimental chemotherapy of human breast carcinomas heterotransplanted in nude mice. Proc. 2nd Int. Workshop on Nude Mice, pp. 475–481. University of Tokyo Press.

Gupta, V. and Krishan, A. (1982). Effect of oxygen concentration of the growth and drug sensitivity of human melanoma cells in soft-agar clonogenic assay. *Cancer Res.* **42,** 1005–1007.

Nowak, K., Peckham, M. J. and Steel, G. G. (1978). Variation in response of xenografts of colorectal carcinoma to chemotherapy. *Br. J. Cancer* **37,** 576–584.

Rice, J. M., Houchens, D. P., Sanchez, M. S. and Ovejera, A. A. (1980). Correlation of drug sensitivity on human tumor cells grown in soft agar and in nude mice. *Proc. Am. Assoc. Cancer Res.* **21,** 274.

Shorthouse, A. J., Peckham, M. J., Smyth, J. F. and Steel, G. G. (1980). The therapeutic response of bronchial carcinoma xenografts: a direct patient–xenograft comparison. *Br. J. Cancer* **41** (Suppl. IV), 142–145.

Steel, G. G. and Peckham, M. J. (1980). Human tumour xenografts: a critical appraisal. *Br. J. Cancer* **41** (Suppl. IV), 133–141.

Taetle, R., Koessler, A. K. and Howel, S. B. (1981). *In vitro* growth and drug sensitivity of tumor colony-forming units from human tumor xenografts. *Cancer Res.* **41,** 1856–1860.

Tveit, K. M., Fodstad, Ø., Olsnes, S. and Pihl, A. (1980). *In vitro* sensitivity of human melanoma xenografts to cytotoxic drugs: correlation to *in vivo* chemosensitivity. *Int. J. Cancer* **26,** 717–722.

Tveit, K. M., Endresen, L., Rugstad, H. E., Fodstad, Ø. and Pihl, A. (1981a). Comparison of two soft agar methods for assaying chemosensitivity of human tumours *in vitro*: malignant melanomas. *Br. J. Cancer* **44,** 539–544.

Tveit, K. M., Fodstad, Ø. and Pihl, A. (1981b). Cultivation of human melanomas in soft agar: factors influencing plating efficiency and chemosensitivity. *Int. J. Cancer* **28,** 329–334.

Tveit, K. M., Fodstad, Ø., Lotsberg, J., Vaage, S. and Pihl, A. (1982). Colony growth and chemosensitivity *in vitro* of human melanoma biopsies: relationship to clinical parameters. *Int. J. Cancer* **29,** 533–538.

**Part III
Laboratory Predictions and
Clinical Correlations**

17. A Review of Methods for Estimating Clinically Achievable Antitumour Drug Levels and Their Association with Studies *in vitro*

S. A. METCALFE

I. Introduction

When designing assays to measure antitumour drug sensitivities *in vitro* so as to obtain clinical correlations, it is important to understand the pharmacokinetic behaviour of the drugs and especially to have information about therapeutically relevant drug concentrations. To estimate clinically achievable drug levels the relationship between pharmacological parameters and physiological variables must be considered. Pharmacokinetic factors influencing clinically achieved drug levels are outlined in Table 1. Furthermore, the apparent activity of the drug may be altered radically by the disease state; for example, drug binding to plasma proteins may be affected by changes in hepatic function, and renal excretion of drug may be reduced when renal function is impaired owing to either the clinical disease state or side-effects of other drug treatment.

II. Pharmacokinetic principles

A. Definitions of pharmacokinetic terms

Pharmacokinetics is the mathematical analysis of the time courses of absorption, distribution, and elimination of drugs. Application of this principle is essential when attempting to develop dosage schedules that provide optimal therapeutic action and reduce toxic side-effects to a minimum. Pharmacokinetics often includes various assumptions, such as applying first-order kinetics to drug absorption and elimination rates, which

Table 1 Pharmacokinetic factors that influence clinically
achieved drug levels

Absorption
  Route of administration
  Extent of bioavailability of drug (expressed as percentage
    of dose administered orally that is available to
    produce pharmacologic action)

Transfer of drugs across membranes
  Receptors
  Physicochemical factors: e.g. passive, pH, etc.

Distribution
  Plasma; cerebrospinal fluid
  Drug reservoirs: binding to plasma proteins;
    cellular reservoirs; fat
  Redistribution

Biotransformation
  Primarily liver, but also other organs
    (microsomal, non-microsomal)

Excretion
  Renal, biliary, faecal, others

---

are described in further detail. The simplest model of the process of absorption
and elimination of drugs is represented in Fig. 1. In this elementary kinetic
model, where the body is considered a single compartment, the rate of drug
absorption is deemed to follow first-order kinetics (i.e. a constant fraction of
drug is absorbed per unit of time); this can be written as a differential
equation:

$$dD/dt = -K_{abs}D$$

which when integrated becomes

$$D_t = De^{-K_{abs}t}$$

where D = amount of drug administered,
       D_t = amount of drug remaining at time t after start of absorption at
             site of administration,
       e = base of natural logarithms, and
    K_{abs} = absorption rate constant. Since

$$D = Q_t + D_t$$

where Q_t = amount of drug already absorbed at time t after start of
absorption,

$$Q_t = D(1 - e^{-K_{abs}t})$$

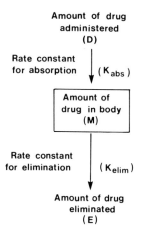

Fig. 1 Simple one-compartment pharmacokinetic model of body.

If only a fraction f of the drug is bioavailable,

$$Q_t = fD(1 - e^{-K_{abs}t})$$

Most drugs are eliminated from the body at a rate that depends on the amount of drug present in the body. In other words, elimination usually follows first-order kinetics, and the rate can be expressed as

$$dM/dt = -K_{elim}M$$

or

$$M_t = M_0 e^{-K_{elim}t}$$

where M_0 = initial amount of drug in body when no more drug is administered or remains to be absorbed, and

M_t = amount of drug remaining in body at time t.

The value of M_t falls exponentially towards zero, and the time for the amount to fall to half of that initially present is termed the half-life ($t_{\frac{1}{2}}$). Thus, by calculation,

$$t_{\frac{1}{2}} = (\ln 2)/K_{elim}$$

and

$$M_t = M_0 2^{-t/t_{\frac{1}{2}}}$$

It is not usually possible to measure the total amount of drug in the body, but the concentration in plasma, C, can be measured for many drugs, and this is related to the total amount of drug in the body, M, by

$$M = CV_d$$

where V_d = apparent volume of distribution of drug.

Thus, by substitution, an equation can be derived that would produce a graph similar to Fig. 2a, expressed in terms of concentration of drug in plasma:

$$C_t = C_0 e^{-(\ln 2)t/t_{\frac{1}{2}}}$$

where C_0 is the initial drug concentration in plasma.

When the logarithmic (to the base 10) concentration of drug is plotted against this, from

$$\log C_t = \log C_0 - 0.301t/t_{\frac{1}{2}}$$

a straight-line graph is produced, the gradient being a function of the half-life (gradient $= -0.301/t_{\frac{1}{2}}$), as shown in Fig. 2b.

In the simple one-compartment model, where it is assumed that absorption and equilibrium distribution are instantaneous,

$$C_0 = fD/V_d$$

where f is now the fraction of administered dose (D) that is absorbed and enters the plasma.

It is assumed that intravenous administration of the drug results in $f = 1$,

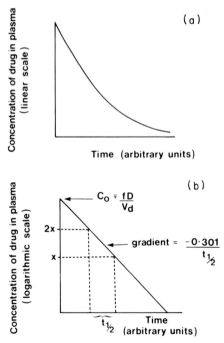

Fig. 2   Time course of drug disappearance from plasma.

and therefore the volume of distribution can be determined from an analysis of elimination kinetics. However, when the rate of reaching equilibrium distribution is slow (as may be the case with oral administration) this model could be grossly inaccurate. In these circumstances, analysis is performed using a two-compartment model, although more complex models have been used. A plot of logarithmic plasma concentration against time no longer gives a straight line but a curve.

Derivation of the equations containing the factors for the amounts of drug in each compartment is complex, the final form for the equation being

$$C_t = A\mathrm{e}^{-\alpha t} + B\mathrm{e}^{-\beta t}$$

where A and B are the intercepts of the two linear components of the curve on the logarithm of concentration axis at $t = 0$, and α and β are the rate constants of these two components. Further details of this derivation are described by Bowman and Rand (1980).

The amount of drug lost from the body during any given period is determined by integrating the plasma concentration with respect to time over that interval. This is equivalent to measuring the area under the curve (AUC) from the graph of plasma concentration against time as in Fig. 2a, i.e. on a linear not a semi-logarithmic plot. The final equation representing this is

$$\mathrm{AUC} = fD/V_\mathrm{d}K_\mathrm{elim}$$

The clearance of a drug is the volume of plasma from which the drug is completely removed per unit time:

$$\mathrm{clearance} = V_\mathrm{d}K_\mathrm{elim}$$

therefore

$$\mathrm{AUC} = fD/\mathrm{clearance}$$

Clearance can be determined only when the fractional availability of the drug, f, is known; thus, to be accurate, clearance must be determined following intravenous administration.

B. Principal pharmacokinetic parameters

There are several pharmacokinetic parameters which are relevant to *in vitro* drug sensitivity studies.

1. *Plasma drug concentration–time product*

This parameter ($C \times T$) is the same as AUC, described previously, and is generally considered to be the most useful pharmacokinetic parameter relating to drug therapeutic action and toxicity (Alberts *et al.*, 1980). In addition to the method of calculation described for AUC (and therefore $C \times T$) another method of measurement is to apply the "trapezoidal rule", i.e. calculate the areas of triangles and rectangles that fit under the drugs' plasma disappearance curves (see Moon, 1980).

2. *Peak plasma drug concentration*
This parameter also is directly related to drug dosage. However, some compounds are metabolized to active products, e.g. cyclophosphamide may be metabolized to phosphoramide mustard (Colvin *et al.*, 1976), so it is the biotransformed moiety that should be analysed in the plasma, not the parent compound.

3. *Plasma drug half-life*
Although this parameter is not usually used in the design or analysis of *in vitro* drug assays, it is relevant because it is involved in determination of the drug's $C \times T$, reflecting the dynamics of its elimination. It is useful for establishing optimal *in vivo* dosing schedules for clinical protocols.

Values for these various parameters for a comprehensive range of antitumour drugs are listed by Alberts and Chen (1980). It should be noted that a range of values are quoted frequently depending on the route of administration and dosage employed. For example, intravenously adminis-tered adriamycin at 30 mg m^{-2} results in peak plasma concentrations in the range 0.36–0.5 μg ml^{-1}, with $C \times T$ values between 1.38 and 2.34 μg h ml^{-1}, and peak plasma concentration of cis-platinum administered intravenously at 100 mg m^{-2} is reported at 2.49 ± 0.41 μg ml^{-1} with a range of $C \times T$ values at 1.45–2.52 μg h ml^{-1}.

4. *Intratumoural drug concentration*
Drug concentration in "solid" tumours is obviously the principal parameter of importance. However, as yet, negligible data have been obtained regarding the rate and amount of drug entering a tumour, concentration and retention of drug within the tumour, and intratumoural drug half-lives, following administration of drug to the patient.

III. Importance of pharmacokinetic principles in drug assay design *in vitro*

The application of pharmacokinetic principles is essential in the design of *in vitro* drug assays, and it appears that plasma drug $C \times T$ and peak plasma concentrations are the two most relevant parameters available for selecting drug concentrations to be used *in vitro*. Results from *in vitro* cell culture experiments and some mouse tumour model systems suggest that an antitumour drug's $C \times T$ is directly related to the degree of its cellular lethal effects (Alberts and van Daalen Wetters, 1976). Other workers have shown that for some anticancer agents, particularly alkylating compounds, the peak plasma concentration and $C \times T$ equivalents of the drugs when used *in vitro* correlated well with cytotoxicity in human xenografts grown in mice *in vivo* (Bateman *et al.*, 1979, 1980).

A range of pharmacological clinically achievable drug concentrations should be used when selecting appropriate concentrations for sensitivity testing *in vitro*. Table 2 lists the range of concentrations of a number of drugs used in such studies. Drug exposure time to be used *in vitro* will be discussed later, but often a 1 hour exposure time is selected for convenience because cell viabilities decrease during prolonged exposures and also because pharmaco-kinetic data for intravenously administered drugs generally suggest that significant exposure to most drugs is greatest during the first hour after administration (see Alberts *et al.*, 1981). Concentrations significantly smaller than the maximum clinically achievable dose should be evaluated since the plasma drug level ($C \times T$ and peak concentration) may not be achieved in the tumour, e.g. regions within the tumour may be poorly perfused and may accumulate less drug. Conversely, some drugs may be retained in tumours resulting in accumulation within the tumours for long periods. Higher drug concentrations also may be tested for studies with tumours exhibiting drug resistance, expecially those from previously treated patients.

Table 2 Concentration ranges of some drugs used in drug sensitivity studies *in vitro* (Von Hoff *et al.*, 1981)

Drug	Range tested ($\mu g\ ml^{-1}$)
Actinomycin D	0.01–0.1
m-AMSA	0.1–10.0
Adriamycin	0.01–04
Bleomycin	0.01–1.0
5-Fluorouracil	0.001–10.0
Interferon	10.0–1000.0 units ml^{-1}
Methotrexate	0.05–5.0
Cis-platinum	0.05–1.0
Vinblastine	0.01–10.0
Vincristine	0.01–0.1

IV. Dose–response in drug assays *in vitro*

Dose–response curves produced from data *in vitro* can be plotted on a linear scale (see Fig. 3a) or semi-logarithmic scale (see Fig. 3b), but the more simple linear plots, e.g. of percentage survival against drug concentration as shown in Fig. 3a, are useful for obtaining an overall impression of response when there is tumour heterogeneity in colony forming assays. If the survival curve produced *in vitro* shows a minimal decrease (curve A) this corresponds to a small percentage of response (lethality) with increasing drug concentration and usually predicts resistance *in vivo*. Conversely, a rapid decrease in the survival curve at low drug concentrations (curve C) demonstrates a degree of sensitivity *in vitro* and may correlate with sensitivity *in vivo*. An intermediate curve (B) indicates moderate response and at higher concentrations may suggest kinetic or biochemical resistance of subpopulations of tumour "stem"

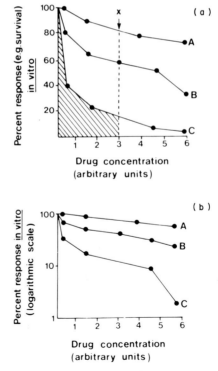

Fig. 3   Dose–response curves produced from drug assays *in vitro*. (Rupniak *et al.*, 1982)

cells to the drug under examination, or indeed may reflect technical problems with the particular assay methodology. Figure 3b shows the form in which most survival data obtained from *in vitro* drug sensitivity studies with cell lines are presented.

Often, quantitation of these survival curves is made by calculating the sensitivity index (Alberts *et al.*, 1980; Moon, 1980). This is defined as the area under the linear survival curve obtained *in vitro*, between 0 and an upper cut-off concentration limit, x (see hatched area under curve C in Fig. 3a). The upper cut-off concentration is determined by clinically achievable $C \times T$ values for each particular drug. Calculation of the sensitivity index is most easily performed by the trapezoidal method (Moon, 1980). From Fig. 3a it can be seen that the sensitivity index for curve C is much smaller than for curve A.

More recently a modified sensitivity index definition has been published. Abel and Kaufmann (1982) suggested that measuring relative, rather than absolute, response might be more valid in comparative studies. Thus

$$S' = (100C_{max} - S)/S$$

where S' = modified sensitivity index,

S = sensitivity index as previously defined, and

C_{max} = upper cut-off limit of drug concentration.

Since pharmacokinetic data for certain drugs and newly developed drugs not tested clinically are not available, an ID_{50} value (concentration of drug causing 50% inhibition of response) has been estimated. These workers, using *in vitro* studies, correlated ID_{50} values with response of human xenografts in mice (Tveit *et al.*, 1980, 1982), thus producing calibration curves ($1/ID_{50}$ *in vitro* versus growth delay *in vivo*).

V. Relationship of dose–response curves *in vitro* with drug pharmacokinetics *in vivo*

On the basis of preliminary experiments, sensitivity limits have been selected for each drug and then patients have been classified as sensitive if the corresponding area is less than the selected limit and resistant if it is greatly above it, with an intermediate area of indeterminate response (Salmon *et al.*, 1978; Moon, 1980). Von Hoff and colleagues (1981) define *in vitro* sensitivity as a 70% or greater reduction in survival of tumour colony-forming units. Indeed this cut-off point may well need to be defined for each tumour type. Statistical analysis of various definitions of sensitivity is discussed by Clark and Von Hoff in Chapter 18.

When *in vitro* drug concentrations (e.g. for melphalan, bleomycin, and methotrexate) and C × T associated with the "sensitive" range of sensitivity index areas were compared to the peak plasma concentrations and C × T for these drugs *in vivo*, the empirically established cut-off concentrations were only 5–10% of those that were clinically achievable (Salmon *et al.*, 1978; Alberts *et al.*, 1980, 1981). These workers have therefore utilized 10% C × T drug levels *in vivo* to select the *in vitro* cut-off limits. Von Hoff's group (1981) have used only one concentration of drug in *in vitro* studies, in order to perform more drug studies per tumour specimen, the concentration chosen being approximately 10% of the peak plasma concentration achievable *in vivo*.

Since a variety of methods has been employed to define sensitivity and resistance, training sets should be established for each of these particular methods.

For clonogenic assays, usually a 1 hour drug exposure time is selected. However, comparative studies of different time-course exposures for tumour cells to single drug concentrations and concentration ranges have been performed. Cis-platinum and adriamycin showed an increasingly greater lethal effect with prolonged exposure times (1, 6, 18 h, and continuous

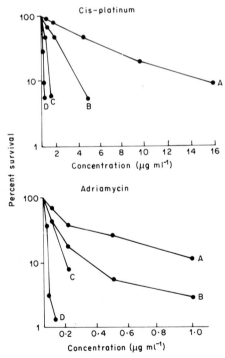

Fig. 4 Survival dose–response curves showing effect of increasing exposure times: (A) 1 hour; (B) 6 hours; (C) 18 hours; (D) continuous exposure. (Rupniak *et al.*, 1983)

exposure; i.e. colony formation assayed in continuous presence of drug), reflecting greater response with increased $C \times T$ *in vitro* (Rupniak *et al.*, 1983) as shown in Fig. 4. Alberts and co-workers (1981) have also demonstrated a similar effect with bleomycin, and suggested that administration by continuous infusion may be clinically useful in some cases (although, of course, toxicity of bleomycin *in vivo* may be altered by continuous infusion). However, Alberts and Salmon and their groups often failed to show reproducibly increased kill with longer exposure times for adriamycin, methotrexate, cis-platinum, and vinblastine, perhaps reflecting differences in methodology between these various studies.

VI. Conclusion

The selection of clinically relevant drug concentrations and exposure times for sensitivity testing *in vitro* is obviously complex. Determination of clinically valid and achievable plasma drug concentration–time products is an important consideration when analysing a "predictive" chemosensitivity assay. Further knowledge of drug concentrations achievable at, and within, the tumour site would be of definite benefit in extending the potential usefulness of *in vitro* antitumour drug assays.

References

Abel, U. and Kaufmann, M. (1982). A methodologically improved definition of chemosensitivity indices. *Cancer Res.* **42,** 1610.

Alberts, D. S. and Chen, G. H.-S. (1980). Tabular summary of pharmacokinetic parameters relevant to *in vitro* drug assay. In *Cloning of Human Tumor Stem Cells* (ed. S. E. Salmon), pp. 351–359. Alan R. Liss, New York.

Alberts, D. S. and van Daalen Wetters, T. (1976). The effect of phenobarbital on cyclophosphamide antitumour activity. *Cancer Res.* **36,** 2785–2789.

Alberts, D. S., Chen, G. H.-S. and Salmon, S. E. (1980). *In vitro* drug assay: pharmacologic considerations. In *Cloning of Human Tumor Stem Cells* (ed. S. E. Salmon), pp. 197–207. Alan R. Liss, New York.

Alberts, D. S., Salmon, S. E., Chen, G. H.-S., Moon, T. E., Young, L. and Surwit, E. A. (1981). Pharmacologic studies of anticancer drugs with the human tumor stem cell assay. *Cancer Chemother. Pharmacol.* **6,** 253–264.

Bateman, A. E., Peckham, M. J. and Steel, G. G. (1979). Assay of drug sensitivity for cells from human tumours: *in vitro* and *in vivo* tests on a xenografted tumour. *Br. J. Cancer* **40,** 81–88.

Bateman, A. E., Selby, P. J., Steel, G. G. and Towse, G. D. W. (1980). *In vitro* chemosensitivity tests on xenografted human melanomas. *Br. J. Cancer* **41,** 189–198.

Bowman, W. C. and Rand, M. J. (eds) (1980). *Textbook of Pharmacology*. Blackwell Scientific Publications, Oxford.

Colvin, M., Brundrett, R. B., Kan, M.-N. N., Jardine, I. and Fenselau, C. (1976). Alkylating properties of phosphoramide mustard. *Cancer Res.* **36,** 1121–1126.

Moon, T. E. (1980). Quantitative and statistical analysis of the association between *in vitro* and *in vivo* studies. In *Cloning of Human Tumor Stem Cells* (ed. S. E. Salmon), pp. 209–221. Alan R. Liss, New York.

Rupniak, H. T., Marks, P., Watkins, S., Bourne, G., Slevin, M., Bancroft-Livingston, G. H., Simmons, C. A. and Hill, B. T. (1982). Drug sensitivities of human tumour cells obtained directly from biopsy material. In *Current Chemotherapy and Immunotherapy* (ed. P. Periti and C. G. Grassi), Vol. II, pp. 1274–1276. Am. Soc. Microbiology.

Rupniak, H. T., Whelan, R. D. H. and Hill, B. T. (1983) Concentration and time dependent inter-relationships for antitumour drug cytotoxicities against tumour cells *in vitro*. *Int. J. Cancer* **32,** 7–12.

Salmon, S. E., Hamburger, A. W., Soehnlen, B., Durie, B. G. M., Alberts, D. S. and Moon, T. E. (1978). Quantitation of differential sensitivity of human-tumor stem cells to anticancer drugs. *New Engl. J. Med.* **298,** 1321–1327.

Tveit, K. M., Fodstad, Ø., Olsnes, S. and Pihl, A. (1980). *In vitro* sensitivity of human melanoma xenografts to cytotoxic drugs: correlation with *in vivo* chemosensitivity. *Br. J. Cancer* **26,** 717–722.

Tveit, K. M., Fodstad, Ø., Lotsberg, J., Vaage, S. and Pihl, A. (1982). Colony growth and chemosensitivity *in vitro* of human melanoma biopsies: relationship to clinical parameters. *Int. J. Cancer* **29,** 533–538.

Von Hoff, D. D., Casper, J., Bradley, E., Sandbach, J., Jones, D. and Makuch, R. (1981). Association between human tumor colony-forming assay results and response of an individual patient's tumor to chemotherapy. *Am. J. Med.* **70,** 1027–1032.

18. Statistical Considerations for *in vitro*/*in vivo* Correlations Using a Cloning System

G. M. CLARK and D. D. VON HOFF

I. Introduction

In vitro human tumour cloning systems have the potential for helping to select the most effective chemotherapy against an individual patient's tumour. These assays may also be useful as a preclinical screen to identify new agents of potential clinical value. For either of these applications there are a variety of ways in which assay results may be expressed, and several factors that may influence these results. In this chapter we will discuss the impact of several of these factors and describe some statistical considerations for human tumour cloning systems. We will illustrate these principles with data from the San Antonio Human Tumour Cloning Laboratory.

II. Experimental design

The two-layer soft agar human tumour cloning assay developed by Hamburger and Salmon (1977a,b) requires the plating of single cell suspensions from tumour specimens both in the presence and in the absence of chemotherapeutic agents. In San Antonio, triplicate plates are used for controls and for each of the drugs tested. The number of tumour colony forming units (TCFU) on each plate is recorded 7–14 days after plating. The average number of TCFU on triplicate drug-treated plates is calculated and the *in vitro* sensitivity of the specimen to that drug is expressed as the average number of TCFU relative to the control average.

225

III. Growth control

An important consideration is the distribution of the number of TCFU on control plates. We consider a specimen evaluable for drug sensitivity testing if the control average is greater than 20 TCFU. Table 1 shows the evaluability rates by tumour type for 6937 specimens assayed in San Antonio. The overall rate was 37.4% but this varied considerably by tumour type. Growth was observed in virtually all tumour types.

One measure of the reproducibility of the assay is the standard deviation of

Table 1   Breakdown by tumour type of the results of the clonogenic assay test

Tumour type	Specimens plated	% Evaluable	Evaluable drug tests	%<30% Survival	%<50% Survival
Adrenal gland	13	38.5	9	0.0	0.0
Bladder	120	43.3	146	14.4	24.0
Brain	114	46.5	181	9.4	18.8
Breast	1430	40.6	2175	6.3	16.2
Colon	432	43.3	941	6.5	15.9
Gall bladder	17	41.2	37	10.8	24.3
Head and neck	295	23.4	181	11.6	24.9
Kidney	213	50.7	461	6.9	19.5
Leukaemia	69	15.9	45	17.8	31.1
Liver	61	37.7	93	0.0	9.7
Lung					
small cell	259	22.4	317	12.0	22.7
non-small cell	647	41.4	1342	8.6	19.1
Lymphoma					
Hodgkin's	101	18.8	75	17.3	44.0
non-Hodgkin's	315	14.9	196	14.8	27.6
Melanoma	168	44.6	478	8.8	19.9
Miscellaneous	11	45.4	33	21.2	36.4
Myeloma	75	20.0	76	21.1	46.1
Neuroblastoma	213	26.3	244	8.6	23.4
Ovary	680	52.6	2226	5.4	14.0
Pancreas	113	46.0	235	10.6	24.3
Prostate	162	34.0	150	0.7	8.7
Sarcoma	218	36.2	302	7.6	19.5
Stomach	92	31.5	124	0.0	5.6
Testes	86	38.4	128	5.5	18.8
Thyroid gland	27	27.0	21	4.8	9.5
Unknown primary	1006	33.8	1330	5.9	16.1
Total	6937	37.4	11546	7.3	17.7

the number of TCFU among the control plates. However, the standard deviation is dependent on the number of TCFU on the plates, and for the control plates in our 2595 evaluable specimens the standard deviations were highly correlated with the mean number of TCFU ($r = 0.72$). This suggests that the coefficient of variation,

$$CV = 100 \times (\text{Standard Deviation/Mean})$$

should be fairly constant and might be useful as a measure of quality control. Figure 1 shows the distribution of the CV for these 2595 specimens. The CV ranged from 0 to 173 with a median of 20. The 95th percentile was 60, indicating that any CV greater than 60 might be considered unusually high and any drug sensitivity results for those specimens might be unreliable.

One of the major problems with the human tumour cloning assay is the preparation of single cell suspensions, and good single cell suspensions are of the utmost importance for performing drug sensitivity testing. To address this problem we initiated a small study to examine serial counts on plates from 18 specimens that did not grow. Of the 18 specimens 5 had completely acceptable background counts on day 0 (less than 20 features). The 13 high background counts were attributed to (i) red blood cell (RBC) clumping (8 cases), (ii) tissue debris (4 cases), and (iii) clumped agar (1 case). Of special note was that, by day 14, 5 of the 8 specimens with RBC clumping had RBC dissolution to acceptable levels. We feel that it is absolutely necessary that all control plates be examined on day zero to ensure excellent single cell suspensions. This can best be accomplished objectively by an image analysis system.

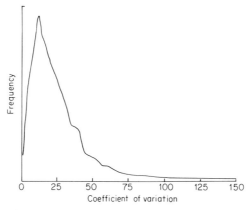

Fig. 1 Frequency distribution of coefficient of variation (CV) of number of colonies in replicate cultures for 2595 specimens.

IV. Percent survival

The percent survival of drug-treated TCFU relative to control plates is the standard sensitivity index for this assay system. A specimen is defined as sensitive to an agent *in vitro* if the percent survival is less than a specified value. The most commonly used cut-offs have been 30% or 50%.

We have performed 11 546 drug sensitivity tests on the 2595 evaluable specimens. Table 1 presents these results by tumour type for all drugs using both the 30% and the 50% survival criteria. Sensitivity results for a number of specific drugs against a variety of tumour types have been previously published (Von Hoff *et al.*, 1981c,d; Cowan *et al.*, 1982).

Most of the antineoplastic agents that have been tested in the human tumour cloning system are soluble in water. However, a few require DMSO, ethanol, or other solvents. We have examined the effect of some of these solvents by calculating the percent survival of vehicle controls relative to water controls. There was a slight inhibition in the median growth for the solvents, but the effect was quite variable among specimens.

It is often useful to estimate the variability associated with a percent survival. The standard error of percent survival cannot easily be calculated, but an approximation can be obtained by expanding the ratio in a Taylor's series:

$$SD = (CV_D^2/N_D + CV_C^2/N_C)^{1/2} \times \text{Percent Survival}$$

where CV_D = coefficient of variation for drug-treated plates, N_D = number of drug-treated plates, CV_C = coefficient of variation for control plates, and N_C = number of control plates.

This quantity can be used to obtain an estimate of the variability associated with a particular assay result. If triplicate control and drug-treated plates are used, and an upper limit of 60 is adopted for CV_C and CV_D, the corresponding upper limit for the CV for percent survival is 49. Therefore drug sensitivities with CV greater than or equal to 50 might be considered unreliable.

V. Other measures of sensitivity

Another criterion for drug sensitivity is percent kill. At first glance this index appears to be interchangeable with percent survival. However, percent kill is usually truncated at 0% when the drug-treated average exceeds the control average. This technique masks possible tumour stimulation. Approximately 10% of all drug tests result in percent survival at least 2 standard errors greater than 100% (Clark and Von Hoff, 1982b). We have found no discernible pattern of apparent stimulation by any combination of drugs or tumour types.

Instead of expressing drug sensitivity as a ratio (e.g. percent survival or percent kill), it might be thought possible to perform a simple two-sample t-test to compare the number of TCFU on control and drug-treated plates. However, since it has already been shown that the standard deviation is highly related to the mean, it would be necessary to use more complex statistics. Logarithmic transformation of the individual counts might improve the power of this procedure although it is not always easy to find a logical basis for such a transformation.

Another method for assessing the effectiveness of a drug *in vitro* might be to compare the size distributions of the drug-treated TCFU relative to control (Clark and Von Hoff, 1982a). It has been suggested that the TCFU population may be comprised of two subpopulations: stem cells and non-stem cells (Steel, 1975; Buick, 1980). In theory stem cells are prolific and have the capacity for self-renewal. This subpopulation of stem cell TCFU would be expected to be large in size but small in number. A drug that reduces the number of non-stem cell TCFU might produce a short-term clinical response, but would not be expected to produce "cures" unless it could also affect stem cells. A measure of a drug's effectiveness in eliminating stem cells might be the shift of the TCFU size distribution toward smaller colonies relative to the control. This concept of size reduction is biologically attractive and might be appropriate for future *in vitro/in vivo* correlative studies.

VI. Clinical correlations

The key to the usefulness of human tumour cloning systems is whether or not they can accurately and reliably predict *in vivo* results. Various statistics can be used to summarize results of correlative trials (Chiang *et al.*, 1956; Staquet *et al.*, 1981). Sensitivity describes the ability of a test to identify patients who will respond clinically, and specificity measures the ability to identify patients who will fail to respond clinically. Using the notation in Table 2, these statistics can be defined as follows:

$$\text{Sensitivity} = SS/(SS + RS)$$
$$\text{Specificity} = RR/(RR + SR)$$

Table 2   Notation for *in vivo/in vitro* correlations

	Responds clinically	Does not respond clinically
Sensitive *in vitro*	S/S	S/R
Resistant *in vitro*	R/S	R/R

For diagnostic tests, Sensitivity is usually the True Positive rate, and Specificity is the True Negative rate. However, when evaluating a predictive test, it is often more important to estimate its predictive value. The predictive value of an *in vitro* sensitive test (PV +) is the probability that a patient with a sensitive test will respond clinically to the same drug. Similarly, the predictive value of an *in vitro* resistant test (PV −) is the probability that a patient with a resistant test will fail to respond clinically. Using the notation in Table 2, these statistics can be defined as follows:

$$PV+ = SS/(SS+RR)$$
$$PV- = RR/(RR+RS)$$

In the "stem" cell drug sensitivity testing literature, the terms True Positive rate and True Negative rate have frequently been used instead of PV + and PV −.

One can easily be deceived by high predictive values. When the *in vitro* and *in vivo* response rates are relatively low, PV − is guaranteed to be high. For example, if both the *in vitro* and *in vivo* response rates are 20%, PV − will be at least 75% in the complete absence of a correlation. This value increases to 90% if the response rates are both 10%. The degree of association between the *in vitro* and *in vivo* results can be measured by the Kappa statistic (Fleiss, 1973) which takes into account agreements that might be expected purely by chance. The usual Chi-square test or Fisher's exact test can be applied to assess the statistical significance of the association.

Salmon and colleagues were the first to correlate drug sensitivity information obtained from the human tumour cloning system with response of an individual patient's tumour to the same drugs (Salmon *et al.*, 1978). These initial studies, as well as additional reports from the Tucson group (Salmon *et al.*, 1980), demonstrated good correlations between *in vitro* assay results and clinical tumour response or lack of response.

Investigators in San Antonio confirmed these results in a retrospective trial of the cloning assay (Von Hoff *et al.*, 1981a). More recently we reported results of a prospective correlative trial (Von Hoff *et al.*, 1981b). In the retrospective study useful *in vitro* information was obtained for only 25% of the patients. This figure increased to 64% in the prospective study owing primarily to greater experience with the culturing technique as well as to improved methods for tumour procurement. Table 3 summarizes results of these studies. The retrospective study included both single agent and combination clinical trials, while the prospective study consisted only of single agent therapies. The overall predictive values for the retrospective study were 71% and 98% respectively for *in vitro* sensitive and resistant specimens. The predictive values for the prospective study were somewhat lower (PV + = 60% and

Table 3 Results showing sensitivity, specificity, and the predictive value of a positive (PV +) and a negative (PV −) test for both the retrospective and the prospective study

	S/S	S/R	R/S	R/R	Sensi-tivity	Speci-ficity	PV +	PV −
Retrospective study								
Single agents	3	6	0	73	1.00	0.92	0.33	1.00
Combinations	12	0	2	27	0.86	1.00	1.00	0.93
Total	15	6	2	100	0.88	0.94	0.71	0.98
Prospective study								
Single agents	26	17	31	172	0.46	0.91	0.60	0.85

PV − = 85%). The Kappa statistics were highly statistically significant ($p < 0.001$) for each of these studies.

Despite the very significant *in vitro/in vivo* correlations in these trials, there are several questions that remain to be answered. It has not yet been determined whether the assay is superior to results that could be achieved by a clinician selecting therapy. In addition, it is also possible that the assay is merely an indicator that a particular patient's tumour is highly responsive *in vivo*. To address these uncertainties a future study should be performed that requires randomization of patients whose tumours had some drug that was effective *in vitro* between a choice of drug by the clinician versus the drug selected by the cloning system. With the present cloning assay such a trial would require a very large number of patients. Additional basic work on improving culture techniques as well as additional prospective clinical trials are needed before routine use of the cloning system for directing drug selection for patients can be recommended.

VII. Strategies for screening new agents

Perhaps the greatest utility of the human tumour cloning system will be the screening of new compounds for potential antitumour activity. Two new drugs, mitoxantrone and bisantrene, have recently been brought into clinical trials based partially on activity demonstrated in this *in vitro* system (Von Hoff *et al.*, 1981c,d).

The standard procedure in our laboratory is to test compounds at approximately one-tenth the peak plasma concentration achievable in humans. Cells are usually exposed to the drug for 1 hour. For investigational agents with little or no pharmacological data, initial screens are performed at $10 \ \mu g \ ml^{-1}$ with a continuous exposure. If activity is seen under these conditions, additional testing is performed at lower concentrations, and with 1 hour exposure. Based on our experience with standard agents and the new compounds, mitoxantrone and bisantrene, we recommend that drugs be considered for clinical trials only if the *in vitro* activity at one-tenth peak plasma concentration exceeds 25%.

It is feasible to use the human tumour cloning system to screen for new antineoplastic agents. One of the major advantages of the cloning assay is the tremendous heterogeneity (in terms of both tumour type and drug sensitivities) that it introduces into a tumour screen. This is theoretically closer to the real world. The major disadvantages are the low growth rates, large amounts of patient's tumours needed, difficulty in obtaining enough cells from an individual patient to provide for re-testing of the drug, and the fact that it is an *in vitro* system which ignores drug metabolism and distribution.

Acknowledgement

These studies were supported in part by contract NCI-CM-07327 and grant CA-30195 from the National Cancer Institute.

References

Buick, R. N. (1980). *In vitro* clonogenicity of primary human tumor cells: quantitation and relationship to tumor stem cells. In *Cloning of Human Tumor Stem Cells* (ed. S. E. Salmon), pp. 15–20. Alan R. Liss, New York.

Chiang, C. L., Hodges, J. L. Jr. and Yerushalmy, J. (1956). Statistical problems in medical diagnoses. In *Proceedings of the Third Berkeley Symposium of Mathematical Statistics and Probability* (ed. J. Neyman), Vol. IV, pp. 121–133. University of California Press, Berkeley.

Clark, G. M. and Von Hoff, D. D. (1982a). Reduction of size of tumor colony forming units (TCFU's) as a measure of drug effectiveness in the human tumor cloning system (HTCS). *Third Conference on Human Tumor Cloning* (ed. S. E. Salmon and J. M. Trent), p. 34. University of Arizona, Tucson.

Clark, G. M. and Von Hoff, D. D. (1982b). Stimulation of tumor growth by anticancer agents in the human tumor cloning system. *Proc. Am. Soc. Clin. Oncol.* **1**, 9.

Cowan, J. D., Von Hoff, D. D., Clark, G. M. and Paque, R. E. (1982). Comparative human tumor sensitivity to adriamycin (A), mitoxantrone (M), and bisantrene (B) as measured by a human tumor cloning assay (HTCA). *Proc. Am. Assoc. Cancer Res.* **23**, 187.

Fleiss, J. L. (1973). *Statistical Methods for Rates and Proportions*, pp. 145–147. John Wiley and Sons, New York.

Hamburger, A. W. and Salmon, S. E. (1977a). Primary bioassay of human myeloma stem cells. *J. Clin. Invest.* **60**, 846–854.

Hamburger, A. W. and Salmon, S. E. (1977b). Primary bioassay of human tumor stem cells. *Science* **197,** 461–463.

Salmon, S. E., Hamburger, A. W., Soehnlen, B., Durie, B. G., Alberts, D. S. and Moon, T. E. (1978). Quantitation of differential sensitivity of human tumor stem cells to anticancer drugs. *New Engl. J. Med.* **298,** 1321–1327.

Salmon, S. E., Alberts, D. S., Meyskens, F. L. Jr., Durie, B. G. M., Jones, S. E., Soehnlen, B., Young, L., Chen, H. S. G. and Moon, T. E. (1980). Clinical correlations of *in vitro* drug sensitivity. In *Cloning of Human Tumor Stem Cells* (ed. S. E. Salmon), pp. 223–245. Alan R. Liss, New York.

Staquet, M., Rozencweig, M., Lee, Y. J. and Muggia, F. M. (1981). Methodology for the assessment of new dichotomous diagnostic tests. *J. Chron. Dis.* **34,** 599–610.

Steel, G. G. (1975). In *Medical Oncology: Medical Aspects of Malignant Disease* (ed. K. D. Bagshawe), p. 49. Blackwell, Oxford.

Von Hoff, D. D., Casper, J., Bradley, E., Sandbach, J., Jones, D. and Makuch, R. (1981a). Association between human tumor colony-forming assay results and response of an individual patient's tumor to chemotherapy. *Am. J. Med.* **70,** 1027–1032.

Von Hoff, D. D., Page, C., Harris, G., Clark, G., Cowan, J. and Coltman, C. A., Jr. (1981b). Prospective clinical trial of a human tumor cloning system. *Proc. Am. Soc. Clin. Oncol.* **22,** 154.

Von Hoff, D. D., Coltman, C. A., Jr. and Forseth, B. (1981c). Activity of mitoxantrone in a human tumor cloning system. *Cancer Res.* **41,** 1853–1855.

Von Hoff, D. D., Myers, W. J., Kuhn, J., Sandbach, J., Pocelinko, R. and Coltman, C. A., Jr. (1981d). Phase I clinical investigation of 9,10-anthracenedicarboxalde-hyde bis-[(4,5-dihydro-1*H*-imidazol-2-yl)hydrazone] dihydrochloride hydrate (CL216,942). *Cancer Res.* **41,** 3118–3120.

19. An Overview of Correlations Between Laboratory Tests and Clinical Responses

B. T. HILL

I. Introduction

Advances in the last decade which have led to increased "cure" rates in certain "solid" tumours including, for example, childhood cancers (Simone *et al.*, 1982), testicular teratomas (Einhorn, 1981), and small cell carcinomas of the lung (Minna *et al.*, 1982), have resulted largely from the integration of combination chemotherapy with optimal local therapy. These effective chemotherapy protocols have been selected empirically by the clinician in the light of prior experience of the management of human malignancies. Such progress, whilst tremendously worthwhile, has not been rapid and the problem of designing effective treatments for the other common "solid" tumours, which are responsible for the majority of cancer deaths, remains. One approach towards improving on clinical empiricism has centred on identifying effective preclinical drug screening systems. This chapter provides an overview of the methodologies employed, emphasizing the necessary requirements of the *ideal* system. These include the mandatory strong correlation between laboratory tests and clinical responses, which are summarized and critically discussed. The chapter ends on an optimistic note by considering the future prospects for clinically relevant laboratory studies using human tumours.

II. Methods used for predictive drug screening tests

The ideal test must be simple, sensitive, specific, easily standardized, cheap, rapid, flexible, *and* provide results that correlate with clinical data (Hamburger, 1981; Weisenthal, 1981). This objective has not been achieved, yet. However, since one of the first publications in 1954 by Black and Speer, which reported a correlation between clinical response and alterations in cellular dehydrogenase activity following *in vitro* drug exposure, experimentalists have continued to tackle this daunting task.

Details of the various methodologies employed have been provided and discussed in earlier chapters of this volume and have been reviewed recently (Tanneberger *et al.*, 1979; Hamburger, 1981; Livingston, 1981; Von Hoff and Weisenthal, 1980; Weisenthal, 1981). Table 1 provides a summary of advantages and disadvantages of these test procedures. The major problems of distinguishing between tumour and normal "stromal" elements in biopsy specimens and coping with tumour cell heterogeneity were initially, and somewhat optimistically, thought to be solved with the introduction of clonogenic assays. Whilst the "stem" cell population within the tumour is obviously of critical importance in terms of continued growth or regrowth, since such poor plating efficiencies are frequently obtained, it is most likely at present that we are not examining this total population. This leaves open the question of whether the colonies observed are truly representative of this crucial subpopulation. Furthermore, recent publications reporting growth of non-malignant cell colonies under clonogenic assay conditions (discussed in Chapter 8 and by Livingston, 1981) introduce a further necessary note of caution when interpreting these results. However, the evidence that clonogenic assays provide currently the only reliable indicator of cellular reproductive capacity is now almost overwhelming, as discussed in Chapter 12. This should not be taken to mean that all other assays should be abandoned, since the possibility remains that (i) different tests may be valuable for specific drugs or groups of drugs with known mechanism(s) of action, and (ii) different tests may be appropriate for individual tumour types. Thus, whilst efforts to improve on the clonogenic assay procedures are encouraged (see Chapter 8), it is hoped that there will also be further investment in developing alternative methodologies. In this respect Weisenthal (1981) draws attention to two recent approaches to "specific" *in vitro* pre-clinical screening involving (i) use of an alkaline elution technique to quantitate the differential formation and removal of DNA cross-links by alkylating agents in drug sensitive or drug resistant cell populations, and (ii) measurement of DNA binding activity of a series of anthracyclines which correlated with *in vitro* cytotoxicity. However, the overriding requirement is that, irrespective of the actual measurement from which data are derived, they must correlate positively with clinical responses, as best judged at the present time.

III. Results of studies reporting laboratory/clinical correlations

An uncritical review of the literature on predictive drug sensitivity testing might well encourage the reader to wonder why any problems remain in

Table 1 Overview of the "pros" and "cons" of the various predictive test measurements *in vitro*

Test measurements	Disadvantages	Advantages
1. *Gross changes in cell morphology*	Difficult to standardize procedures, and liable to observer bias. Semiquantitative at best. Subjective element in identifying which cells are tumour cells. Changes in cellular morphology may not reflect those that render cells reproductively sterile. May fail to detect any "delayed cell killing" effects which permit several rounds of cell division before death.	Successful growth of tumour in culture not required.
2. *Inhibition of cellular metabolism*	May fail to detect any "delayed cell killing" effects of drugs. No distinction made between tumour and non-tumour cells. No distinction made between altered metabolism of cells in the "clonogenic" fraction of the tumour as opposed to those constituting the bulk of the tumour mass.	Successful growth of tumour in culture not required. Fast and simple. Tumour disaggregation unnecessary. May be applied to tumour and normal tissues to investigate any selectivity of drug action.
3. *Drug effects on a defined enzyme or metabolic pathway*	Frequently involve cumbersome and technically exacting systems unsuitable for general screening. Not applicable unless primary site(s) of drug action is known (which may differ with tumour type). If a radioactively labelled drug is employed, after metabolism, the cytotoxic moiety may not contain the label.	Successful growth of tumour in culture not required. Complete cell dispersal into a "single cell suspension" unnecessary.
4. *Radioactive nucleotide incorporation*	Uncertain influence of drug-induced alterations in nucleoside transport and/or intracellular nucleotide pool sizes. Influence of drug-induced alterations in synthesis of dTMP via the "salvage" pathway vis à vis the *de novo* pathway. Radionuclides may be toxic to the cells being assayed and thus artifactually potentiate results of cytotoxicity assay.	Relatively simple. Complete cell dispersal into a "single cell suspension" not mandatory since assay may be carried out on tumour pieces. Does not require cells to maintain

[Table continued overleaf]

Table 1 (*cont.*)

Test measurements	Disadvantages	Advantages
5. *Labelling index* (LI)	Variable rates of DNA synthesis may occur in tumour tissue related to its blood supply and/or degree of oxygenation. Misleading low incorporation of label may occur in cells destined to recover from depressed cellular metabolism after receiving "potentially lethal damage". Drug-induced alterations in nucleoside transport and/or intracellular nucleotide pool sizes. If labelling is delayed to allow recovery from the potential artifacts associated with drug exposure, a misleadingly high LI may result since "killed" cells may have degenerated. Difficulty of distinguishing between labelled tumour as opposed to non-tumour stromal cells. Grain counting is tedious and poorly suited for large-scale screening programmes. Questionable reliability of a 2-fold change, if LI is only of the order of 1%. No distinction possible between labelled cells with intact reproductive potential and those destined to die after one or two divisions.	DNA synthesis for more than 1 or 2 days in culture. Data available within 1 week. Morphology of tumour cells studied verifiable. Successful growth of tumour in culture not necessary. Complete cell dispersal into a "single cell suspension" not mandatory since assay may be carried out on tumour pieces.
6. *Cell viability*	No distinction between clonogenic and non-clonogenic cells. Timing of experiment is critical since lethally exposed cells may not show dye uptake for 2–4 days following drug treatment and/or in a rapidly proliferating population the dead cells may be diluted out with time, hence providing an underestimate of viability. In monolayers, non-viable cells tend to detach and may be washed away resulting in a predominantly viable population remaining attached.	Simple and rapid. Not dependent on cell growth *in vitro*. Simultaneous testing on normal and control non-tumour cells possible.

Table 1 (*cont.*)

7. *Cellular reproductive capacity*	Only a subpopulation of the heterogeneous tumour sample evaluated, which may or may not be truly representative. Poor plating efficiencies obtained. Large number of tumour cells necessary for successful drug evaluations ($>5 \times 10^6$). Dispersal of tumour into a "single cell suspension" often difficult and may cause cell injury. Less successful on "solid" tumours than ascites and effusions. Some colonies of "stromal" origin have been identified. Time-consuming and costly. Colony counting manually very tedious. $C \times T$ is not necessarily a constant even for a single drug in a single cell culture assay system.	Fibroblast overgrowth effectively markedly reduced or prevented. Morphologic and histochemical criteria can be used to confirm that colonies consist of cells with the same characteristics as the original tumour. Applicable to most, if not all, tumour types studied.
8. *Xenografted tumours*	Latent period of 10 to >30 days before transplanted tumour becomes apparent in the mouse. Need 3–6 weeks to evaluate drug effects. ? Altered growth kinetics of xenograft. ? Influence of altered blood supply to tumour related to inoculation site. Serial passage of tumour may alter responsiveness to specific drugs. Problems of sterile handling and housing.	Plentiful supply of tumour material. Allows testing of drugs requiring *in vivo* metabolic activation.

establishing optimal use of individualized chemotherapy programmes for cancer patients. However, a closer inspection of these data will reveal that in most cases accuracy is claimed in predicting drug resistance and hence treatment failure. The value of such studies should not be dismissed or denigrated; indeed, as Cline (1969) stated, "In this era of escalating chemotherapy, even this modest goal is desirable". However, clearly the task of identifying drug sensitivity and hence aiding *successful* therapy remains our overwhelming future goal.

Table 2 provides a summary of those studies in which attempts have been made to correlate results derived from laboratory tests, using different assay methods, with those obtained clinically following drug administration to the patient. Several general points are illustrated by these data:

1. Most of these studies present results on less than 50 patients.
2. Claims of 100% correlation of sensitivity refer only to evaluations on 5 or fewer patients, whilst frequently correlations of resistance of the order of 90–100% relate to evaluations on at least 50–100 patients.
3. Only one group claimed significantly better correlations for sensitivity than resistance (Daidone *et al.*, 1981; and see Chapter 23).

Table 2 Survey of studies attempting to correlate laboratory and clinical studies relating to human tumour drug sensitivities

Method	Patients (tests)	Tumour type	Clinical value: % correlations of Sensitivity	Resistance	References
Cell suspension/ enzyme assay	76	Various	50	100	DiPaolo and Dowd (1961)
Explant cultures/ morphology	131	Various	44 (36/81) (excludes 29% equivocal)	78 (39/50)	Wright *et al.* (1962)
Explant cultures/ morphology	(373)	Various	Overall 65% (but 35% S/R*)		Hurley and Yount (1965)
Cell cultures/ morphology	88	Various	Overall 63%		Tanneberger and Bacigalupo (1970)
Cell suspension/ enzyme assay	18	Various	78 (11/14)	100 (4/4)	Kondo (1971)
Tumour slices/ autoradiography	148	Various	No correlation		Wolberg and Ansfield (1971)
Tumour slices/ pretreatment LI	25	Various	75 (6/8)	88 (15/17)	Sky-Peck (1971)
Cell suspension/ morphology	48	Various	Overall 73%		Dendy *et al.* (1973)
Cell culture/ radionuclide incorp.	85	Gynaecol.	Overall 65%		Limburg (1973)
Cell culture/ cell counting	12 (13)	Various	100 (5/5)	88 (7/8)	Holmes and Little (1974)
Cell culture/ autoradiography	53	AL*	Overall 77%		Zittoun *et al.* (1975)

Table 2 (*cont.*)

Method	Patients (tests)	Tumour type	Clinical value: % correlations of		References
			Sensitivity	Resistance	
Bone marrow/ specific enzyme assays	10	AL and Burkitt's lymphoma	100 (3/3)	100 (7/7)	Bender *et al.* (1976)
Bone marrow/ specific enzyme assays	29	AML*	No correlation		Smyth *et al.* (1976)
Bone marrow/ specific enzyme assays	51	AL*	No correlation		Chang *et al.* (1977)
Bone marrow/ pretreatment LI	71	AL*	Good correlation		Hart *et al.* (1977)
Biopsy/ specific enzyme assay	23	Head and neck	"Strong correlation"		Muller (1977)
Tumour slice/ autoradiography	26	Leukaemia	93 (13/14)	83 (10/12)	Raich (1978)
Cell suspension/ dye exclusion	11	NHL*	100 (3/3)	100 (8/8)	Durkin *et al.* (1979)
Cell suspension/ clonogenic assay	40 (95)	Ovary	63 (13/21)	99 (73/74)	Alberts *et al.* (1980)
Cell suspension/ LI change	11	Various	Overall 79% (18% false +*)		Livingston *et al.* (1980)
Cell suspension/ DNA or RNA synthesis	48 31 15	NHL* Breast Testis	96 (22/23) 79 (11/14) 90 (9/10)	56 (14/25) 76 (13/17) 80 (4/5)	Daidone *et*
Cell culture/ cell counting	14	Glioma	67 (6/9)	100 (5/5)	Kornblith *et al.* (1981)
Cell suspension/ clonogenic assay	41 (48)	Melanoma	63 (12/19) (includes MR* as S *in vivo*)	86 (25/29)	Meyskens *et al.* (1981)
Cell culture/ clonogenic assay	12	Glio-blastomas	60 (3/5)	100 (7/7)	Rosenblum *et al.* (1981)
Cell suspension/ DNA or RNA synthesis	155 (115)	Various	69 (40/58) (36 no change clinically, 19S and 17R *in vitro*)	98 (56/57)	Volm *et al.* (1981)
Cell suspension/ clonogenic assay	(123) (246)	Various	(a) 71 (15/21) (b) 60 (26/43)	98 (100/102) 85 (172/203)	Von Hoff *et al.* (1981a,b, 1983)
Cell suspension/ dye exclusion	33 (92)	Various	86 (6/7)	100 (16/16)	Weisenthal and Marsden (1981)
Cell culture/ ^{3}H-leucine incorp.	15	Ovary	100% for 1st line drugs 57% for 2nd line drugs		Wilson and Neal (1981)
Cell suspension/ clonogenic assay	32 (37)	Various	82 (9/11)	96 (25/26)	Mann *et al.* (1982)
Cell culture/ ^{35}S-methionine uptake	5 (15)	Glioma	Close correlation noted		Thomas *et al.* (1982)
Cell suspension/ ^{3}H-thymidine incorp.	20	Ovary	86 (12/14) (includes SD* as S *in vivo*)	67 (4/6)	Trope and Sigurdsson (1982)
Cell suspension clonogenic assay	39 (49)	Melanoma	Good overall correlations (1 false +)		Tveit *et al.* (1982)
Cell suspension/ clonogenic assay	(65)	Myeloma	79 (22/28)	95 (35/37)	Durie *et al.* (1983)

AL = acute leukaemia; AML = acute myeloid leukaemia; MR = mixed response; NHL = non-Hodgkin's lymphoma; SD = stable disease; S/R = sensitive *in vitro* but resistant *in vivo*, i.e. false +.

4. Results are available from investigators from several different institutions employing clonogenic assays which suggest some reproducibility of such data, but reports using other methodologies in general come only from individual research groups employing specific tests, so no comment can be made on their reproducibility from laboratory to laboratory.
5. No group has compared clinical correlations obtained using different methodologies.

It was also perhaps significant that, whilst reports of no correlations were acceptable for publication in the 1970s, either such negative studies are a thing of the past or only positive success merits publication today. However, it should be noted that endpoints for sensitivity range from as low as 25% cell kill (e.g. Kornblith *et al.*, 1981), or $>25\%$ inhibition of radionuclide incorporation (e.g. Kaufmann, 1982), to $\geqslant 75\%$ tumour colony inhibition (e.g. Mann *et al.*, 1982). Clearly, if the endpoint is selected after the correlation, success can be guaranteed.

Correlative studies on reasonably large series of patients are still in their infancy. One way of increasing the number of tumours evaluated is to set up collaborative studies. Von Hoff's group have already attempted this by receiving and processing tumour specimens from other centres, and they have recently published details of suitable procedures for collecting, storing, and transporting such specimens (Von Hoff *et al.*, 1982). Alternatively, data may be accumulated from tests carried out in a number of centres, a practice adopted by Volm's group, but it is then critical that the procedures be standardized. At present, observer bias is an acknowledged problem not only in evaluating endpoints of laboratory assays but also in clinical evaluation of tumour response. It has been suggested that the former difficulty may be alleviated by automation, and Salmon's group make use of an automated colony counter, the Bausch and Lomb FAS II Image Analysis System (see Chapter 24). However, this is an extremely expensive item of equipment and any definite advantage in its use remains to be established. Indeed, its ability to distinguish accurately between clusters, colonies, clumps, or debris remains controversial.

Criteria for defining *in vitro* and *in vivo* sensitivity for specific drugs also vary depending not only on the assay method adopted but also on the tumour type being studied and from laboratory to laboratory. These have been discussed briefly in Chapter 8, and the methods employed by individual investigators are included in Chapters 18 and 21–25. In most cases, whilst the opposite ends of the spectrum, namely, sensitivity and resistance, can be clearly identified, there is inevitably a great area of intermediate response. However, this must be taken into account when overall correlative values are quoted. These equivocal or mixed responses are also a problem in clinical studies (see e.g. Tveit *et al.*, 1982; Meyskens *et al.*, 1981; Volm *et al.*, 1981). Indeed, problems associated with clinical evaluation of tumour response are legion, as discussed by Simon (1982). They are extremely relevant to a consideration of the validation of laboratory and clinical correlation studies, and may be a highly significant factor in explaining the divergent results and success rates being reported by different investigators. In this respect it is also absolutely essential that, for each drug and each tumour type, every laboratory obtains their "training set" of data under their experimental and clinical conditions. It is only in this way that correlations can be considered valid. The tendency of investigators at various institutions using clonogenic assays to utilize the "training set" data of Salmon *et al.* (see Chapter 24) in this respect should be discouraged.

Other critical factors which require further investigation include selection of drug concentrations, exposure time, and conditions of drug exposure for *in vitro* tests that correspond most appropriately to clinical drug administration. The immensity of this task should not be overlooked. The dose and schedule dependence of antitumour drugs is well recognized both clinically and from experimental animal studies. It should be appreciated that application of $C \times T = $ constant does not in any way solve this problem since in most cases this simple relationship has not been found to be valid (as discussed in Chapter 17). It is hoped that, by increasing our knowledge of the pharmacokinetics of antitumour agents, laboratory testing can be carried out under realistic and representative conditions. Powis *et al.* (1981) have reviewed the dose dependent pharmacokinetics of antitumour agents, and certain aspects of this have been discussed in Chapter 17, with emphasis placed on the time dependent cell killing effects of certain drugs which have been clearly demonstrated in some studies but not in others.

The fact that cytotoxic effects of antitumour drugs show both time and dose dependence adds weight to the argument that *in vitro* tests should provide a full dose–response curve from which sensitivity or resistance can be assessed, rather than be based on a single drug concentration with a fixed exposure time. However, this latter approach is obviously more suitable for a rapid screening procedure, and when quantities of tumour cells available for testing are small it allows a larger number of drugs to be evaluated. Again, the true test of each procedure will depend on the strength of the correlations with clinical data.

Most of the studies summarized in Table 2 have provided data from retrospective clinical trials, i.e. a series of *in vitro* assays have been carried out and compared retrospectively with what happened in the clinic. However, recently a few prospective studies have been carried out employing clonogenic assays (Alberts *et al.*, 1980; Meyskens *et al.*, 1981; Von Hoff *et al.*, 1983; Durie *et al.*, 1983). In general, results agree with those from earlier studies, although Von Hoff has pointed out that predictive values were somewhat lower for prospective studies. The fact that resistance is predicted more accurately than sensitivity must also be remembered, and it remains to be established whether the clonogenic system, or indeed any other, is truly cost effective, providing superior results not only as measured by response rate but also by response duration and/or survival. Further prospective clinical trials are necessary, and Carter (1981) has described his ideal experimental design for a prospective clinical trial in which patients for whom the *in vitro* assay can be performed are randomized to be treated either empirically with a specified protocol or according to the assay results. Patients for whom the assay could not be performed would also receive the specified protocols. The endpoint of the trial would be to see whether patients treated according to the assay had the highest response rates and the lonest survival times. Clearly this is the direction in which to move in the future.

IV. Recent developments and future prospects

Whilst accepting the need for new and better methodologies, for more data supporting the validity of present assay systems, and especially for prospective clinical trials assessing survival, we can still expand our horizons using present technology. Recent developments in clinical applications of *in vitro* tests include the following.

Screening new antitumour agents and analogues to predict clinical efficacy
For example, Von Hoff *et al.* (1981b) have utilized the human tumour cloning system to screen for antitumour effects *in vitro* of a new anthracene derivative (CL 216,942). Evaluations were possible in 273 tumours covering a wide range of tumour types, and a broad spectrum of *in vitro* activity was noted. These data will be retrospectively compared with results of Phase II clinical trials. A similar study has been reported by Ahmann *et al.* (1982) evaluating mAMSA, but in addition this group provides preliminary encouraging prospective *in vitro/in vivo* correlations in 8 patients. If these data are confirmed, the use of *in vitro* Phase II studies would have major advantages since large numbers of varied tumour types could be studied, results could be available within a month, and tests could be carried out on untreated tumours and not just on those from extensively pretreated patients.

Providing prognostic indicators for resistance and/or survival
In multiple myeloma, tumour cell mass and labelling index correlate with subsequent survival duration, but do not predict the response to treatment. However, Hofmann *et al.* (1981) have shown that high *in vitro* incorporation of ^{3}H-thymidine, as expressed by the grain count over bone marrow myeloma

cells, is correlated with both *in vivo* and *in vitro* (as judged by clonogenic assay) resistance to treatment with drugs commonly used in multiple myeloma. Two further examples are provided from studies with clonogenic assays. Von Hoff *et al.* (1981c) reported an inverse relationship between cloning efficiency and patient survival times for both neuroblastoma and head and neck tumours, although it remains to be established whether this holds true for other tumour types. Rosenblum *et al.* (1982), using a modified assay system developed for brain tumour cells, have reported an age-related chemosensitivity of "stem" cells from malignant brain tumours, with patient age inversely correlated with *in vitro* cell kill and the younger patients surviving longest.

Monitoring bone marrow for tumour involvement
The clonogenic assay has been used successfully to document marrow involvement by small cell lung cancer and neuroblastoma (Von Hoff *et al.*, 1981d).

These aspects merit further investigation, but at the same time it should be possible to explore the use of *in vitro* test systems (i) to optimize the scheduling of "standard" antitumour agents and newer drugs, (ii) to screen for antagonistic and/or synergistic drug combinations, (iii) to monitor drug therapy, if repeated biopsies or samples can be taken, and in this respect the use of peritoneal washings advocated by Ozols *et al.* (1980) in ovarian cancer may be valuable, and (iv) to study the development of clinical drug resistance.

Several of these newer and potential applications involve moving away from the idea of predicting individual drug sensitivities for each patient. This is probably a more realistic approach at the present time in view of the limitations of our present methodologies. One of the major problems is the time required before a test result is obtained, particularly with a clonogenic assay. Another problem relates to the fact that combination chemotherapy is now frequently employed clinically and at the present time even the most enthusiastic investigator is likely to be daunted by the thought of testing drug combinations *in vitro*. However, we should be encouraged by the major developments that have occurred even within the last 5 years in this area of predictive drug sensitivity testing. The establishment of closer links between experimental laboratory and clinical staff can only be beneficial. It is hoped that these clinically orientated studies will continue and can be paralleled by the more basic studies of the biology of human tumours using these *in vitro* culture methods. This might lead to the identification of agents that interfere with tumour cell proliferation by mechanisms other than direct cytotoxicity.

Acknowledgements

I am indebted particularly to Dr J. R. W. Masters and also to Mr J. Darling for comments and constructive criticisms during the preparation of the manuscript.

References

Ahmann, F. R., Meyskens, F. L., Moon, T. E., Durie, B. G. M. and Salmon, S. E. (1982). *In vitro* chemosensitivities of human tumor stem cells to the Phase II drug 4'-(9-acridinylamino)methanesulfon-*m*-anisidide and prospective *in vivo* correlations. *Cancer Res.* **42,** 4495–4498.

Alberts, D. S., Salmon, S. E., Chen, H. S. G., Surwit, E. A., Soehnlen, B., Young, L. and Moon, T. E. (1980). *In vitro* clonogenic assay for predicting response of ovarian cancer to chemotherapy. *Lancet* **ii,** 340–342.

Bender, R. A., Gieger, W. A., Drake, J. C. and Ziegler, J. L. (1976). *In vitro* correlates of clinical response to methotrexate in acute leukaemia and Burkitt's lymphoma. *Br. J. Cancer* **34,** 484–492.

Black, M. M. and Speer, F. D. (1954). Further observations on the effects of cancer chemotherapeutic agents on the *in vitro* dehydrogenase activity of cancer tissue. *J. Nat. Cancer Inst.* **14,** 1147–1158.

Carter, S. K. (1981). Predictors of response and their clinical evaluation *Cancer Chemother. Pharmacol.* **7,** 1–4.

Chang, P., Wiernik, P., Bachur, N., Stoller, R. and Chabner, B. (1977). Failure to predict response of acute non-lymphocytic leukaemia (ANLL) using assays for deoxycytidine kinase, cytidine deaminase and daunorubicin reductase. *Proc. Am. Assoc. Cancer Res.* **18,** 352.

Cline, M. (1969). *In vitro* test systems for anticancer drugs. *New Engl. J. Med.* **208,** 955.

Daidone, M. G., Silvestrini, R. and Sanfilippo, O. (1981). Clinical relevance of an *in vitro* antimetabolite assay for monitoring human tumour chemosensitivity. In *Adjuvant Therapy of Cancer*. III (ed. S. E. Salmon and S. E. Jones), pp. 25–32. Grune and Stratton, New York.

Dendy, P. P., Dawson, M. P. A. and Honess, D. J. (1973). Studies on the drug sensitivity of human tumour cells in short-term culture. In *Aktuelle Probleme der Therapie maligner Tumoren* (ed. G. Wüst), pp. 34–44. Georg Thieme, Stuttgart.

DiPaolo, J. A. and Dowd, J. E. (1961). Evaluation of inhibition of human tumor tissue by cancer chemotherapeutic drugs with an *in vitro* test. *J. Nat. Cancer Inst.* **27,** 807–815.

Durie, B. G. M., Young, L. and Salmon, S. E. (1983). Human myeloma stem cell culture: relationship between *in vitro* drug sensitivity and kinetics and patient survival duration. *Blood*, **61,** 929–934.

Durkin, W. J., Ghanta, V. K., Balch, C. M., Dorris, D. W. and Hiramoto, R. N. (1979). A methodological approach to the prediction of anticancer drug effects in humans. *Cancer Res.* **39,** 402–407.

Einhorn, L. H. (1981). Testicular cancer as a model for a curable neoplasm. *Cancer Res.* **41,** 3275–3280.

Hamburger, A. W. (1981). Use of *in vitro* tests in predictive cancer chemotherapy. *J. Nat. Cancer Inst.* **66,** 981–988.

Hart, J. S., George, S. L., Frei, E., Bodey, G. P., Nickerson, R. C. and Freireich, E. J.

(1977). Prognostic significance of pretreatment proliferative activity in adult acute leukemia. *Cancer* **39**, 1603–1617.

Hofmann, V., Salmon, S. E. and Durie, B. G. M. (1981). Drug resistance in multiple myeloma associated with high *in vitro* incorporation of ^{3}H-thymidine. *Blood* **58**, 471–476.

Holmes, H. and Little, J. (1974). Tissue-culture micro test for predicting response of human cancer to chemotherapy. *Lancet* **ii**, 985–987.

Hurley, J. and Yount, L. (1965). Selection of anticancer drug for palliation using tissue culture sensitivity studies. *Am. J. Surg.* **109**, 39–42.

Kaufmann, M. (1982). Nucleic acid precursor incorporation assay for testing tumour sensitivity and clinical applications. *Drugs Exp. Clin. Res.* **8**, 335–358.

Kondo, T. (1971). Prediction of response of tumour and host to cancer chemotherapy. *Nat. Cancer Inst. Monogr.* **34**, 251–256.

Kornblith, P. L., Smith, B. H. and Leonard, L. A. (1981). Response of cultured human brain tumors to nitrosoureas: correlation with clinical data. *Cancer* **47**, 255–265.

Limburg, H. (1973). Selektion von Zytostatika bei gynäkologischen Tumoren in der Gewebekultur. In *Aktuelle Probleme der Therapie maligner Tumoren* (ed. G. Wüst), pp. 7–17. Georg Thieme, Stuttgart.

Livingston, R. B. (1981). Methods to predict response to chemotherapy. In *Breast Cancer. IV. Advances in Research and Treatment* (ed. W. L. McGuire), pp. 1–32. Plenum Press, New York.

Livingston, R. B., Titus, G. A. and Heilbrum, L. K. (1980). *In vitro* effects on DNA synthesis as a predictor of biological effect from chemotherapy. *Cancer Res.* **40**, 2209–2212.

Mann, B. D., Kern, D. H., Giuliano, A. E., Burk, M. W., Campbell, M. A., Kaiser, L. R. and Morton, D. L. (1982). Clinical correlations with drug sensitivities in the clonogenic assay. *Arch. Surg.* **117**, 33–36.

Meyskens, F. L., Moon, T. E., Dana, B., Gilmartin, E., Casey, W. J., Chen, H. S. G., Hood Franks, D., Young, L. and Salmon, S. E. (1981). Quantitation of drug sensitivity by human metastatic melanoma colony-forming units. *Br. J. Cancer* **44**, 787–797.

Minna, J. D., Higgins, G. A. and Glatstein, E. J. (1982). Cancer of the lung. In *Cancer: Principles and Practice of Oncology* (ed. V. T. DeVita, S. Hellman and S. A. Rosenberg), pp. 396–474. J. B. Lippincott Co., Philadelphia.

Muller, W. E. G. (1977). Bleomycin-sensitivity test application for human cell carcinoma. *Cancer* **40**, 2787–2792.

Ozols, R. F., Wilson, J. K. V., Grotzinger, K. R. and Young, R. C. (1980). Cloning of human ovarian cancer cells in soft agar from malignant effusions and peritoneal washings. *Cancer Res.* **40**, 2743–2747.

Powis, G., Ames, M. M. and Kovach, J. S. (1981). Dose dependent pharmacokinetics and cancer chemotherapy. *Cancer Chemother. Pharmacol.* **6**, 1–9.

Raich, P. C. (1978). Prediction of therapeutic response in acute leukaemia. *Lancet* **i**, 74–76.

Rosenblum, M. L., Dougherty, D. V., Reese, C. and Wilson, C. B. (1981). Potentials and possible pitfalls of human stem cell analysis. *Cancer Chemother. Pharmacol.* **6**, 227–235.

Rosenblum, M. L., Gerosa, M., Dougherty, D. V., Reese, C., Barger, G. R., Davis, R. L., Levin, V. A. and Wilson, C. B. (1982). Age-related chemosensitivity of stem cells from human malignant brain tumours. *Lancet* **i**, 885–887.

Simon, R. M. (1982). Design and conduct of clinical trials. In *Cancer: Principles and Practice of Oncology* (ed. V. T. DeVita, S. Hellman and S. A. Rosenberg), pp. 198–225. J. B. Lippincott Co., Philadelphia.

Simone, J. V., Cassady, J. R. and Filler, R. M. (1982). Cancers of childhood. In *Cancer: Principles and Practice of Oncology* (ed. V. T. DeVita, S. Hellman and S. A. Rosenberg), pp. 1254–1330. J. B. Lippincott Co., Philadelphia.

Sky-Peck, H. (1971). Effect of chemotherapy on the incorporation of ^{3}H-thymidine into DNA of human neoplastic tissue. *Nat. Cancer Inst. Monogr.* **34**, 197–205.

Smyth, J. F., Robins, A. B. and Leese, C. L. (1976). The metabolism of cytosine arabinoside as a predictive test for clinical response to the drug in acute myeloid leukaemia. *Eur. J. Cancer* **12**, 567–573.

Tanneberger, St. and Bacigalupo, G. (1970). Einige Erfahrungen mit der individuellen Zytostatischen Behandlung maligner Tumoren nach prätherapeutischer Zytostatika-Sensibilitätsprufung *in vitro* (Onkobiogramm). *Arch. Geschwulstforsch.* **35**, 44–53.

Tanneberger, St., Nissen, E. and Schalicke, W. (1979). Prediction of drug efficacy potentialities and limitations. In *Advances in Medical Oncology, Research and Education.* V. *Basis for Cancer Therapy* 1 (ed. B. W. Fox), pp. 197–211. Pergamon Press, Oxford.

Thomas, D. G. T., Darling, J. L. and Bullard, D. E. (1982). The chemosensitivity of human gliomas: an *in vitro* assay and correlation with clinical response. *Eur. J. Cancer Clin. Oncol.* (Suppl. 3), 83–89.

Trope, C. and Sigurdsson, K. (1982). Use of tissue culture and predictive testing of drug sensitivity in human ovarian cancer: correlation between *in vitro* results and the response *in vivo*. *Neoplasma* **29**, 309–314.

Tveit, K. M., Fodstad, Ø., Lotsburg, J., Vaage, S. and Pihl, A. (1982). Colony growth and chemosensitivity *in vitro* of human melanoma biopsies: relationship to clinical parameters. *Int. J. Cancer* **29**, 533–538.

Volm, M. and The Group for Sensitivity Testing of Tumors (KSST) (1981). *In vitro* short-term test to determine the resistance of human tumors to chemotherapy. *Cancer* **48**, 2127–2135.

Von Hoff, D. D. and Weisenthal, L. (1980). *In vitro* methods to predict patient response to chemotherapy. In *Advances in Pharmacology and Chemotherapy* (ed. S. Garattini, A. Goldin, F. Hawking and I. J. Kopin), pp. 133–156. Academic Press, New York.

Von Hoff, D. D., Casper, J., Bradley, E., Sandbach, J., Jones, D. and Makuch, R. (1981a). Association between human tumor colony-forming assay results and response of an individual patient's tumor to chemotherapy. *Am. J. Med.* **70**, 1027–1032.

Von Hoff, D. D., Coltman, C. A. and Forseth, B. (1981b). Activity of 9,10-anthracenedicarboxaldehyde bis-[(4,5-dihydro-1*H*-imidazol-2-yl)hydrazone] dihydrochloride (CL 216,942) in a human tumor cloning system: leads for phase II trials in man. *Cancer Chemother. Pharmacol.* **6**, 141–144.

Von Hoff, D. D. Cowan, J., Harris, G. and Reisdorf, G. (1981c). Human tumor cloning: feasibility and clinical correlations. *Cancer Chemother. Pharmacol.* **6**, 265–271.

Von Hoff, D. D., Swenerton, K. D., Hetanen, L., Rivkin, S., Schuchart, S. and Coltman, C. A. Jr (1982). Long distance transportation of specimens for human tumor cloning. *Stem Cells* **2**, 122–128.

Von Hoff, D. D., Clark, G. M., Stogdill, B. J., Sarosdy, M. F., O'Brien, M. T., Casper,

J. T., Mattox, D. E., Page, C. P., Cruz, A. B. and Sandbach, J. F. (1983). Prospective clinical trial of a human tumor cloning system. *Cancer Res.* **43,** 1926–1931.

Weisenthal, L. M. (1981). *In vitro* assays in preclinical antineoplastic drug screening. *Semin. Oncol.* **8,** 362–376.

Weisenthal, L. M. and Marsden, J. (1981). A novel dye exclusion assay for predicting response to cancer chemotherapy. *Proc. Am. Assoc. Cancer Res.* **22,** 155.

Wilson, A. P. and Neal, F. E. (1981). *In vitro* sensitivity of human ovarian tumours to chemotherapeutic agents. *Br. J. Cancer* **44,** 189–200.

Wolberg, W. H. and Ansfield, F. J. (1971). The relation of thymidine labelling index in human tumors *in vitro* to the effectiveness of 5-fluorouracil chemotherapy. *Cancer Res.* **31,** 448–450.

Wright, J. E. C., Plummer-Cobb, J., Gumport, S. L., Safadi, D., Walker, D. G. and Galomb, F. M. (1962). Further investigations of the relation between the clinical and tissue culture response to chemotherapeutic agents on human cancer. *Cancer* **15,** 284–293.

Zittoun, R., Bouchard, M., Gacquet-Davis, J., Percie-du-Sert, M. and Bousser, J. (1975). Prediction of the response to chemotherapy in acute leukemia. *Cancer* **35,** 507–513.

20. Results Obtained Using a Short Term Radionuclide Assay and Clinical Correlations

M. VOLM, M. KAUFMANN and J. MATTERN

I. Introduction

There are a number of methods for determining the sensitivity or resistance of tumours to antineoplastic agents; for reviews see Kaufmann (1980) and Hamburger (1981).

For routine clinical work predictive assays should be simple, standardized, and reproducible. Our group has developed a simple test in which a tumour cell suspension is prepared and uptake of radioactive nucleic acid precursors is determined after drug addition (Volm *et al.*, 1970, 1975a,b; see also Chapter 6). This assay is standardized for "solid" tissues and for tumour cells from body fluids. Results for freshly prepared tumour cell suspensions, using standard anticancer drugs, can be obtained within a few hours.

The success rate of the test varies for each "solid" tumour type, being highest with ovarian and lung carcinomas (90–95%) because cell suspensions or cell fragments with a high proportion of viable cells are easy to prepare from these "solid" tumours. With breast tumours the success rate was approximately 70%.

Tests on a series of ovarian and lung carcinomas after treatment with adriamycin showed that each tumour exhibited a different dose–response curve (Fig. 1). Some carcinomas were very markedly affected by adriamycin, whereas others showed either only intermediate effects or negligible responses. This variation was most clearly seen at adriamycin concentrations of 0.01 mg ml^{-1} (1.7×10^{-5} M).

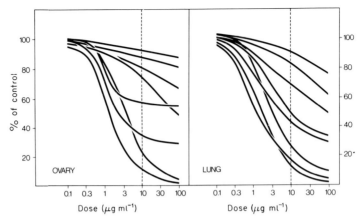

Fig. 1 Incorporation of ^{3}H-uridine *in vitro* after addition of adriamycin at different concentrations to tumour cell suspensions of individual ovarian and lung carcinomas.

II. Results of laboratory/clinical correlations

A. Pilot study for *in vitro/in vivo* correlations of drug sensitivities

In a clinical pilot study (Volm *et al.*, 1979), patients with inoperable ovarian and lung carcinomas were treated by chemotherapy and the effectiveness of the treatment was compared with results of *in vitro* tests (Fig. 2). Patients were distributed into different groups according to the therapeutic regime adopted. Tumours that responded to clinical therapy are represented in Fig. 2 by closed symbols and non-responding tumours are denoted by open symbols. These data illustrate that tumours showing only a weak response to adriamycin treatment ($< 30\%$ inhibition at 0.01 mg ml^{-1}) in the *in vitro* test also failed to respond to chemotherapy in the clinic. Tumours that are strongly inhibited *in vitro* by adriamycin ($> 30\%$ inhibition) generally show some degree of remission clinically.

B. Controlled clinical trial for *in vitro/in vivo* correlations of drug sensitivities

Results of this first clinical study encouraged our group to start a controlled clinical trial predominantly in lung and ovarian cancers but also in other tumour types, using defined standard chemotherapy schedules to compare clinical responses with *in vitro* test results.

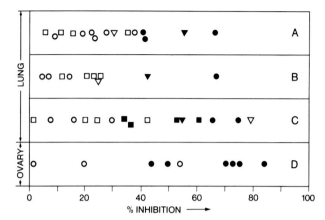

Fig. 2 Comparison of the results of *in vitro* tests and therapy of inoperable lung carcinomas (A–C) and ovarian carcinomas (D). Symbols for lung carcinomas: ○ small cell; ▽ adenocarcinoma, □ epidermoid. Values represent the inhibition (%) of uridine incorporation in the tumour cells *in vitro* due to adriamycin (10^{-2} mg ml^{-1}). Closed symbols: tumours that responded to clinical therapy. Open symbols: tumours that showed no reaction to chemotherapy. Schemes of therapy: group A, monotherapy with adriamycin; groups B–D, combination therapy.

In a cooperative study (KSST, 1981)* conducted by nine different hospitals between 1975 and 1979, results of the short-term test *in vitro* were compared with results of drug therapy in 155 patients. Seventy-two patients with ovarian carcinomas, 24 patients with lung carcinomas, and 18 patients with mammary carcinomas were treated according to a uniform therapy schedule. The remaining patients received alternative schedules.

In vitro drugs routinely used were tested at a range of concentrations, and, depending on the mode of action of the particular agent, an appropriate radioactive nucleic acid precursor was employed in the biochemical assay (see Chapter 6).

In Fig. 3 the *in vitro* test results, in which the effects of 4-hydroperoxycyclophosphamide (instead of cyclophosphamide, which is inactive *in vitro*) and

* This study was conducted by the Cooperative Study Group for Sensitivity Testing of Tumors (KSST). The following institutions (and investigators) participated in the study: German Cancer Research Center, Heidelberg (K. Goerttler, J. Mattern, M. Volm, K. Wayss, E. Weber); Departments of Obstetrics and Gynaecology of the Universities of Frankfurt (G. Bastert, H. Schmidt-Matthiesen), Freiburg (A. Pfleiderer, G. Teufel), Hamburg (M. Albrecht, G. Trams), Heidelberg (M. Kaufmann, F. Kubli), Mainz (R. Kreienberg, F. Melchert), Tübingen (J. Neunhoeffer), and Ulm (G. Geier, R. Schuhmann); Biology Chemistry Center, University of Frankfurt (H. J. Hohorst); Dept. Internal. Med., University of Münster (G. Segeth, G. Wüst); Rohrbach Hospital, Heidelberg (P. Drings, M. Kleckow, I. Vogt-Moykopf).

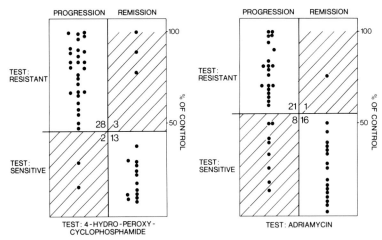

Fig. 3 Correlation between test results after addition of 4-hydroperoxycyclophos-phamide or adriamycin and results of therapy (cyclophosphamide, 5-fluorouracil) in solid ovarian carcinomas (stages III and IV).

adriamycin were determined, are compared with those of clinical therapy for solid non-pretreated ovarian carcinomas. All ovarian cancer patients were treated with a combination of cyclophosphamide and 5-fluorouracil. Tumours that responded only slightly in the *in vitro* test were also clinically progressive. Twenty-eight of 30 tumours that progressed clinically were resistant *in vitro* to 4-hydroperoxycyclophosphamide, whereas 13 of 16 tumours in remission were sensitive *in vitro*. In the tests with adriamycin, similar correlations were obtained between the "sensitive" and "resistant" *in vitro* results and clinical responses. The test was most accurate in predicting resistance of tumour detected by testing with adriamycin. Thus, out of 22 "solid" tumours that were resistant to the test, only one tumour showed a clinical remission. According to these results, a test using adriamycin only would appear to be sufficient to predict resistance of non-pretreated tumours to chemotherapy.

The *in vitro/in vivo* correlations of the clinical trial are summarized in Tables 1 and 2. Good correlations were observed between results *in vitro* using 4-hydroperoxycyclophosphamide and adriamycin and the *in vivo* responses of the different tumours, but the best correlations were obtained with the adriamycin–uridine test system.

To summarize the overall results, there were 151 comparisons of *in vitro* test results using adriamycin and results of clinical therapy (KSST, 1981). Of these 151 tumours, 76 were judged resistant and 75 sensitive in the *in vitro* test. Of these 76 "resistant" tumours, 56 were clinically progressive (73%), 2 (2%) were

Table 1 *In vitro/in vivo* correlation of chemosensitivity (S) and chemoresistance (R) for cells treated *in vitro* with 4-hydroperoxycyclophosphamide and patients treated with combination chemotherapy; patients showing neither remission nor progression of the disease have been excluded

Tumour sites	Patients	S/S	R/R	S/R	R/S
Ovarian carcinomas					
Solid tumours	46	13	28	2	3
Ascites and pleural effusions	12	5	3	2	2
Recurrences	15	2	9	2	2
Solid lung tumours	15	7	2	4	1
Various solid tumours	25	4	17	1	3
	113	31	59	11	12

For explanation of the notation S/S etc., see Table 2 of Chapter 18.

in remission, and 19 (25%) showed no change. Whilst in the 75 "sensitive" tumours 18 (24%) progressed clinically, 40 (53%) were in clinical remission and 17 (23%) were unchanged. The threshold between sensitivity and resistance differs between various tumour types (solid tumours, effusions) as well as between different drugs. Therefore, if only the definite progression or remission evaluations are compared with the *in vitro* results, 55 of the 57 tumours that were resistant in the test were clinically progressive (96%), and

Table 2 *In vitro/in vivo* correlation of chemosensitivity (S) and chemoresistance (R) for cells treated *in vitro* with adriamycin and patients treated *in vivo* with combination therapy; patients showing neither remission nor progression of disease have been omitted

Tumour sites	Patients	S/S	R/R	S/R	R/S
Ovarian carcinomas					
Solid tumours	46	16	21	8	1
Ascites and pleural effusions	11	6	3	2	0
Recurrences	14	3	8	3	0
Solid lung tumours	15	9	4	2	0
Various solid tumours	29	6	19	3	1
	115	40	55	18	2

40 of 58 tumours that were sensitive in the test showed clinical remission (69%). Thus resistant tumours are predictable with high accuracy and instances of *in vitro* resistance but sensitivity *in vivo* occurred in only a few cases.

In Fig. 4 survival times of the patients divided into two groups according to their test results (i.e. resistant or sensitive) are shown. There is good agreement between the *in vitro* test results and survival. Patients whose tumours were "resistant" in the test generally died sooner than patients with "sensitive" tumours.

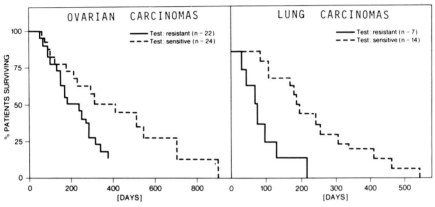

Fig. 4 Life tables for patients separated into either resistant or sensitive groups according to test results. The differences in the survival times are significant.

This cooperative trial confirmed that it is possible to predict chemo-resistance *in vitro*, and this is relevant for *in vivo* treatment. However, it is still not possible to predict with the same degree of accuracy drug specific chemosensitivity in primary non-pretreated advanced human carcinomas with this short-term test system.

A new study design has now been started for primary advanced ovarian carcinomas (FIGO stages III and IV). Chemotherapy is randomized between a choice of cis-platinum, adriamycin, and cyclophosphamide, or cis-platinum and cyclophosphamide, or cyclophosphamide alone. Stratification is carried out according to *in vitro* adriamycin test results (sensitive or resistant), and *in vitro/in vivo* correlations will be analysed for clinical response and survival.

C. Comparison of various trials with biochemical short-term assays

In Table 3 our *in vitro* test and clinical results are compared with results of other authors obtained using short-term incubations of cell suspensions with

Table 3 *In vitro/in vivo* correlation of chemosensitivity (S) and chemoresistance (R), and predictive accuracy (%) of correct positive (A) or correct negative (B) results.

S/S	R/R	S/R	R/S	A	B	Patients	Reference
19	25	5	0	79	100	49	Volm *et al.* (1979)
40	55	18	2	69	96	115	KSST (1981)*
24	57	13	0	65	100	94	Possinger *et al.* (1980)
42	31	5	16	89	66	94	Daidone *et al.* (1981)
125	168	41	18	75	90	352	

A = Correct positive prediction $[(S/S)/(S/S + S/R)] \times 100$.
B = Correct negative prediction $[(R/R)/(R/R + R/S)] \times 100$.
* Excluding cases where there was no change in the patient's condition.

drugs. In most studies described, chemoresistance is shown to be more successfully predicted than chemosensitivity, with the frequency of correct prediction being 75% for "sensitive" tumours but 90% for "resistant" tumours.

These results are based almost exclusively on retrospective investigations. It is necessary to emphasize that only prospective, randomized studies will definitely prove whether and to what extent results from predictive tests can be extrapolated to provide clinically suitable individual tumour therapy.

III. Discussion

No model system has yet been developed that is capable of exact simulation of the effects of a drug in the human body. Chemosensitivity of tumour cells detected outside the organism need not necessarily comply with the specific situation of a patient under the applied chemotherapy. Effective levels of antineoplastic agents in tumour tissues, for instance, may not be attained if the tumour or its metastases are poorly vascularized. Differing biotransformation of drugs or interaction between drugs may also play a role. For these reasons, false positive results (sensitivity *in vitro* but resistance *in vivo*) should be found more frequently than the converse. This has been confirmed in many analyses relating to attempted *in vitro/in vivo* correlations.

There are currently too few investigations and analyses to answer firmly the question of whether chemoresistance established *in vitro* is generally responsible for the failure of a range of cytotoxic chemotherapy protocols or whether there are actually drug-specific resistances that can also be predicted. Data now available from results obtained *in vitro* with survival times after corresponding chemotherapy tend to suggest that it is not drug-specific resistance that can be detected. Indeed, one essential factor for successful chemotherapy seems first and foremost to be a high proliferative activity of individual tumour cells.

In conclusion, the short-term test described here is not used to find the most effective drug, but merely to determine whether the tumour responds to any chemotherapy at all. According to our investigations, a test using adriamycin would appear to be sufficient to detect proliferation-dependent tumour resistance.

References

Daidone, M. G., Silvestrini, R. and Sanfilippo, O. (1981). Clinical relevance of an *in vitro* antimetabolic assay for monitoring human tumor chemosensitivity. In *Adjuvant Chemotherapy of Cancer*. III (ed. S. E. Salmon and S. C. Jones), pp. 25–32. Grune and Stratton, New York.

Hamburger, A. W. (1981). Use of *in vitro* tests in predictive cancer chemotherapy. *J. Nat. Cancer Inst.* **66,** 981–988.

Kaufmann, M. (1980). Clinical applications of *in vitro* chemosensitivity testing. In *Ovarian Cancer* (ed. C. E. Newman, C. H. J. Ford and J. A. Jordan). *Advances in the Biosciences*, Vol 26, pp. 189–210. Pergamon Press, Oxford.

KSST (Group for Sensitivity Testing of Tumors) (1981). *In vitro* short-term test to determine the resistance of human tumors to chemotherapy. *Cancer* **48,** 2127–2135.

Possinger, K., Hartenstein, R. and Ehrhart, H. (1980). In vitro Resistenztestung von Tumoren gegenüber Zytostatika. *Onkologie* **3,** 291–300.

Volm, M., Kaufmann, M., Hinderer, H. and Goerttler, K. (1970). Schnellmethode zur Sensibilitätstestung maligner Tumoren gegenüber Cytostatika. *Klin. Wochenschr.* **48,** 374–376.

Volm, M., Kaufmann, M., Mattern, J. and Wayss, K. (1975a). Möglichkeiten und Grenzen der prätherapeutischen Sensibilitätstestung von Tumoren gegen Zytostatika im Kurzzeittest. *Schweiz. Med. Wochenschr.* **105,** 74–82.

Volm, M., Kaufmann, M., Mattern, J. and Wayss, K. (1975b). Sensitivity tests of tumors to cytostatic agents. I. Comparative investigations on transplanted tumors *in vivo* and *in vitro*. *Z. Krebsforsch.* **83,** 85–96.

Volm, M., Wayss, K., Kaufmann, M. and Mattern, J. (1979). Pretherapeutic detection of tumour resistance and the results of tumour chemotherapy. *Eur. J. Cancer* **15,** 983–993.

21. Results Obtained Using a Vital Dye Exclusion Assay and Clinical Correlations

W. J. DURKIN, V. K. GHANTA and R. N. HIRAMOTO

I. Introduction

Measurement of tumour cell sensitivity has been an unrealized goal of cancer therapy for decades. A human bone marrow aspirate mistakenly taken several hours after drug administration was carefully reviewed as a protocol violation. This sensitive human tissue exhibited marked megaloblastosis less than 24 hours after drug administration. This observation suggested that cytotoxic drugs exert powerful effects on sensitive cells over a short time scale; also, the possibility of quantifying a predictive effect occurring shortly after drug exposure seemed feasible.

Numerous microcytotoxicity assays have been described. The most widely employed clinical assay is the vital dye exclusion assay employed for the HLA assay (Terasaki *et al.*, 1978). Since cell death is a clear endpoint, studies were done *in vitro* to correlate this endpoint with drug levels in cancer patients. If the drug concentration in plasma is plotted as a function of time, the area under the curve (AUC) provides estimates of the duration of contact by cancer cells with the drug *in vivo*. Conditions that correlated with response and resistance to drug therapy initially were defined in tumour models. Human neoplastic cells were then investigated. A good correlation was noted in these studies between *in vivo* responsiveness and *in vitro* chemotherapy results in both animal models and human neoplasms (Durkin *et al.*, 1979).

II. Materials and methods

A. Tissue culture conditions and drugs

All *in vitro* experiments were performed in medium 199 containing glutamine

(0.7 mM), Hepes (25 mM), foetal calf serum (10% FCS), penicillin (50 U ml^{-1}), and streptomycin (50 μg ml^{-1}), at 37°C unless otherwise specified.

Adriamycin (Adria Laboratories, Wilmington, Delaware) and vinblastine (Lilly and Company, Indianapolis, Indiana) were procured commercially. BCNU and cis-platinum were obtained from the National Cancer Institute, Bethesda, Maryland.

B. Cytotoxicity assay

Cytotoxicity was measured with the trypan blue dye exclusion test. Cells were incubated for 4 min with 0.167% trypan blue and 5% foetal calf serum. Viable cells were identified by their ability to exclude dye. At least 100 cells were counted for each experimental value recorded. The cytotoxicity index (CI) is defined as:

$$CI = \left(1 - \frac{\% \text{ Viable Treated Cells}}{\% \text{ Viable Control Cells}}\right) \times 100$$

C. Drug concentration studies

Tumour cells were incubated in tissue culture media containing a range of drug concentrations. After 24 hours of drug exposure the cytotoxicity index was measured. A log range of drug concentrations associated with a CI $\geqslant$ 20 (i.e. less than 80% control values) was identified. This log range was then further investigated at intermediate values. The lowest drug concentration associated with measurable cytotoxicity (CI $\geqslant$ 20) after 24 hours of drug exposure was identified for further study.

D. Duration of drug exposure studies

To determine the duration of drug exposure required to affect cytotoxicity, tumour cells were incubated for variable time periods with drug at the lowest cytotoxic (CI $\geqslant$ 20) concentration. The drug was then removed, tumour cells were incubated in a drug-free environment for 48 hours, and the cytotoxicity index was measured. A dose–response curve was defined involving three variables: (i) concentration of drug; (ii) duration of drug exposure; (iii) cytotoxicity due to drug exposure.

E. Clinical studies

1. *Patient characteristics*

Patients were studied provided that (a) a pathologic diagnosis of malignant lymphoma was established, (b) malignant tissue was available for study, (c) measurable parameters of disease were present, and (d) the patient was a candidate for single agent therapy with either BCNU or adriamycin. Prior chemotherapy and radiotherapy were allowable provided that none of the agents under study had been previously administered. All prior antineoplastic treatment was terminated at least 30 days before study entry.

2. *In vitro studies*

After surgical removal, a pathologically enlarged lymph node was cut into two pieces. One piece was processed for pathological examination. The other half was teased aseptically in tissue culture medium to make a single cell suspension. This suspension was centrifuged and the supernatant discarded. The cell pellet was washed, suspended in medium, and carefully layered on top of Ficoll-Isopaque in a test tube according to the method of Böyum (1967). The preparation was then centrifuged at 400 *g* for 40 min at room temperature. Cells located at the interface were carefully removed, washed twice, and suspended in tissue culture medium. Cells were exposed to antineoplastic agents *in vitro* as described earlier. Two days later the CI was measured. These experiments were conducted in quintuplicate and results were reported as the mean $\pm$ standard error. It was not ethically possible to study tumour preparations repetitively on different days, since each study requires freshly biopsied human tumour tissue.

3. *Treatment programme*

BCNU was given at a dosage of 150 mg m^{-2} every 6 weeks. Adriamycin was given at a dosage of 60 mg m^{-2} every 3 weeks or 20 mg m^{-2} weekly. Concurrent steroid therapy was permitted if the patient had received corticosteroids for more than 2 months prior to the study.

III. Results

In selected referred patients with non-Hodgkin's lymphoma, biopsy is necessary when the clinical course conflicts with the original tissue diagnosis or when original tissue is unavailable for histologic review. These patients generally have been extensively treated with combination drug therapy, usually cyclophosphamide, vincristine, and prednisone, or are appropriately treated with single agent BCNU or adriamycin, two of the *in vitro* drugs studied. Cis-platinum, an investigational drug, and vinblastine, an inactive drug, could not be justified for use in our preliminary studies. Eleven single agent clinical trials were conducted in seven patients whose tumours were studied *in vitro*. In each instance *in vitro* cytotoxicity results paralleled results of *in vivo* human drug treatment.

A. Selection of *in vitro* dosage

The *in vivo* serum level of all four antineoplastic agents has been reported (see Table 1). The *in vitro* dosage that produced 50% cell death in drug-sensitive tumour cells did not conflict with available clinical pharmacokinetic data.

Table 1 Comparison of derived *in vitro* concentration and time of exposure with reported *in vivo* values (Durkin *et al.*, 1979)

Drug	*In vitro* exposure time (min)	*In vitro* concentration (μg ml^{-1})	Drug concentration (μg ml^{-1}) × exposure time (min)		References
			in vitro	*in vivo*	
Adriamycin	42	2.0	84	94	Benjamin *et al.* (1977)
Vinblastine	51	0.4	20	20	Owellen *et al.* (1977)
Cis-platinum	33	20.0	660	500–1000	Conran (1974)
BCNU	25	20.0	500	200–1200	DeVita *et al.* (1967) Ogawa *et al.* (1973)

Measurable cytotoxicity occurred with clinical dose levels for the sensitive tumour cells in an *in vitro* environment. This measure of cytotoxicity was postulated to be less in resistant neoplasms.

B. Lymphoma treatment results

Seven patients with a diagnosis of malignant non-Hodgkin's lymphoma were studied. Although all the patients had received prior treatment, none had been treated with any of the agents under study. Only one drug was administered during a single treatment period. The age range was 42–71 years. No patient had a Karnofsky performance score below 80 at the start of therapy. All patients had measurable and progressive disease.

Response criteria were conventional (Table 2). Three patients achieved partial remission status. Two patients responded to BCNU and one patient responded to adriamycin. No patient experienced complete disappearance of all measurable evidence of disease. There were eight instances in which patients did not respond. Full-dosage drug therapy was continued for 6 weeks before a patient was considered a non-responder.

Table 2 Effects of adriamycin and BCNU on human malignant lymphomas *in vivo* and *in vitro* (Durkin *et al.*, 1979)

Trial	Patient	Drug	*In vitro* % CI*	*In vivo* treatment†	Correlation‡	Diagnosis (Rappaport classification§)
1	1	Adriamycin	46 ± 2	PR	+	Poorly differentiated lymphocytic lymphoma, diffuse
2	2	BCNU	46 ± 3	PR	+	Poorly differentiated lymphocytic lymphoma, nodular
3	3	Adriamycin	4 ± 2	NR	+	Poorly differentiated
4	3	BCNU	42 ± 2	PR	+	lymphocytic lymphoma, nodular, with transformation to diffuse histiocytic lymphoma
5	4	Adriamycin	22 ± 2	NR	+	Well differentiated
6	4	BCNU	36 ± 2	NR	+	lymphocytic lymphoma, diffuse
7	5	Adriamycin	0 ± 1	NR	+	Poorly differentiated
8	5	BCNU	14 ± 6	NR	+	lymphocytic lymphoma, diffuse
9	6	Adriamycin	0 ± 4	NR	+	Well differentiated
10	6	BCNU	19 ± 5	NR	+	lymphocytic lymphoma, diffuse
11	7	BCNU	18 ± 4	NR	+	Poorly differentiated lymphocytic lymphoma, diffuse

* Mean $\pm$ S.E.

† PR, partial remission (a 50% or greater reduction in measured tumour surface area, unassociated with the development of new lesions, lasting 1 month or longer); NR, no remission (a patient not meeting partial response criteria).

‡ A positive correlation associated *in vitro* cytotoxicity of $>40\%$ with an active *in vivo* antineoplastic agent and *in vitro* cytotoxicity of $<40\%$ with an inactive *in vivo* antineoplastic agent ($P<0.01$).

§ Banks and Berard, 1977.

Toxicity was predictable and generally mild. Dosage reduction was necessary in only one case, since the patient had extensive marrow involvement and a compromised haematologic status. In one patient receiving full dose BCNU, severe myelosuppression (an absolute granulocyte count below 1000 mm^{-3} and resulting sepsis) occurred. There were no drug associated deaths.

C. Clinical correlation of *in vitro* studies

Malignant human tissue was studied before clinical drug therapy was undertaken. All tumour tissues were studied *in vitro* with each of the four drugs. In no instance was there evidence of tumour susceptibility to cis-platinum or vinblastine. In three instances a high CI was recorded. In one instance the high CI was due to adriamycin, while in the other two instances elevation was associated with BCNU.

A clinical correlation was demonstrable. The three instances of *in vitro* tumour susceptibility were paralleled by tumour regression with treatment. The eight demonstrated instances of *in vitro* tumour resistance correlated to the clinical instance by tumour progression with treatment ($P < 0.1$) (Table 2). There were seven instances in which *in vitro* studies demonstrated no activity for vinblastine, which conforms to reports of a lack of disease activity for this drug. No definitive statements have been made regarding a clinical correlation of seven consecutive negative *in vitro* studies with cis-platinum, since trials with cis-platinum in non-Hodgkin's lymphoma have not been completed. When all tests in animals and man were combined, a positive correlation was found associating *in vitro* cytotoxicity of $> 40\%$ with an active antineoplastic agent *in vivo* ($P < 0.00001$).

IV. Discussion

A. Considerations for use of *in vitro* cytotoxicity testing

Chemotherapeutic agents while effective in some patients with malignant diseases are totally ineffective in others. Clinical drug therapy of malignant disease is rooted today in the probabilities and statistics of benefit based on large numbers of similarly treated patients. Definition of methods for prediction of drug efficacy for individual neoplasms would be of enormous benefit.

Most cancer chemotherapeutic agents have been demonstrated to have relatively steep dose–response curves. This implies that all mammalian cells may be killed if an excessive dosage is employed. Conversely, if the dosage is inadequate, no mammalian cell may even be injured. An *in vitro* dosage must therefore be defined that kills susceptible cells but minimally affects resistant tumour cells. This determination should correspond to clinical measurements of serum drug concentration and half-life.

B. Dosage

A major limitation of previous studies has been the inability to determine an *in vitro* drug dosage that corresponds to the *in vivo* situation. Present pharmacologic principles suggest that, within limits, the following equation holds true *in vivo*: $C \times T = K$ (Vessel, 1974, Oliverio, 1971; discussed in Chapter 17), where C is concentration, T is time, and K is a specific pharmacologic effect. While it is difficult to duplicate the fluctuating curve of *in vivo* drug exposure, it is possible to integrate mathematically the total drug exposure curve.

To ensure that *in vitro* studies are relevant to *in vivo* treatment, two essential criteria must be fulfilled. The *in vivo* and *in vitro* doses should correspond and dosage effects must be quantifiable and comparable. Dose–response curves should be established and compared. An *in vitro* dosage can then be determined that (i) produces effects similar to *in vivo* therapeutic effects and (ii) correlates with the known *in vivo* data of serum drug level and half-life. Measuring effects of such an *in vitro* dosage would then predict the drug treatment to be used on the cancer-bearing host. Dosages to be selected for *in vitro* testing should be based on the pharmacokinetic data of the drug used in man. Drug levels are measured from the area under the serum level–time curve (AUC) given in μg min ml^{-1} (as discussed in Chapter 17 by Metcalfe).

C. Drug metabolism

Metabolic drug alteration is a phenomenon that has been well described. Tissue culture study of anticancer agents can only be relevant to the *in vivo* situation if (i) the drug is directly cytotoxic and (ii) the drug has not been demonstrated to have a metabolite more active than the parent compound. Adriamycin (Drewinko and Gottlieb, 1973), cis-platinum (Rosenberg, 1975), BCNU (Ogawa *et al.*, 1973), and vinblastine (Tucker *et al.*, 1977) are directly cytotoxic and no metabolite has been identified that is more active than the parent compound.

D. *In vitro* quantitation of drug effect

Cytotoxic effects have been primarily studied *in vitro* through either biochemical or viability measurements. Biochemical efforts have centred on metabolic studies. Cytotoxic studies inhibit the synthesis of DNA, RNA, protein, glycolysis, aerobic metabolism, or other parameters. Viability

W. J. Durkin, V. K. Ghanta and R. N. Hiramoto

measurements have emphasized either proliferative capacity or surface membrane integrity (Hodges, 1976). Measures of growth inhibition and surface membrane injury have been considered to be representative of tumour cell death.

Since tumour cell death occurs *in vivo* after drug therapy, an *in vitro* viability measure would correspond closely to the *in vivo* situation. However, it should be remembered that the goal of predictive testing is not to define the optimal *in vitro* measure of "viability" but rather to define a clinically employable methodology to predict anticancer drug effects in man. A clinical viability test would involve quantitation of either proliferative function or surface membrane function. Many authors currently consider the former more exact, but the latter tends to have been more widely used. Tests of proliferative capacity generally quantitate colony formation after inoculation with specific tumour cell numbers in cell cultures. Cell surface membrane integrity can be assessed easily with either chromium release or vital dye staining. Inhibition of colony formation, cell staining, and chromium release are all quantifiable measures of drug effect. Recent advances have demonstrated that cloning studies do have the capacity to predict tumour sensitivity in certain instances (Salmon *et al.*, 1978, and Chapter 25).

Trypan blue dye exclusion is considered to be a measure of cell surface membrane integrity. Uptake of dye by a cell indicates a loss of surface membrane function and cell death by membrane criteria (Phillips, 1973).

Whilst most studies have centred on growth inhibition or reproductive cell death as an endpoint, it has been emphasized that drug dosage that inhibits replication often does not affect membrane cell death. However, it has not been emphasized that a reproductively dead cell may still be living. A good example of reproductively dead but living cells includes all red cells, granulocytes, and platelets in the blood stream. Reproduction and physical death are different endpoints.

The trypan blue viability test has been successfully adapted for clinical use. The microcytotoxicity test for HLA tissue-typing successfully uses the trypan blue viability test as a rapid means of providing predictive information. The trypan blue study has also provided useful experimental data (Kataoka *et al.*, 1978; Markland *et al.*, 1978; Kosloski *et al.*, 1978). Recent investigations have, however, criticized this trypan blue method, since it has been pointed out that cells inhibited from proliferation may retain their capacity to exclude the dye. Indeed, the drug dosage that inhibits colony formation is inadequate to effect cell death as measured by trypan blue. However, it should be borne in mind that clonogenicity and dye exclusion do not measure the same cellular function.

The goal of cancer chemotherapy is to provide the patient with effective drug treatment. A practical and accurate methodology must be identified if predictive testing is to be clinically employed. It has been shown that viability studies of proliferative function can predict tumour sensitivity. Likewise our studies have shown that viability studies of surface membrane function can predict drug sensitivity. Since cloning and dye exclusion testing are measures of different cell functions, experimental conditions necessary to predict drug efficacy should not be expected to be identical.

V. Summary

Recent advances have made it possible to treat cancer cells *in vitro* with a drug dosage bearing resemblance to the *in vivo* situation. Pharmacologic procedures have defined the *in vivo* pharmacokinetic behaviour of many antineoplastic agents, providing a basis for *in vivo* and *in vitro* drug dosage comparison.

While dosage is an obviously critical factor, mechanisms of drug action are also important. Suspending tumour cells in tissue culture medium can alter tumour cell kinetics. Altering kinetics may affect tumour sensitivity to cycle-specific agents. Alternatively, sensitive tumours are thought to be susceptible to non-cycle-specific agents regardless of kinetic alterations. These considerations suggest that *in vitro* drug treatment would correspond to the *in vivo* situation if (i) the studied drug is cycle-non-specific in action, (ii) *in vivo* and *in vitro* drug dosages are equivalent, (iii) the studied drug does not have a metabolite more active than the parent compound, and (iv) *in vivo* and *in vitro* treatment endpoints are similar.

Based on fundamental considerations, we studied *in vitro* effects of adriamycin, BCNU, vinblastine, and cis-platinum. We devised a series of *in vitro* tests that agreed with the known non-cycle-specificity of the agents studied, the known facts of intercellular drug transport, and the known *in vivo* measurements of serum drug level and drug half-life. Seven human tumours were studied. The *in vitro* cytotoxicity correlated closely with subsequent *in vivo* results of drug therapy in all patients.

Acknowledgements

This work was supported by research grants from the National Cancer Institute, National Institutes of Health, R01-CA-27765, CA-25965, and CA-16699.

References

Banks, P. M. and Berard, C. E. (1977). Histopathology of the malignant lymphomas. In *Hematology* (ed. W. Williams, E. Beutler, A. Ersley and R. Rundles), pp. 1026–1037. McGraw Hill, New York.

Benjamin, R. S., Riggs, C. E. and Bachur, N. R. (1977). Plasma pharmacokinetics of adriamycin and its metabolites in humans with normal hepatic and renal function. *Cancer Res.* **37**, 1416–1420.

Böyum, A. (1967). Separation of leukocytes from blood and bone marrow. *Scand. J. Clin. Invest.* **21**, 9–109.

Conran, P. B. (1974). Pharmacokinetics of platinum compounds. *Recent Results Cancer Res.* **48**, 124–136.

DeVita, V. T., Denham, C. and Davidson, J. D. (1967). The physiological disposition of the carcinostatic 1,3-bis-(2-chloroethyl)-1-nitrosourea (BCNU) in man and animals. *Clin. Pharmacol. Therap.* **8**, 566–577.

Drewinko, B. and Gottlieb, J. A. (1973). Survival kinetics of cultured human lymphoma cells exposed to adriamycin. *Cancer Res.* **33**, 1141–1145.

Durkin, W. J., Ghanta, V. K., Balch, C. M., Davis, D. W. and Hiramoto, R. N. (1979). A methodological approach to the prediction of anticancer drug effect in humans. *Cancer Res.* **39**, 402–407.

Hodges, G. M. (1976). An overview of tissue culture procedures in tumor biopsy studies. In *Human Tumors in Short Term Culture* (ed. P. P. Dendy), pp. 3–14. Academic Press, New York.

Kataoka, T., Kobayashi, H. and Sakurai, Y. (1978). Potentiation of concanavalin A bound L1210 vaccine *in vivo* by chemotherapeutic agents. *Cancer Res.* **38**, 1201–1207.

Kosloski, M. J., Rosen, F., Millholland, R. J. and Papahadjopoulos, D. (1978). Effect of lipid vesicle (liposome) encapsulation of methotrexate on its chemotherapeutic efficacy in solid rodent tumors. *Cancer Res.* **38**, 2848–2853.

Markland, F. S., Chopp, R. T., Cosgrove, M. D. and Howard, E. B. (1978). Characterization of steroid hormone receptors in the Dunning R-3327 rat prostatic adenocarcinoma. *Cancer Res.* **38**, 2818–2826.

Ogawa, M., Bergasgel, D. E. and McCulloch, E. A. (1973). Chemotherapy of mouse myeloma: quantitative cell cultures predictive of response *in vivo*. *Blood* **41**, 7–15.

Oliverio, V. T. (1971). Pharmacology in the chemotherapy drug development program of the National Cancer Institute. *Cancer Chemother. Rep.* **2**, 73–79.

Owellen, R. J., Bortke, C. A. and Hains, F. (1977). Pharmacokinetics and metabolism of vinblastine in humans. *Cancer Res.* **37**, 2597–2602.

Phillips, H. J. (1973). Dye exclusion tests for cell viability. In *Tissue Culture* (ed. P. F. Kruse and M. K. Patterson), p. 406. Academic Press, New York.

Rosenberg, B. (1975). Possible mechanisms for the antitumor activity of platinum coordination complexes. *Cancer Chemother. Rep.* **59**, 589–598.

Salmon, S. E., Hamburger, A. W., Soehnlen, B., Durie, B., Alberts, D. and Moon, P. (1978). Quantitation of differential sensibility of human-tumor stem cells to anticancer drugs. *New Engl. J. Med.* **298**, 1321–1327.

Terasaki, P. I., Bernoco, D., Park, M., Ozturk, G. and Iwaki, Y. (1978). Micro-droplet testing for HLA A, B, C, and D antigens. *Am. J. Clin. Pathol.* **69**, 103–120.

Tucker, R. W., Owellen, R. J. and Harris, S. B. (1977). Correlation of cytotoxicity and mitotic spindle dissolution by vinblastine in mammalian cells. *Cancer Res.* **37**, 2346–4351.

Vessel, E. S. (1974). Relationship between drug distribution and therapeutic effects in man. *Ann. Rev. Pharmacol.* **14**, 249–271.

22. Results Obtained Using Assays of Intermediate Duration and Clinical Correlations

J. L. DARLING and D. G. T. THOMAS

I. Introduction

Chemosensitivity assays fall into three broad groups (Dendy, 1981): tests where the residual viability of tumour cells is measured within a few minutes of drug treatment (Mattern *et al.*, Chapter 6); long-term tests where viability is determined after 14–21 days in culture (these are usually tests where the clonogenicity of drug treated cells is determined; Salmon, Chapter 24); tests of intermediate duration where viability is measured within 1–3 days of drug removal.

Tests of the third type have a number of attractive features. For example, the degree of cytotoxicity can be measured by isotopic uptake or cell counts, both techniques that can be automated quite easily. They also frequently utilize microtitration plates which greatly simplifies handling of 60 or 96 replicate cultures. With a large number of replicate cultures derived from a relatively small amount of tumour material it is possible to produce dose–response curves over a large range of drug concentrations, to test a statistically acceptable number of replicates, and to test drug combinations *in vitro*.

The principles of these types of test have been examined by Freshney and Dendy in Chapter 7, so only brief mention of the technical aspects will be made here and this chapter will be concerned predominantly with their clinical application.

II. Assays utilizing cell counts or visual assessment of cytotoxicity

From the earliest days of drug sensitivity testing, visual assessments have been used to quantify drug effects. A number of early workers used this approach

269

(Easty and Wylie, 1963; Dendy, 1968) although until relatively recently no clinical correlations had been made. Dendy and his colleagues (Dendy et al., 1970) reported three case studies where the results of drug sensitivity tests carried out on serial tumour biopsies in vitro accurately predicted the clinical findings. This same group later studied the clinical progress of a larger series of patients (Wheeler et al., 1974). In this study the patients were divided into two groups. The treatment of patients in group A followed the test results closely in that when only one drug was recommended it was used or when more than one agent was recommended at least two were used. Patients in group B received treatment that did not follow the test closely; for example, when more than one drug was recommended only one drug was used. Careful examination of the data was carried out to ensure that patients in group A were not favourably biased in respect of the site of their primary tumour, the hospital where they were treated, or the nature of the specimen used for chemosensitivity testing. There was little difference between the two groups in terms of age distribution, clinical stage, or histological grading. The results indicated that more group A patients survived in the early months of treatment. However, after 2 years the number of patients surviving in both groups was the same. Using a larger group of 88 patients all with ovarian carcinoma, Dendy (1981) has been able to produce survival curves for group A and group B patients (Fig. 1). They show clearly that in early months survival was better when treatment closely followed test predictions, and the median survival of these patients was almost twice as long as for those who did not follow the test prediction. However, this advantage was transient and was lost within 2 years.

Holmes and Little (1974) described a microtitration test in which cells were treated for 72 hours with drugs before being trypsinized and counted with a Coulter counter. A 40% reduction in cell numbers, compared with control cultures, was considered a significant in vitro response. No attempt was made to influence therapy and all correlations were made retrospectively. In 11/12 patients response was accurately predicted. The twelfth patient was treated clinically with chlorambucil, to which he responded, and tested against chlorambucil (no response in vitro) and nitrogen mustard (response in vitro). The authors suggest that the alkylating effect of activated chlorambucil resembles that of nitrogen mustard. An alternative approach was adopted by Lickiss et al. (1974) who assessed the degree of cell confluence after drug treatment using a Chalkley graticule. They reported a single clinical correlation where an osteolytic rib lesion was tested in vitro and found to be sensitive to vincristine and cyclophosphamide, but insensitive to 5-fluorouracil, methotrexate, and procarbazine. The patient was treated pragmatically with nitrogen mustard, vincristine, procarbazine, and prednisone, and responsed to chemotherapy. The main objection to observations of this kind is that it is difficult to assess which drug initiates the response. Although it seems

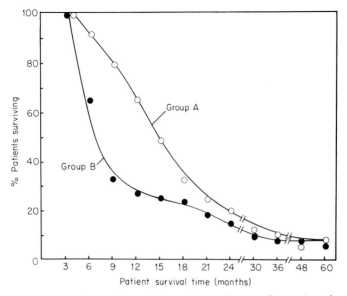

Fig. 1 Survival curves for patients with ovarian carcinoma. Group A patients (open symbols) were treated with chemotherapy in accordance with the chemosensitivity assay and Group B patients (solid symbols) were treated pragmatically. (Dendy, 1981)

attractive to suppose that the tumour responded to vincristine, it may have actually responded to nitrogen mustard which was not tested *in vitro*.

Terasaki plates have recently been used for measurement of brain tumour chemosensitivity. Kornblith *et al.* (1981) compared chemosensitivities of a panel of 14 gliomas with the clinical response of the patients to BCNU. The assay used a 1 hour exposure to BCNU followed by a 20–24 hour recovery period after which cells were fixed, stained, and counted under a microscope (Kornblith and Szypko, 1978). All patients had histologically confirmed high grade astrocytomas, and all had undergone postoperative radiotherapy (4500–5000 rads), at least two courses of BCNU or CCNU, and had two or more CT scans during chemotherapy. In reality only one of the 14 patients described had been treated with BCNU, and that was only one course followed by eight courses of CCNU. Another patient had been treated with CCNU, vincristine, and procarbazine, and one had been treated with CCNU and methotrexate. The remaining 11 patients had all been treated with CCNU. The present authors (Thomas and Darling, 1981) have found CCNU to be satisfactory in chemosensitivity assays, even considering its relative insolubility in aqueous solutions. It has been suggested, however, that cellular sensitivity (Rosenblum, 1980) and tumour response (Fewer *et al.*, 1972) are equivalent for BCNU and CCNU. *In vitro* response was defined as a 25% or greater cell kill at a clinically achievable dose of BCNU; the results are shown in Table 1. There was correct prediction in 10/13 patients (5 true positives, 5 true negatives). There were 3 false positives (cases where the *in vitro* test suggested sensitivity, but where there was no clinical response). There were no false negatives. Using a similar microtitration assay Yung *et al.* (1982) have found considerable heterogeneity in sensitivity to BCNU and cis-diammine-dichloroplatinum (CDDP) between six karyotypically distinct clonal cell lines isolated from two malignant gliomas. This finding confirms the observation that gliomas are heterogeneous with regard to many phenotypic character-istics (Bigner *et al.*, 1981), not only between tumours of similar histology but even within the same tumour. It may also explain the relative lack of efficacy of single agents in chemotherapy of glioma.

III. Assays using isotopic uptake as an index of cytotoxicity

A. ^{35}S-Methionine assay

Over half the brain tumours diagnosed in adults prove to be malignant gliomas of the cerebral hemispheres (Graham, 1980). Treatment of these tumours by surgery and radiotherapy alone is ineffective; the median survival is 5–6 months from operation, and fewer than 10% of patients are alive at 2 years (Walker and Gehan, 1976). There is therefore considerable interest in developing effective chemotherapy.

Table 1 *In vitro/in vivo* correlations of 14 patients with malignant gliomas, using a cell counting assay (Kornblith *et al.*, 1981)

	Patients	Sensitive *in vitro* Sensitive *in vivo*	Sensitive *in vitro* Resistant *in vivo*	Resistant *in vitro* Resistant *in vivo*	Resistant *in vitro* Sensitive *in vivo*
Astrocytoma (grade III)	3*	2	0	0	0
Astrocytoma (grades III–IV)	5	1	1	3	0
Astrocytoma (grade IV)	6	2	2	2	0

* One tumour could not be evaluated because no evidence of tumour on postoperative CT scan.

Nitrosoureas are among the most effective drugs in the treatment of glioma, their success being partly due to their lipid solubility which allows them to cross the blood brain barrier (BBB). Some authors have argued that the BBB is severely disrupted within the tumour and that any drug should be able to pass into the neoplasm (Vick et al., 1977). Others, however, have suggested that the concentration of drug passing through a "leaky" capillary tends to fall rapidly within the tumour by diffusing down a steep concentration gradient into normal brain or cerebrospinal fluid. This effectively reduces the exposure of the tumour to high drug concentrations. Alternatively, it may be that, although within the body of the tumour the BBB is defective, the aggressive growing outer edge has a partially intact barrier and is therefore not effectively treated. In any case, all nitrosoureas tested as single agents have been found effective, with remission rates of up to 50% of patients, and this benefit may be sustained for up to 9 months. It would therefore be of importance to predict those patients who would benefit from nitrosourea therapy and from the small number of alternative drugs that are suitable for glioma chemotherapy. The present authors have been working with a microtitration plate assay in which the degree of drug sensitivity is measured by ^{35}S-methionine uptake (Freshney and Morgan, 1978; Thomas et al., 1979; Morgan et al., 1983). The methodology is described in detail by Freshney and Dendy in Chapter 7.

Patients in this study all had high grade astrocytomas (Kernohan grades III or IV) and were treated with a combination of surgery, radiotherapy and chemotherapy. A combination regimen comprising orally administered CCNU in combination with procarbazine and vincristine (PCV protocol) was used. In a preliminary investigation of this regimen Shapiro and Young (1976) attained a projected median survival of over 50 weeks in their patients.

In the protocol adopted by the present authors, patients underwent surgery, ranging from formal lobectomy to simple burr hole biopsy. Radiation was administered to the whole head in fractionated doses until a total dose of 4000–5000 rads was achieved. From 2 to 6 weeks after completion of radiation therapy, patients began chemotherapy with vincristine (1.4 mg m^{-2} i.v. as a single dose), CCNU (110 mg m^{-2} as a single oral dose), and procarbazine (orally, 60 mg m^{-2} per day for 10 days). They were then monitored clinically and haematologically on an outpatient basis at 6 week intervals. Patients had 12 cycles of treatment over an 18 month period, and during this time CT scanning was performed every 3 months. The time course until disease progression, defined as a marked deterioration in clinical status usually accompanied by a worsening of the CT scan, was determined for all patients. The time between operation and relapse was termed the relapse free interval. This was chosen as the endpoint rather than survival since extensive use of high-dose glucocorticoids to control cerebral oedema can prolong survival considerably even in the face of obvious tumour recurrence. The survival time was also recorded.

In order to test the correlation between *in vitro* sensitivity and clinical progress, cultures were treated as previously described (Freshney and Dendy, Chapter 7; Thomas *et al.*, 1979) against each of the three drugs used clinically. Cultures were treated with drugs on three consecutive days and uptake of ^{35}S-methionine was determined at various time intervals during recovery. Cultures were designated as responders if the ID_{50} (dose of drug that inhibited protein synthesis by 50%) fell or remained stable during recovery, or as non-responders if the ID_{50} rose. In a preliminary analysis of the study, a direct comparison was made between the relapse free interval and *in vitro* sensitivity. It was found that, of three patients with grade III astrocytomas who survived longer than 2 years following operation, two had responses to 3/3 drugs and one to 2/3 drugs whereas one patient who survived only 17 weeks had no response to any drug. In two patients with grade IV astrocytomas, one patient responded to 3/3 drugs and survived over 1 year while another patient had no response to any drug and survived only 24 weeks (Darling and Thomas, 1981; Thomas *et al.*, 1982). In a larger series of 99 patients treated with the PCV protocol it has been possible to make a retrospective correlation with 33 patients. Relapse free interval curves were produced for responders and non-responders to each of the three drugs (Fig. 2). The result suggests that *in vitro* response to CCNU and procarbazine may be of clinical importance but that any response to vincristine seems to make little difference to the relapse free interval. Although the number of responders is small, these are interesting preliminary findings.

B. ^{3}H uptake assays

Although a number of authors have produced methodologies based on residual protein synthesis measured by ^{3}H uptake (Freshney *et al.*, 1975), only recently have any *in vitro* clinical correlations been reported. Wilson and Neal (1981) have described the sensitivity of ovarian carcinoma to a number of cytotoxic drugs. In their assay tumour cells were exposed to drugs for 48 hours and then allowed a period of 24 hours recovery. After a 3-hour pulse of ^{3}H-leucine the endpoint was determined by scintillation spectrometry (Freshney *et al.*, 1975). As might be expected, tumour specimens exhibited considerable heterogeneity in their response to cytotoxic drugs. In 15 patients, who all had stage III or stage IV ovarian carcinoma, it was possible to compare *in vitro* data with clinical response. Two subgroups of patients were considered; the first contained 8 patients who had only received first line chemotherapy, and the second comprised 7 patients who had relapsed on first line chemotherapy and were now undergoing second line chemotherapy. A clinical response was defined as "complete" if there was alleviation of

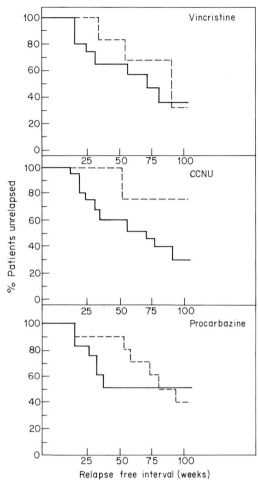

Fig. 2 Relapse-free interval curves for patients with malignant glioma. Sensitivity measured with the ^{35}S-methionine uptake assay. Dashed lines represent responders *in vitro* and solid lines represent non-responders *in vitro*.

symptoms, disappearance of palpable masses, and absence of ascitic fluid accumulation for at least 3 months, and "partial" if there was alleviation of symptoms, subjectively or objectively, for more than 3 months on first line chemotherapy and more than 1 month with second line chemotherapy. Sensitivity *in vitro* was defined as $> 50\%$ inhibition of ^{3}H-leucine uptake and resistance as $< 50\%$ ^{3}H-leucine uptake at clinically achievable drug doses. The results of this study are summarized in Table 2. Two of the three patients who received first line chemotherapy and were apparently sensitive *in vitro* but did

Table 2 *In vitro/in vivo* correlations of 15 patients with stages III and IV ovarian carcinoma, using a ^{3}H-uptake assay (Wilson and Neal, 1981)

	Sensitive *in vitro*		Resistant *in vitro*	
	1st line chemotherapy	2nd line chemotherapy	1st line chemotherapy	2nd line chemotherapy
Clinical responder	6 (complete) 1 (partial)	3 (partials)	0	0
Clinical non-responder	0	3*	1	1

* Equivocal cases; see text.

not respond clinically were said to be equivocal cases because combinations of drugs with differing *in vitro* activities were used in their treatment. There was generally greater drug resistance in tumour cells taken from treated patients than in those taken from previously untreated ones. This confirmed Percival's (1974) observation that the first course of chemotherapy for ovarian carcinoma is often the most effective.

C. ^{3}H-thymidine uptake assays

The use of tritiated thymidine as an index of cytotoxicity in leukaemic cells has been assessed by Raich (1978). In this microtitration plate assay, 10^5 leukaemic cells in 100 μl were added to 100 μl of cytosine arabinoside (ara-C) solution (0.5 μg ml^{-1}) to yield a final concentration of 0.25 μg ml^{-1}, a dose well below that clinically attainable (Alberts and Chen, 1980). After 36 hours incubation, 2 μCi of ^{3}H-thymidine was added to each well and the cells were labelled for 8 hours. Residual uptake was measured with an automated precipitator and counts were expressed as a percentage of control uptake. It was possible to correlate the *in vitro* results with clinical response in 26 patients: 9 patients with acute lymphocytic leukaemia (ALL), 7 patients with myelocytic leukaemia (AML), 6 patients with myelomonocytic leukaemia (AMML), 3 patients with monocytic leukaemia (AMOL), and 1 patient with a blastic crisis of chronic myelocytic leukaemia (BC-CML). Patients with ALL were treated with prednisone, vincristine, methotrexate, and 6-mercapto-purine (POMP regimen), or with cyclophosphamide, vincristine, ara-C, or prednisone (CoAP regimen). Most non-ALL patients were treated with ara-C alone or in combination with thioguanine and/or daunomycin. Table 3 shows the comparison of *in vitro* and *in vivo* data re-tabulated in the manner of Salmon *et al.* (1978), using 85% inhibition of isotope uptake as the cut-off

Table 3 *In vitro/in vivo* correlations of 26 patients with leukaemia, using a ^{3}H-thymidine uptake assay (Raich, 1978)

Leukaemia	Patients	Sensitive *in vitro* Sensitive *in vivo*	Sensitive *in vitro* Resistant *in vivo*	Resistant *in vitro* Resistant *in vivo*	Resistant *in vitro* Sensitive *in vivo*
AML*					
AMML*	13	6	1	4	2
ALL*	9	7	0	2	0
Others	4	0	0	4	0

* For abbreviations, see text.

point. For the whole group 13/14 patients with inhibitions of 85% or greater achieved complete or partial remission, while 10/12 patients with inhibitions of less than 85% did not achieve remission.

Dendy and his colleagues (1973, 1976) have suggested the use of an assay based on ^{3}H-thymidine to quantitate the percentage of cells proceeding through S phase after drug treatment. This is done by determining the labelling index. However, the relevance of labelling index to cell proliferation has been questioned by Streffer *et al.* (1980). A second assay that has been used measures the ability of drug treated cells to incorporate ^{125}I-iododeoxyuridine (^{125}IUdR). Using this method, Warenius (1976) was able to chart the increase of acquired resistance in patients with ovarian carcinoma who had multiple draining of recurrent ascites. The use of ^{125}IUdR in combination with ^{75}Se-methionine in a dual isotope assay for drug sensitivity has been proposed by Dendy (1981). Although no clinical correlations have been reported, this type of assay may be important in distinguishing reversible from irreversible damage.

IV. Conclusions

Assays of intermediate duration are capable of generating drug sensitivity data on a large number of clinical samples rapidly. There are, however, a number of problems, both in the laboratory and in the clinic, which must still be resolved. First, any approach that uses monolayer cultures will only be useful if the cultures are representative of the original tumour. It has been shown that cell cultures from human glioma are made up of dividing aneuploid astrocyte-like cells which display many malignant characteristics both in short-term culture (Guner *et al.*, 1977; Freshney, 1980; Freshney *et al.*, 1980; Morgan and Freshney, 1980) and in long-term culture (Bigner *et al.*, 1981; Bullard *et al.*, 1981). These cultures are only rarely overgrown by stromal fibroblasts, in contrast to many other tumour cell cultures (Billiau *et al.*, 1975). Much more work needs to be done to define accurately characteristics of tumour cells in culture or to produce ways of separating malignant cells from stromal material by cultural or physical methods. Assay systems will also need to be refined since the question of endpoint is as critical in tests of intermediate duration as in any other type of assay. Two important questions remain to be answered: what level of residual viability should be used to determine *in vitro* response?; at what point in the assay should the endpoint determination be made? Our own work suggests that the assay should be allowed to continue for as long as possible after drug treatment before growth limitation becomes apparent. At this point, correlation between the ^{35}S-methionine assay and a monolayer cloning assay is very good (Morgan *et al.*, 1983).

The most important questions to be answered are clinical. Although there appears to be an interesting correlation between *in vitro* sensitivity measured by intermediate duration assays and clinical response, there is clearly a need for large prospective clinical trials to be carried out. The assay systems are quite capable of producing *in vitro* information on a large number of patients, but there is a need for a large input of patients for such a trial. It may be that no one centre has sufficient patients to carry this out and multicentre trials will be necessary.

Acknowledgements

We are grateful to the Cancer Research Campaign, Brain Research Trust, London, and the National Cancer Institute for support for work carried out in our laboratories. We are also grateful to Dr D. E. Bullard, Duke University Medical Center, for help with the chemosensitivity studies, and to Dr R. I. Freshney for helpful discussions. We are indebted to the neurosurgeons at the National Hospitals, Queen Square and Maida Vale, the Hospital for Sick Children, Great Ormond Street, and Atkinson Morley's Hospital, Wimbledon, for the supply of tumour biopsies for our studies on *in vitro* chemosensitivity.

References

Alberts, D. S. and Chen, H. S. G. (1980). Tabular summary of pharmacokinetic parameters relevant to *in vitro* drug assay. In *Cloning of Human Tumour Stem Cells* (ed. S. Salmon), pp. 351–359. Alan R. Liss, New York.

Bigner, D. D., Bigner, S. H., Ponten, J., Westermark, B., Mahaley, M. S., Ruoslahti, E., Herschman, H., Eng, L. F. and Wikstrand, C. J. (1981). Heterogeneity of genotypic and phenotypic characteristics of fifteen permanent cell lines derived from human gliomas. *J. Neuropathol. Exp. Neurol.* **41**, 210–229.

Billiau, A., Cassiman, J. J., Willems, D., Verhelst, M. and Hermans, H. (1975). *In vitro* cultivation of human tumour tissues. *Oncology* **31**, 257–272.

Bullard, D. E., Bigner, S. H. and Bigner, D. D. (1981). The morphological response of cell lines derived from human gliomas to dibutryl adenosine 3′,5′-cyclic monophosphate. *J. Neuropathol. Exp. Neurol.* **40**, 230–246.

Darling, J. L. and Thomas, D. G. T. (1981). Evaluation of the *in vitro* response of human gliomas to chemotherapeutic agents and its correlation with clinical response. *Br. J. Cancer* **43**, 734–735.

Dendy, P. P. (1968). Responses of freshly cultured tumours to certain selected chemotherapeutic agents. *J. Obstet. Gynaec. Br. Cwlth.* **75**, 1256–1261.

Dendy, P. P. (1981). Cell cultures and their use in drug sensitivity prediction. *Arch. Geschwulstforsch.* **51**, 111–118.

Dendy, P. P., Bozman, G. and Wheeler, T. K. (1970). *In vitro* screening test for human malignant tumours before chemotherapy. *Lancet* **2**, 68–72.

Dendy, P. P., Dawson, M. P. A. and Honess, D. J. (1973). Studies on the drug sensitivity of human tumors in short term culture. In *Aktuelle Probleme der Therapie Maligner Tumoren* (ed. G. Wüst), pp. 34–45. Thieme Verlag, Stuttgart.

Dendy, P. P., Dawson, M. P. A., Warner, D. M. A. and Honess, D. J. (1976). Quantitative assays of *in vitro* drug damage. In *Human Tumours in Short Term Culture: Techniques and Applications* (ed. P. P. Dendy), pp. 139–149. Academic Press, London.

Easty, D. M. and Wylie, J. A. H. (1963). Screening of 12 gliomata against chemotherapeutic agents *in vitro*. *Br. Med. J.* **2**, 1589–1592.

Fewer, D., Wilson, C. B., Boldrey, E. B. and Enot, K. J. (1972). Phase II study of 1-(2-chloroethyl)-3-cyclohexyl-1-nitrosourea (CCNU; NSC-79037) in the treatment of brain tumours. *Cancer Chemother. Rep.* **56**, 421–427.

Freshney, R. I. (1980). Tissue culture of glioma of the brain. In *Brain Tumours: Scientific Basis, Clinical Investigation and Current Therapy* (ed. D. G. T. Thomas and D. I. Graham), pp. 21–50. Butterworths, London.

Freshney, R. I. and Morgan, D. (1978). Radioisotopic quantitation in microtitration plates by an autofluorographic method. *Cell Biol. Int. Rep.* **2**, 375–380.

Freshney, R. I., Paul, J. and Kane, I. M. (1975). Assay of anticancer drugs in tissue culture: conditions affecting their ability to incorporate ^{3}H-leucine after drug treatment. *Br. J. Cancer* **31**, 89–99.

Freshney, R. I., Sherry, A., Hassanzadah, M., Freshney, M., Crilly, P. and Morgan, D. (1980). Control of cell proliferation in human glioma by glucocorticoids. *Br. J. Cancer* **41**, 857–866.

Graham, D. I. (1980). Primary malignant tumours of the cerebral hemispheres of adults. In *Brain Tumours: Scientific Basis, Clinical Investigation and Current Therapy* (ed. D. G. T. Thomas and D. I. Graham), pp. 268–300. Butterworths, London.

Guner, M., Freshney, R. I., Morgan, D., Freshney, M. G., Thomas, D. G. T. and Graham, D. I. (1977). Effects of dexamethasone and betamethasone on *in vitro* cultures from human astrocytoma. *Br. J. Cancer* **35**, 439–447.

Holmes, H. L. and Little, J. M. (1974). Tissue culture microtest for predicting response of human cancer to chemotherapy. *Lancet* **2**, 985–987.

Kornblith, P. L. and Szypko, P. E. (1978). Variations in response of human brain tumours to BCNU *in vitro*. *J. Neurosurg.* **48**, 580–586.

Kornblith, P. L., Smith, B. H. and Leonard, L. A. (1981). Response of cultured human brain tumors to nitrosoureas: correlation with clinical data. *Cancer* **47**, 255–265.

Lickiss, J. N., Cane, K. A. and Baikie, A. G. (1974). *In vitro* drug selection in antineoplastic chemotherapy. *Eur. J. Cancer* **10**, 809–814.

Morgan, D. and Freshney, R. I. (1980). Dexamethasone effect on glial cell surface glycoproteins. *Cell. Biol. Int. Rep.* **4**, 756.

Morgan, D., Freshney, R. I., Darling, J. L., Thomas, D. G. T. and Celik, F. (1983). Assay of anticancer drugs in tissue culture: cell cultures of biopsies of human astrocytoma. *Br. J. Cancer* **47**, 205–214.

Percival, R. (1974). Cancer and the ovary. *Proc. Roy. Soc. Med.* **67**, 381–387.

Raich, P. C. (1978). Prediction of therapeutic response in acute leukaemia. *Lancet* **1**, 74–76.

Rosenblum, M. L. (1980). Chemosensitivity testing of human brain tumors. In *Cloning of Human Tumor Stem Cells* (ed. S. Salmon), pp. 259–276. Alan R. Liss, New York.

Salmon, S. E., Hamburger, A. W., Soehnlen, B., Durie, B. G. M., Alberts, D. S. and Moon, T. E. (1978). Quantitation of differential sensitivity of human tumor stem cells to anticancer drugs. *New Engl. J. Med.* **298**, 1321–1327.

Shapiro, W. R. and Young, D. F. (1976). CCNU alone and combined with vincristine sulfate (VCR) and procarbazine (PCZ) as chemotherapy for malignant glioma. *Proc. Am. Soc. Clin. Oncol.* **17**, 258.

Streffer, C., van Beuningen, D., Molls, M. and Zamboglou, N. (1980). How relevant is the labelling index for cell proliferation? *Br. J. Cancer* **41** (Suppl IV), 205.

Thomas, D. G. T. and Darling, J. L. (1981). The use of human glioma cell cultures in evaluating the clinical efficacy of nitrosoureas. In *Nitrosoureas in Cancer Treatment* (ed. B. Serrou, P. S. Schein and J. L. Imbach), pp. 239–246. Elsevier/North Holland Biomedical Press.

Thomas, D. G. T., Darling, J. L., Freshney, R. I. and Morgan, D. (1979). *In vitro* chemosensitivity assay of human glioma by scintillation autofluorography. In *Multidisciplinary Aspects of Brain Tumor Therapy* (ed. P. Paoletti, M. D. Walker, G. Butti and R. Knerich), pp. 19–35. Elsevier/North Holland Biomedical Press.

Thomas, D. G. T., Darling, J. L. and Bullard, D. E. (1982). The chemosensitivity of human gliomas: an *in vitro* assay and correlation with clinical response. *Eur. J. Cancer Clin. Oncol.* (Suppl. 3), 83–89.

Vick, N. A., Khandekar, J. D. and Bigner, D. D. (1977). Chemotherapy of brain tumors: the blood–brain barrier is not a factor. *Arch. Neurol.* **34**, 523–526.

Walker, M. D. and Gehan, E. A. (1976). Clinical studies in malignant gliomas and their treatment with the nitrosoureas. *Cancer Treat. Rep.* **60**, 713–716.

Warenius, H. M. (1976). Detection of acquired resistance to cytotoxic drugs *in vivo* by short term *in vivo* cultures of human tumours. In *Human Tumours in Short Term Culture: Techniques and Applications* (ed. P. P. Dendy), pp. 311–327. Academic Press, London.

Wheeler, T. K., Dendy, P. P. and Dawson, A. (1974). Assessment of an *in vitro* screening test of cytotoxic agents in the treatment of advanced malignant disease. *Oncology* **30**, 362–476.

Wilson, A. P. and Neal, F. E. (1981). *In vitro* sensitivity of human ovarian tumours to chemotherapeutic agents. *Br. J. Cancer* **44**, 189–200.

Yung, W. K. A., Shapiro, J. R. and Shapiro, W. R. (1982). Heterogeneous chemosensitivities of subpopulations of human glioma cells in culture. *Cancer Res.* **42**, 992–998.

23. An Attempt to Use Incorporation of Radioactive Nucleic Acid Precursors to Predict Clinical Response

R. SILVESTRINI, O. SANFILIPPO and M. G. DAIDONE

I. Introduction

The use of an antimetabolic assay *in vitro* to predict the clinical activity of drugs was proposed some decades ago and has been used by various groups (Dendy, 1976; Wolberg, 1971). However, the results have not always been encouraging, perhaps owing to a lack of adequate standardization of technical conditions or to insufficiently rigorous and correct evaluation of patient follow-up. The main advantages of the antimetabolic assay are relative simplicity, potential applicability to almost all tumours, and the short time needed to obtain information, in accordance with clinical requirements. The antimetabolic assay is feasible on cell suspensions (Costa *et al.*, 1977) as well as on tumour fragments (Sanfilippo *et al.*, submitted for publication), and the main limitation is availability of sufficient and adequate tumour material. The possibility to perform the *in vitro* test on fragments of solid tumours obviates criticisms related to the possible selection of cells during mechanical or enzymatic procedures used to obtain cell suspensions and the danger of consequent changes in chemosensitivity of the original tumour. This feature may be of particular importance in view of recent observations suggesting that chemosensitivity may change unless cell-to-cell contact is maintained (Heppner and Miller, 1982).

The antimetabolic assay therefore appears to be a potentially reliable method for routine evaluation of the chemosensitivity of individual tumours. However, there are still many aspects that have to be investigated and accurately defined to guarantee its reproducibility and reliability. Specifically, the most crucial points relate to the use of labelled nucleic acid precursors and the possible changes induced by drugs on transport and intracellular pools of nucleosides.

II. Methodology

Our standard *in vitro* assay procedure is shown schematically in Fig. 1. The
assay is normally performed on cell suspensions from effusions and systemic
diseases such as non-Hodgkin's lymphomas (NHL), for which complete cell
release can be obtained easily by gentle mechanical disaggregation. For
"solid" tumours the assay is performed on pooled fragments (about 1 mm³)
sampled from different areas of the tumour. For each tumour, some randomly
selected fragments are submitted for histological verification of correct
tumour sampling. If there is no evidence of tumour material or if the
pathological diagnosis is not confirmed, the case is excluded from the study.
Tumour material is processed immediately after surgery, since we have
observed variations in chemosensitivity patterns in stored tissue (either frozen
or maintained at different temperatures) relative to fresh tumour material.
For *in vitro* treatment, samples containing a minimum of eight fragments or

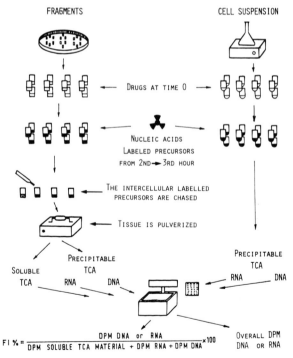

Fig. 1   Flow chart for the antimetabolic assay. The effect of the drug is calculated as
percentage variation in the precursor incorporation of treated samples in relation to
untreated samples.

between 2 and 10×10^6 viable cells, generally in triplicate, are incubated for 3 hours at 37°C in a Dubnoff shaker water bath.

Drugs are individually tested, and the basic dose ($\mu g\ ml^{-1}$) for each is calculated from the single dose used in clinical treatment, according to the formula of Tisman *et al.* (1973), as $(mg \times m^2 \times 100)/(kg \times 60)$. Whenever possible a range of doses around the pharmacologically relevant value is tested. Labelled precursors (^{3}H-thymidine and ^{3}H-uridine) are added from the second to the third hour of incubation with the concentration of labelled precursor chosen from pool equilibration plots defined for each tumour type (Costa *et al.*, 1977). In the case of tumour fragments, label present in intercellular spaces at the end of the incubation is chased with a 100-fold concentration of unlabelled precursor. Nucleic acids are extracted directly from cell suspensions or after pulverization of tissue fragments according to a modification of the method of Schneider (Costa *et al.*, 1977). Precursor incorporation into RNA and DNA is evaluated as total dpm for cell suspensions and as fractional incorporation (FI) according to Tew and Taylor (1978) for tumour fragments. The effect of the drug is expressed as percentage change of the radioactive incorporation in treated versus untreated samples.

III. Potentiality of the assay

The potentiality of the antimetabolic assay, for routine use on individual patients, is shown in Table 1. The percentage of tumours for which the assay is feasible, as well as the number of drugs tested, is high and depends essentially on the tumour material available, as shown by data for operable as opposed to

Table 1 Potential of the antimetabolic assay according to the experience of the Istituto Nazionale Tumori of Milan

	Tumours received by laboratory	Tumours in which *in vitro* assay possible (%)	Median number of drugs tested	Tumours in which assay evaluable (%)
NHL	423	60	7	95
Breast	1430	15*–71†	3	93
Testis	187	79	4	85
Colorectal	79	92	6	93
Ovarian	53	54	5	80

* Operable cancers (stage T2-T3).
† Advanced cancers (stage T3b-T4).

locally advanced breast cancers. The percentage of *in vitro* cultures for which an assay is possible is very high for all tumour types tested.

IV. *In vitro* studies

A. Dose–effect plots

Dose–effect plots were studied to investigate the specificity of *in vitro* behaviour. For tumours that responded to the equivalent clinical dose, typical dose-related effects on ^{3}H-thymidine incorporation were observed for adriamycin (Fig. 2a). Similar behaviour was observed with other typical phase-non-specific drugs such as 4-hydroperoxycyclophosphamide (4-OHC) or the nitrosoureas. Conversely, for bleomycin (Fig. 2b) and for vincristine, the exponential plateau type response characteristic of phase-specific agents was observed within the dose ranges used. For all drugs, plots of ^{3}H-uridine incorporation resembled the respective plots of ^{3}H-thymidine incorporation. Standard deviations around the mean values for each concentration of both

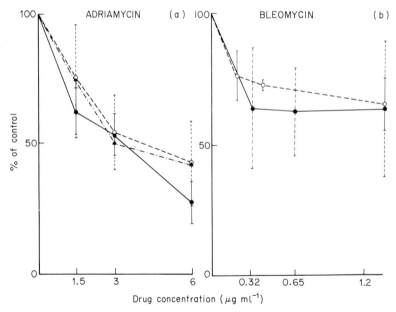

Fig. 2 (a) Effect of adriamycin on ^{3}H-thymidine incorporation in NHL (– – – –), breast cancer (–·–·–·), and testicular tumours (———); vertical bars represent standard deviations. (b) Effect of bleomycin on ^{3}H-thymidine incorporation in NHL (– – – –) and testicular tumours (———).

drugs (see Figs. 2a and 2b) clearly indicate broad variability of *in vitro* responses among individual tumours of the same type.

The relationship between the changes in ³H-thymidine and ³H-uridine incorporation was analysed to define further the mechanism of action of drugs in this *in vitro* system. The effect on incorporation of the two nucleic acid precursors was similar for adriamycin, 4-OHC, cis-platinum, and mitomycin C, whereas for other drugs such as bleomycin, vincristine, actinomycin D, and VP-16-213 the effects were not significantly correlated (Sanfilippo *et al.*, submitted for publication). For the latter group of drugs it remains to be established from analyses of *in vitro*/clinical correlations whether the effect on the DNA or the RNA precursor is more indicative of clinical response.

B. Definition of *in vitro* sensitivity

Since in our assay, as well as in other assays that provide a quantitative evaluation of *in vitro* drug effects (Daidone *et al.*, 1982), response to drugs can be considered as a continuous variable, ranging from no effect to different degrees of inhibition of the biological event being studied (i.e. cytocidal or antimetabolic), definition of *in vitro* sensitivity is critical. One possibility is to define the "cut-off" point of sensitivity to a particular drug by relating the *in vitro* drug effect to the corresponding clinical response for individual tumours. This criterion has been used by many authors including ourselves in retrospective correlative studies to investigate specificity of *in vitro* data (Daidone *et al.*, 1981; Kaufmann, 1982; Moon, 1980; Sanfilippo *et al.*, 1981a, 1982). However, to be accurate numerous samples would have to be analysed *in vitro*, and subsequent clinical response in individual patients submitted to monochemotherapy regimens would be necessary.

To try and overcome these difficulties we proposed a definition of sensitivity on the basis of the frequency distribution of the *in vitro* effect of each drug on each tumour type. This criterion takes into account (i) multiple factors that influence the distribution of drug effects (in this particular *in vitro* system these include the mechanism of action of each drug, the time of exposure to the drug, and the specific sensitivity of different tumour types to each drug), and (ii) the wide range of variability of drug effects observed for individual tumours within each tumour type. Once it has been shown that the frequency distribution of drug effects is normal, regions of different *in vitro* sensitivities can be defined by considering the distribution parameters; we have taken the median value as the lower sensitivity boundary, and the standard deviation units as sensitivity categories (Fig. 3). This analysis should be performed for each drug on each tumour type since different sensitivity boundaries were observed for the same drug in different tumour types. The criterion based on

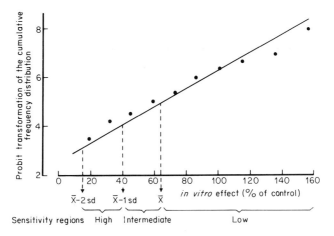

Fig. 3 Analysis of the frequency distribution of ^{3}H-thymidine incorporation in NHL following drug treatment, expressed as a percentage of the control. $\bar{X}$, median value; sd, standard deviation.

the frequency distributions studied for the different drugs was utilized in the present study for analysing the clinical correlations.

V. Clinical correlations

A. Specificity for predicting "tumour type" sensitivity

Information on the specificity of the antimetabolic assay for predicting the clinical outcome has been sought by analysing the relationship between the frequency of *in vitro* responses, determined with our assay, and the frequency of clinical responses reported by other authors for the same drugs and for the same tumour type. *In vitro* response rates for the drugs more extensively studied (Table 2) appear to reflect the general clinical sensitivity of the different tumour types (Bolis *et al.*, 1980; Bonadonna and Monfardini, 1974; Bonadonna *et al.*, 1976; Hoogstraten and Fabian, 1979; Issell and Crooke, 1979; Prestayko, 1981; Wasserman *et al.*, 1975). An overall higher *in vitro* chemosensitivity was observed for NHL and testicular tumours compared with breast cancers. Moreover, the response rates for most of the drugs within each tumour type were very similar to the percentage of tumours for which an objective clinical response has been observed using monochemotherapy regimens. For some drugs, such as VP-16-213, on all the tumour types studied, and nitrosoureas on NHL, *in vitro* sensitivity usually appeared somewhat

Table 2 *In vitro* response rates* of different tumour
types† to drugs

Drug tested	NHL (%)	Testis (%)	Breast (%)	Ovarian (%)
Adriamycin	49	29	32	39
Vincristine	25	—	19	—
Bleomycin	20	37	—	—
4-OHC	58	53	31	43
Nitrosourea	65	—	9	—
VP-16-213	45	64	43	—
Cis-platinum	—	36	15	50

* *In vitro* positive responses were defined as all significant inhibitions exceeding the median values.
† Including previously treated and untreated tumours,
except breast tumours which were all previously untreated.

higher than that reported clinically. *In vitro* sensitivity may have to be
redefined for these particular situations.

B. Specificity for predicting "individual tumour" sensitivity

The most direct analysis of the specificity of the antimetabolic assay in
predicting the clinical effect of drugs on the individual patient is obtained by
comparing *in vitro* and clinical sensitivity of the same tumour to the same
drugs. We made the assessment by a retrospective study of 132 cases including
NHL, testicular tumours, and breast cancer (Table 3). All the drugs used in
the patient's treatment were generally tested *in vitro*, except for cyclophosphamide on NHL since its *in vitro* active form (4-OHC) was available only for the
last 10% of the cases included in the study. The overall correlation between *in
vitro* and clinical findings was 76%. The overall predictive accuracy of
sensitivity was very high (83%), ranging from 94% for testicular tumours to
80% for NHL and 75% for breast cancer. Conversely, the overall predictive
accuracy of resistance was generally lower (63%), ranging from 40% for
testicular tumours to 55% for NHL and 80% for breast cancer.

The poor prediction of resistance for testicular tumours in this series could
be explained on the basis of differences in chemosensitivity (for the same
drugs) observed between the primary tumour and tumour from metastatic
sites (Sanfilippo *et al.*, 1981b) and by the observed correlation between the
metastatic tumour sensitivity but not primary tumour sensitivity and the
clinical outcome evaluated on metastatic sites after induction chemotherapy.

Table 3   Correlation between *in vitro* and clinical chemosensitivity on 132 advanced
tumours

	In vitro sensitive (S) or resistant (R)/clinical S or R				
	S/S	S/R	R/R	R/S	
NHL	36	8	10	8	$P = 0.003$
Breast	15	5	17	4	$P = 0.00016$
Testicular	18	1	4	6	$P = 0.018$
Overall	69	14	31	18	$P < 0.00003$
		83%		63%	
	True positive rate		True negative rate		

In vitro sensitivity: sensitivity (i.e. inhibition greater than the median value defined for each tumour type) to at least one of the drugs used for therapy.

Clinical sensitivity: complete or partial response greater than 50% of tumour volume reduction after induction chemotherapy. Treatment consisted of: alternating courses of ABP and CVP, or BACOP, for NHL; a combination of adriamycin and vincristine for breast cancer; and cis-platinum, bleomycin, and vincristine for testicular tumours. The correlation between *in vitro* and clinical data was studied using the kappa test.

For NHL the modest predictive accuracy of resistance could be due to a lack of information of *in vitro* effect of 4-OHC for about 90% of the cases (Sanfilippo *et al.*, 1981a), since cyclophosphamide is very effective *in vivo*.

Results of this analysis are in agreement with those previously reported using slightly different criteria for defining *in vitro* sensitivity (Daidone *et al.*, 1981; Sanfilippo *et al.*, 1982). When the analysis was extended to the long-term responses to chemotherapy there was evidence of a significant correlation between *in vitro* sensitivity, disease-free survival, and overall survival (Daidone *et al.*, 1981; Sanfilippo *et al.*, 1981a).

VI. Conclusions

The efforts made to optimize each step of the methodologic procedure and the statistical approach used to define *in vitro* sensitivity indices seem to have improved the accuracy of the antimetabolic assay in predicting clinical activity of drugs. At the same time, the fact that the antimetabolic assay can be completed successfully on a very high percentage of tumours, together with the short time required to obtain information, makes this test a potential tool for individualized chemotherapy. The high accuracy of our *in vitro* system for predicting sensitivity, besides providing further evidence of drug specificity, emphasizes its clinical relevance compared with other *in vitro* systems for selecting active drugs.

False positives could possibly be due to insufficient drug concentrations reaching the target cells *in vivo* or to inadequate clinical treatment in relation to the proliferative activity of the tumours and the capacity of cells to repair the metabolic damage observed during the short time period of the assay. Accuracy in predicting resistance to drugs is less satisfactory. In this respect, besides the exclusion of the drug–host interaction from the *in vitro* system, there are other reasons such as the difficulty in measuring the effect of phase-specific drugs over a few hours or the possible additive or synergistic effects when two or more drugs are used in clinical treatment. Finally, differences in sensitivity between the primary and metastatic tumours cannot be discounted.

Good progress with predictive testing has already been made, but many basic studies remain to be done to establish the reliability of the assay for all the drugs, particularly antimetabolites, for which the most relevant measure of drug action has still to be determined. We are also convinced that definitive and conclusive answers on the potential and limitations of the test can be derived only from prospective utilization of the *in vitro* information in monochemotherapy regimens.

Acknowledgements

This study was supported in part by a grant, Progetto Finalizzato, Control of Neoplastic Growth, from the Consiglio Nazionale delle Ricerche, Rome. We thank Dr N. Zaffaroni, Miss C. De Marco, and Miss R. Motta for technical assistance, and Miss B. Johnston for editing and preparing the manuscript.

References

Bolis, G., Bortolozzi, G., Carinelli, G., D'Incalci, M., Gramellini, F., Morasca, L. and Mangioni, C. (1980). Low-dose cyclophosphamide versus adriamycin plus cyclophosphamide in advanced ovarian cancer. *Cancer Chemother. Pharmacol.* **4,** 129–132.

Bonadonna, G. and Monfardini, S. (1974). Chemotherapy of non-Hodgkin's lymphomas. *Cancer Treat. Rev.* **1,** 167–181.

Bonadonna, G., Lattuada, A. and Banfi, A. (1976). Perspectives in cancer research: recent trends in the treatment of non-Hodgkin's lymphomas. *Eur. J. Cancer* **12,** 661–673.

Costa, A., Piazza, R., Sanfilippo, O. and Silvestrini, R. (1977). A quantitative test for chemosensitivity of short-term cultures of human lymphomas. *Tumori* **63,** 237–247.

Daidone, M. G., Silvestrini, R. and Sanfilippo, O. (1981). Clinical relevance of an *in vitro* antimetabolic assay for monitoring human tumor chemosensitivity. In

Adjuvant Therapy of Cancer. III (ed. S. E. Salmon and S. E. Jones), pp. 25–32. Grune and Stratton, New York.

Daidone, M. G., Sanfilippo, O., Zaffaroni, N. and Silvestrini, R. (1982). Definition of *in vitro* sensitivity: a critical point in analyzing the clinical relevance of *in vitro* antimetabolic assays (Abstract). 13th International Cancer Congress, Seattle.

Dendy, P. P. (1976). *Human Tumors in Short Term Culture.* Academic Press, London.

Heppner, G. and Miller, B. E. (1982). Therapeutic consequences of heterogeneity (abstract). 13th International Cancer Congress, Seattle.

Hoogstraten, B. and Fabian, C. (1979). A reappraisal of single drugs in advanced breast cancer. *Cancer Clin. Trials* **2**, 101–109.

Issell, B. F. and Crooke, S. T. (1979). Etoposide (VP-16-213). *Cancer Treat. Rev.* **6**, 107–124.

Kaufmann, M. (1982). Nucleic acid precursor incorporation assay for testing tumour sensitivity and clinical applications. *Drugs Exp. Clin. Res.* **8**, 345–358.

Moon, T. E. (1980). Quantitative and statistical analysis of the association between *in vitro* and *in vivo* studies. In *Cloning of Human Tumor Stem Cells* (ed. S. E. Salmon), pp. 209–222. A. R. Liss, New York.

Prestayko, A. W. (1981). Cisplatin and analogues: a new class of anticancer drugs. In *Cancer and Chemotherapy.* Vol. III. *Antineoplastic Agents* (ed. S. T. Crooke and A. W. Prestayko), pp. 133–154. Academic Press, New York.

Sanfilippo, O., Daidone, M. G., Costa, A., Canetto, R. and Silvestrini, R. (1981a). Estimation of differential *in vitro* sensitivity of non-Hodgkin's lymphomas to anticancer drugs. *Eur. J. Cancer* **17**, 217–226.

Sanfilippo, O., Silvestrini, R. S., Zaffaroni, N. and Pizzocaro, G. (1981b). *In vitro* chemosensitivity of testicular tumors and its clinical perspectives (Abstract). UICC Conference on Clinical Oncology, Lausanne.

Sanfilippo, O., Silvestrini, R., Daidone, M. G. and Monfardini, S. (1982). *In vitro* antimetabolic assay for the prediction of human tumor chemosensitivity. *Proc. Am. Soc. Clin. Oncol.* **1**, 24.

Sanfilippo, O., Silvestrini, R., Daidone, M. G. and Zaffaroni, N. (submitted for publication). A short-term *in vitro* antimetabolic assay for the evaluation of the sensitivity of human solid tumors to anticancer drugs. *Cancer Treat. Rep.*

Tew, K. D. and Taylor, D. M. (1978). The relationship of thymidine metabolism to the use of fractional incorporation as a measure of DNA synthesis and tissue proliferation. *Eur. J. Cancer* **14**, 153–168.

Tisman, G., Herbert, V. and Edlis, H. (1973). Determination of therapeutic index of drugs by *in vitro* sensitivity tests using human host and tumor cell suspensions. *Cancer Chemother. Rep.* **57**, 11–19.

Wasserman, T. H., Comis, R. L., Goldsmith, M., Handelsman, H., Penta, J. S., Slavik, M., Soper, W. T. and Carter, S. K. (1975). Tabular analysis of the clinical chemotherapy of solid tumors. *Cancer Chemother. Rep.* **6**, 399–419.

Wolberg, W. H. (1971). Biochemical approaches to prediction of response in solid tumors. *Nat. Cancer Inst. Monogr.* **34**, 189–195.

24. Clinical Correlations of *in vitro* Drug Sensitivity Using the Clonogenic Assay

S. E. SALMON

I. Introduction

In 1977 our group reported the development of an *in vitro* soft agar clonogenic assay suitable for cultivating human tumour cells from fresh biopsy samples (Hamburger and Salmon, 1977a). Methodological aspects and basic growth features are summarized in Chapter 10. The assay has proven applicable to most types of solid tumours (Salmon, 1980a) with different cloning efficiencies as a function of intrinsic features of the tumour, frequency of contamination of the specimen, and cultural procedures. One of the central objectives in this work was to develop a reliable *in vitro* technique with which drug sensitivity of the clonogenic subpopulation of human tumours could be estimated. Clonogenic tumour cells, as evaluated *in vitro*, are considered to be closely related to the key subpopulation of tumour stem cells present *in vivo*, which are considered responsible for the self-renewal of the tumour cell population, as well as recurrence and metastasis after subcurative local or systemic treatment (Bruce *et al.*, 1966; Steel, 1977). After developing useful culture conditions, the next focus was on standardizing methods for *in vitro* drug testing. These techniques are detailed elsewhere (Salmon, 1980a). Some aspects of the approach are commented on in Chapters 17 and 18. Our overall objectives in drug sensitivity testing were to develop a reproducible, pharmacologically based assay system that would prove useful for prospectively predicting (i) response and survival of cancer patients treated with specific drug regimens, (ii) effects of new Phases I–II anticancer drugs in the course of drug development, and (iii) potential antitumour effects of entirely new compounds referred for new drug screening (Salmon *et al.*, 1980; Salmon, 1980b). This chapter will focus particularly on a brief summary of prospective clinical correlations obtained to date at the University of Arizona Cancer

Center in relation to *in vitro* assay in multiple myeloma, ovarian cancer, and metastatic melanoma. Details of these studies have been published (Salmon *et al.*, 1978, 1980; Durie *et al.*, 1983; Alberts *et al.*, 1980, 1981a,b; Meyskens *et al.*, 1981). Von Hoff's group in San Antonio (Von Hoff *et al.*, 1981) and others (Mann *et al.*, 1982) have also applied this cloning method to chemosensitivity studies with qualitatively similar results.

Methodological aspects of the testing procedure, illustrations of typical *in vitro* survival curves, and exploration of some pharmacological principles as assessed in this assay system will also be briefly addressed. Overall, our drug sensitivity testing studies have provided substantial evidence for patient-to-patient heterogeneity in sensitivity to individual anticancer drugs (even among tumours of the same histopathology) as well as evidence that the assay may have prognostic implications with respect to defining prospectively inherent sensitivity of clonogenic tumour cells to selected anticancer drugs.

II. Methods

The soft agar procedure of Hamburger and Salmon (1977a,b) was utilized for studies of multiple myeloma and various solid tumours tested. Solid tumour biopsies were disaggregated into single cell suspensions by mechanical (Hamburger *et al.*, 1978) or enzymatic methods (Pavelic *et al.*, 1980; Hamburger *et al.*, 1981). Drug exposures were performed either with a 1 hour exposure prior to plating or by continuous exposure by incorporating the agent into the agar (Salmon *et al.*, 1980; Alberts *et al.*, 1981b). The exposure mode was selected to simulate the likely clinical drug dosing or disposition for the specific drug tests. Drugs were obtained from the National Cancer Institute or the pharmaceutical industry. Whenever available, the clinical formulation of the drug was utilized, and reconstituted in appropriate diluents and further diluted into complete tissue culture medium. Stable drugs were stored in replicate single use tubes at suitable dilutions at $-80°C$. Aliquots of cells were exposed at $37°C$ to at least two drug concentrations so that a one-log dose–response curve could be constructed. Drugs were studied at low concentrations (each in triplicate) generally ranging up to 1.0 μg ml^{-1}. Procedures for cell plating have been detailed previously (Hamburger and Salmon, 1977a; Hamburger *et al.*, 1978; Salmon *et al.*, 1978; Salmon, 1980a). Spleen-conditioned medium (Hamburger and Salmon, 1977b) is required only for myeloma cultures.

All plates were examined by inverted microscopy on the day of plating, and experiments with excessive number of aggregates (greater than 15 per plate) were discarded. Positive controls, in which all proliferation was blocked, have included fixation of additional control plates with 3% glutaraldehyde on the day of plating, or refrigeration. Most recently the plant lectin abrin (10 μg ml^{-1}) has been used as a positive control. Proliferation controls were counted simultaneously with normally incubated control plates. Plates are scanned every few days by inverted microscopy, and colonies usually counted on days 10–16 using a Bausch and Lomb FAS II image analysis system optimized for counting tumour colonies and excluding artifacts (Kressner et al., 1980). Currently we accept colonies on the FAS II to be those proliferative cellular units of relatively circular shape and density with a diameter of at least 60 microns. The FAS II routinely discriminates up to ten size classes as specified by the operator. Since testing is non-destructive, serial counts may be obtained throughout the period of culture. In our laboratory, definition of adequate in vitro growth for evaluation of drug effects is a minimum of 30 colonies per 35 mm Petri dish in the controls. Tumour colony formation is linear with the number of tumour cells plated. The median number of tumour colonies from a large series of countable experiments was 108 colonies per control dish (500 000 nucleated cells plated). Thus the cloning efficiencies in this system are low but provide sufficient growth for drug evaluation in 40–70% of cells cultivated from various tumour types. Criteria for defining in vitro sensitivity for specific drugs were based on calculation of percentage survival of drug exposed plates relative to the control at "boundary" concentrations that could be calculated to be readily achievable (generally 10% of the plasma concentration–time product). In initial studies, in vitro survival–concentration curves were ranked for sensitivity using an "area under the curve" technique (Salmon et al., 1978; Moon, 1980). More recently a mathematically simpler ranking of % survival data up to empirically derived "cut-off" drug concentrations has been used (Moon et al., 1981). In each instance correlations are drawn between in vitro and in vivo data in order to form a "training set" (for drugs as well as tumour types), for prospective application thereafter (Moon, 1980; Moon et al., 1981). At present we classify tumours as sensitive to specific drugs if survival of tumour colony forming units (TCFU) is reduced to 30% of control or less, and as intermediate in the range 30–50%. When TCFU survival is greater than 50% of control at the cut-off concentration, the tumour is considered resistant to the specific drug tested. The first report of clinical correlations in myeloma and ovarian cancer represented an initial training set for a number of standard agents (Salmon et al., 1978). Subsequent prospective clinical trials have been of two types: (i) prospective correlative trials, or (ii) prospective decision-aiding trials (Salmon, 1980b). In the prospective correlative trial the laboratory tests the specific drugs the patient is scheduled to receive after the biopsy is performed; treatment is thus independent of the laboratory result and carried out without knowledge of it. In the prospective decision-aiding trial the patient's specific treatment is predicated on evidence of in vitro sensitivity to a specific drug or drugs. In all instances laboratory results are obtained by laboratory technical staff without influence from clinicians responsible for patient treatment who independently assess the patient's clinical response. Criteria for clinical response that were utilized were those of the Southwest Oncology Group. Clinical correlations at the University of Arizona are being gathered from a variety of tumour types in tumour specific protocols, but have thus far been reported only in ovarian cancer, myeloma, and melanoma. Effects of new agents in this assay have been reported for a variety of tumour types (e.g. Ahmann *et al.*, 1982; Salmon *et al.*, 1981, 1983).

III. Results

A. *In vitro* sensitivity of TCFU

After 1 hour exposure, survival curves for tumours exposed to cycle non-specific drugs generally show progressively increasing lethality with increasing drug dosage. However, substantial heterogeneity in sensitivity was observed from patient to patient. Examples of this phenomenon are depicted in Figs 1 and 2 (Salmon, 1982; Meyskens *et al.*, 1981). Drugs that are schedule dependent often manifest flat survival–concentration curves with 1 hour exposure, but steep inhibition curves at substantially lower doses when the drug is added to the agar for continuous exposure studies. An example of this phenomenon with bleomycin in ovarian cancer is illustrated in Fig. 3 (Alberts *et al.*, 1981b). Thus far we have observed such schedule dependent curves with bleomycin, VP-16-213, and vinblastine, but not with doxorubicin, cis-platinum, or alkylating agents (Ludwig *et al.*, 1982). With cycle non-specific agents, greater sensitivity is observed with continuous exposure than for 1 hour, but the difference is generally less than 10-fold. In contrast, with schedule dependent drugs the degree of inhibition may be greater than 100-fold that observed with a 1 hour exposure. A common phenomenon observed with many standard anticancer drugs is that most solid tumour specimens exhibit resistance to the agent up to dose levels that exceed pharmacologically achievable plasma concentrations. For example, colorectal carcinoma specimens only occasionally exhibit *in vitro* sensitivity to 5-fluorouracil, alkylating agents, or vinblastine, whereas sensitivity is more often observed with these drugs when tested against ovarian cancer. Since marked sensitivity to achievable concentrations of standard agents is relatively infrequent, it is clear that relatively large tumour specimens are preferable to increase the probability that sensitivity to one or more agents will be observed. As depicted in Table 1, we have seen precisely this phenomenon in myeloma, melanoma, and ovarian cancer (Moon *et al.*, 1981). Whenever possible we therefore attempt to test at least 7–8 drugs (at two

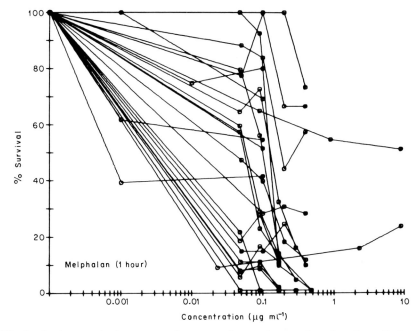

Fig. 1 *In vitro* survival–concentration curves for myeloma colony forming cells from a series of 26 patients tested with various doses of melphalan for 1 hour prior to culture. Marked heterogeneity in sensitivity is apparent from patient to patient. Those curves with reduction in survival to 30% or less at the 0.1 μg ml^{-1} dose level would be classed as sensitive. (Salmon, 1982)

concentrations) to increase the probability of identifying at least one active drug. In ovarian cancer the frequency of *in vitro* sensitivity to common agents such as cis-platinum, doxorubicin, and bleomycin was greater in patients who had received no prior chemotherapy than in those who were in relapse (Fig. 4) (Alberts *et al.*, 1981a). However, this phenomenon was not observed in melanoma (Meyskens *et al.*, 1981), a tumour type for which it is more difficult to define effective drugs (even for previously untreated patients).

Serial *in vitro* studies have also been evaluated in a series of 12 patients who underwent 45 sequential tumour biopsies before, and at various stages after, initiation of therapy (Salmon *et al.*, 1980), summarized in Table 2. Overall we observed that tumours that initially exhibited sensitivity to a specific drug *in vitro* prior to therapy frequently showed resistance *in vitro* on re-biopsy after the patient had relapsed (at least 50% increase in the area under the survival–concentration curve) after treatment with that agent, and none showed increased sensitivity. In contrast, patients who received no therapy or

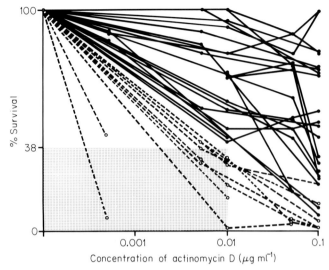

Fig. 2   Chemosensitivity of melanoma colony forming units to actinomycin D. In this study the shaded zone was considered to reflect the relevant range of *in vitro* survival and drug concentrations to reflect *in vitro* sensitivity. Each line represents a different tumour biopsy tested. Lines that pass through the shaded zone of sensitivity are dashed. (Meyskens *et al.*, 1981)

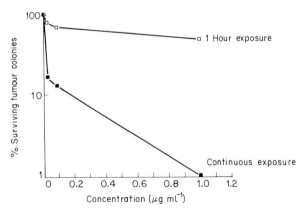

Fig. 3   Effect of *in vitro* bleomycin exposure duration on ovarian TCFU survival. Upper curve represents TCFU survival following a 1 hour drug incubation. Lower curve represents TCFU survival on continuous contact with the drug in the agar gel matrix. (Alberts *et al.*, 1981b)

Table 1 Identification of drugs to which sensitivity was shown *in vitro* related to the number of drugs tested (Moon *et al.*, 1981)

Drugs tested *in vitro*	Patients sensitive*	Patients resistant†	Patients tested
≤3	13 (0.42)	18	31
4–7	82 (0.77)	24	106
7+	19 (1.00)	0	19
Total	114 (0.73)	42	156

* Sensitive means sensitive *in vitro* to at least one of the drugs tested.
† Resistant means resistant to all drugs tested *in vitro*.

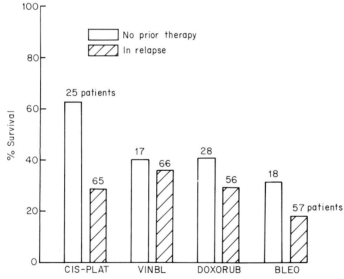

Fig. 4 Effect of clinical therapy status on the frequency of *in vitro* sensitivity of ovarian cancer cells, in the human tumour clonogenic assay, to cis-platinum, vinblastine, doxorubicin, and bleomycin. Differences in the frequency of *in vitro* sensitivity were significant for cis-platinum and doxorubicin. (Alberts *et al.*, 1981a)

Table 2 Correlations of 45 serial *in vitro* studies in 12 patients
(Salmon, 1980a)

Clinical information	Number of instances	Area under survival–concentration curve		
		decrease ($>50\%$)	no change ($<50\%$)	increase ($>50\%$)
No therapy, or unrelated therapy	25	0	22	3
Specific drug given was tested *in vitro*	20	0	11	9*

* Acquisition of resistance (increase in the area under the curve)
was more common when the patient received the specific drug
tested *in vitro* ($P=0.03$).

unrelated therapy did not have a significant increase in the frequency of
resistance in the follow-up *in vitro* tests ($P=0.03$) (Salmon, 1980a).

B. Prospective clinical correlations

A series of prospective clinical trials for specific tumour types have been
carried out in our centre in patients with myeloma, melanoma, and ovarian
cancer, with the results recently reported (Durie *et al.*, 1983; Meyskens *et al.*,
1981; Alberts *et al.*, 1981a). Correlations between *in vitro* sensitivity and *in vivo*
response from these trials are summarized in Table 3. With respect to
prediction of objective response, overall the clonogenic assay had a 67% true
positive rate and a 93% true negative rate for these three tumour types. For
ovarian cancer alone the true positive rate was 67% and the true negative rate
99%, whereas for myeloma the true positive rate was 73% and the true
negative rate 83%. It is important to note that the criteria of response utilized
were less stringent for melanoma than for myeloma or ovarian cancer, since
"mixed responses" (wherein some tumour nodules continue to grow while
others regress) were classified as objective responses in melanoma. If mixed
responses are included for melanoma, the true positive rate was 63% and the
true negative rate 86%. If mixed responses were classified as progressive
disease, the accuracy of identification of true positivity fell to 42% (8/19 trials)
in melanoma. Responses induced by drugs selected from *in vitro* assay were of
longest duration in myeloma, intermediate in ovarian cancer, and relatively
short in melanoma.

Table 3 Clinical correlations of *in vitro* sensitivity.
(Durie *et al.*, 1983; Meyskens *et al.*, 1981; Salmon *et al.*,
1980)

Tumour type	Trials	S/S	S/R	R/S	R/R
Myeloma	33	11	4	3	15
Melanoma	48	12*	7	4	25
Ovarian	95	14	7	1	73
Total	176	37	18	8	113

67% true positive   93% true negative

$p < 0.00001$

S/S = sensitive *in vitro* and sensitive *in vivo*.
S/R = sensitive *in vitro* and resistant *in vivo*, etc.
* Mixed responses included for melanoma.

In addition to these prospective trials for specific tumour types, we have also utilized the assay prospectively with various new agents such as 4′-(9-acridinylamino)methanesulfon-*m*-anisidide (mAMSA) (Ahmann *et al.*, 1982). A total of 140 tumour biopsies from 20 different tumour types were tested with mAMSA, and *in vitro* sensitivity was seen at the 0.1 μg ml^{-1} level (1 hour) in 29 tumours (14%). Prospective correlative trials were conducted in 8 patients, of whom 3 were sensitive *in vitro* and all three responded clinically (partial responses in a lymphoma and a cervical carcinoma, and a mixed response in a melanoma patient) (Ahmann *et al.*, 1982). We found these results encouraging and concluded that this approach warranted additional study with other new agents in Phase I–II clinical trials.

IV. Discussion

Viewed overall, data from our laboratory provide strong evidence that *in vitro* chemosensitivity testing with the human tumour clonogenic assay provides a potentially important new prognostic factor with which to evaluate patients with cancer who are treated with chemotherapy. *In vitro* data that we have obtained on acquisition of drug resistance to specific classes of agents is consistent with prior observations in animal tumour systems, but this is one of the first direct measurements of this phenomenon in cancer patients. The relative infrequency of marked *in vitro* sensitivity to pharmacologically achievable concentrations of many of the currently available anticancer drugs is also concordant with clinical experience in a variety of solid tumours. We selected myeloma, melanoma, and ovarian cancer for our initial correlative studies because it is relatively easy to obtain tumour biopsies in these disorders without major invasive procedures. Additionally, there are some standard agents that are active in myeloma and ovarian cancer, thereby increasing the likelihood that clinical correlations can be sought for agents that manifest *in vitro* activity. The prospective clinical correlations that we have obtained provide evidence that the human tumour clonogenic assay is able to predict correctly clinical chemosensitivity with reasonable accuracy, and chemoresistance with a high degree of accuracy. These findings are analogous to those obtained with antibiotic sensitivity testing for bacterial infections. However, there are still difficulties in routinely applying clonogenic assays for chemosensitivity testing of human tumours. Most important, inadequate *in vitro* growth is still observed overall in about 50% of tumour specimens, although our success rates in ovarian cancer and melanoma are higher (60–75%). Even for those tumours that have grown, cloning efficiencies have been low, and limit the extent of experimentation feasible (and the survival curves to 1–2 logs). However, the population of clonogenic cells that we have been testing *in vitro* clearly appears relevant to the tumour cell population *in vivo* as reflected by clinical correlations obtained to date. All investigative groups are interested in obtaining better *in vitro* growth. Hopefully some of the methodological details used in the culture procedure described by Courtenay in Chapter 9 will prove useful for enhancing clonogenicity of TCFU without adversely affecting clinical correlations of *in vitro* chemosensitivity. Our initial efforts have been directed towards correlating *in vitro* chemosensitivity with clinical response, since this is the most immediate measure that one can assess in relation to *in vitro* testing. We recognize that, in the long run, measurement of the duration of freedom from relapse and overall survival will be more important measures upon which *in vitro* chemosensitivity assays will be evaluated. Such correlations are now being obtained in our centre and others, for various tumour types. Our experience with *in vitro* testing and survival analysis in myeloma suggests that the assay can prospectively identify patients with a good or bad prognosis for overall survival (Durie *et al.*, 1983). Specifically, patients whose clonogenic myeloma cells exhibit *in vitro* sensitivity to at least one of three major agents used in treatment (BCNU, doxorubicin, melphalan) have a better prognosis than those patients whose cells are resistant to all three of these agents ($P < 0.05$). It should be evident from these comments that we recognize that additional developmental and clinical efforts are needed. For example, additional studies are necessary to determine whether the assay identifies patients more likely to respond to treatment in a general sense or those specifically responsive to the selected agent. Nonetheless we believe that clinical correlations obtained by our group and others already provide a reasonable basis for optimism about the applicability of human tumour clonogenic assays in clinical cancer research and therapy. Optimism can have a salutary effect on research efforts, since it is likely to increase the pace of science in a field. The pace has already quickened in relation to clonogenic assays and chemosensitivity, and a large number of centres have become engaged in this pursuit within the past few years. The stage is therefore set for large-scale testing and multicentre clinical trials which are essential to major progress in clinical cancer research. It should also be apparent that effective implementation of a selective chemosensitivity assay is dependent on availability of effective anticancer drugs. The available agents at present are "first generation" drugs and lack efficacy in a number of common tumour types. In that regard, use of human tumour clonogenic assays for new drug development and screening may prove a most useful application.

Acknowledgements

I wish to thank my colleagues David S. Alberts, Brian G. M. Durie, Frank Meyskens, A. H. Ahmann, and Thomas Moon for their participation in these studies, and Laurie Young, Joyce Leibowitz, and Barbara Soehnlen for technical assistance. These studies were supported in part by grants CA-17094, CA-21839, and CA023074 from the National Institutes of Health, Bethesda, Maryland.

References

Ahmann, F. R., Meyskens, F. L., Moon, T. E., Durie, B. G. M. and Salmon, S. E. (1982). *In vitro* chemosensitivities of human tumor stem cells to the phase II drug m-AMSA, and prospective *in vivo* correlations. *Cancer Res.* **42,** 4495–4498.

Alberts, D. S., Salmon, S. E., Chen, H. S. G., Surwit, E. A., Soehnlen, B., Young, L. and Moon, T. E. (1980). *In vitro* clonogenic assay for predicting response of ovarian cancer to chemotherapy. *Lancet* **ii,** 340–342.

Alberts, D. S., Chen, H. S. G., Salmon, S. E., Surwit, E. A., Young, L., Moon, T. E. and Meyskens, F. L. (1981a). Chemotherapy of ovarian cancer directed by the human tumor stem cell assay. *Cancer Chemother. Pharmacol.* **6,** 279–285.

Alberts, D. S., Salmon, S. E., Chen, H. S. G., Moon, T. E., Young, L. and Surwit, E. A. (1981b). Pharmacologic studies of anticancer drugs using the human tumor stem cell assay. *Cancer Chemother. Pharmacol.* **6,** 253–264.

Bruce, W. R., Meeker, B. E. and Valeriote, F. A. (1966). Comparison of the sensitivity of normal hematopoietic and transplanted lymphoma colony-forming cells to chemotherapeutic agents administered *in vivo. J. Nat. Cancer Inst.* **37,** 233–245.

Durie, B. G. M., Young, L. and Salmon, S. E. (1983). Human myeloma stem cell culture: relationship between *in vitro* drug sensitivity and kinetics and patient survival duration. *Blood* **61,** 929–934.

Hamburger, A. W. and Salmon, S. E. (1977a). Primary bioassay of human tumor stem cells. *Science* **197**, 461–463.

Hamburger, A. W. and Salmon, S. E. (1977b). Primary bioassay of human myeloma stem cells. *J. Clin. Invest.* **60**, 846–854.

Hamburger, A. W., Salmon, S. E., Kim, M. B., Trent, J. M., Soehnlen, B., Alberts, D. S. and Schmidt, H. J. (1978). Direct cloning of human ovarian carcinoma cells in agar. *Cancer Res.* **38**, 3438–3443.

Hamburger, A. W., White, C. P. and Tencer, K. (1981). Effect of enzymatic disaggregation on proliferation of human tumor cells in soft agar. *J. Nat. Cancer Inst.* **68**, 945–948.

Kressner, B. E., Morton, R. R. A., Martens, A. E., Salmon, S. E., Von Hoff, D. D. and Soehnlen, B. (1980). Use of an image analysis system to count colonies in stem cell assays of human tumors. In *Cloning of Human Tumor Stem Cells* (ed. S. E. Salmon), pp. 179–193. Alan R. Liss, New York.

Ludwig, R., Alberts, D. S., Miller, T. P., Salmon, S. E. and Wood, D. A. (1982). Schedule dependency of anticancer drugs in the human tumour stem cell assay. *Proc. Am. Assoc. Cancer Res.* **23**, 183.

Mann, B. D., Kern, D. H., Giuliano, A. E., Burk, M. W., Campbell, M. A., Kaiser, L. R. and Morton, D. L. (1982). Clinical correlations with drug sensitivities in the clonogenic assay. *Arch. Surg.* **117**, 33–36.

Meyskens, F. L., Moon, T. E., Dana, B., Gilmartin, E., Casey, W. J., Chen, H. S. G., Franks, D. H., Young, L. and Salmon, S. E. (1981). Quantitation of drug sensitivity by human metastatic melanoma colony forming units. *Br. J. Cancer* **44**, 787–797.

Moon, T. E. (1980). Quantitative and statistical analysis of the association between *in vitro* and *in vivo* studies. In *Cloning of Human Tumor Stem Cells* (ed. S. E. Salmon), pp. 209–221. Alan R. Liss, New York.

Moon, T. E., Salmon, S. E., White, C. S., Chen, H. S. G., Meyskens, F. L., Durie, B. G. M. and Alberts, D. S. (1981). Quantitative association between the *in vitro* human tumor stem cell assay and clinical response to cancer chemotherapy. *Cancer Chemother. Pharmacol.* **6**, 211–218.

Pavelic, Z. P., Slocum, H. K., Rustum, Y. M., Creavin, P. J., Karakousis, C. and Takita, H. (1980). Colony growth in soft agar of human melanoma, sarcoma and lung carcinoma cells disaggregated by mechanical and enzymatic methods. *Cancer Res.* **40**, 2160–2164.

Salmon, S. E. (1980a). *Cloning of Human Tumor Stem Cells* (ed. S. E. Salmon), Alan R. Liss, New York.

Salmon, S. E. (1980b). Applications of the human tumor stem cell assay to new drug evaluation and screening. In *Cloning of Human Tumor Stem Cells* (ed. S. E. Salmon), pp. 291–312. Alan R. Liss, New York.

Salmon, S. E. (1982). *In vitro* cloning and chemosensitivity of human myeloma stem cells. In *Myeloma and Related Disorders* (ed. S. E. Salmon), pp. 47–63. W. B. Saunders Company, London.

Salmon, S. E., Hamburger, A. W., Soehnlen, B., Durie, B. G. M., Alberts, D. S. and Moon, T. E. (1978). Quantitation of differential sensitivity of human tumor stem cells to anticancer drugs. *New Engl. J. Med.* **298**, 1321–1327.

Salmon, S. E., Alberts, D. S., Meyskens, F. L., Durie, B. G. M., Jones, S. E., Soehnlen, B., Young, L., Chen, H. S. G. and Moon, T. E. (1980). Clinical correlations of *in vitro* drug sensitivity. In *Cloning of Human Tumor Stem Cells* (ed. S. E. Salmon), pp. 223–245. Alan R. Liss, New York.

Salmon, S. E., Liu, R. M. and Casazza, A. M. (1981). Evaluation of new anthracycline analogs with the human tumor stem cell assay. *Cancer Chemother. Pharmacol.* **6,** 103–109.

Salmon, S. E., Durie, B. G. M., Young, L., Liu, R. M., Trown, P. W. and Stebbing, N. (1983). Effects of cloned human leukocyte interferons in the human tumor stem cell assay. *J. Clin. Oncol.* **1,** 217–225.

Steel, G. G. (1977). Growth and survival of tumour stem cells. In *Growth Kinetics of Tumors*, pp. 217–262. Clarendon Press, Oxford.

Von Hoff, D. D., Casper, J., Bradley, E., Sandbach, J., Jones, D. and Makuch, R. (1981). Association between human tumor colony-forming assay results and response of an individual patient's tumor to chemotherapy. *Am. J. Med.* **70,** 1027–1032.

25. Evaluation of the Courtenay Assay for Drug Sensitivity Prediction *in vivo*

K. M. TVEIT

I. Introduction

The eventual outcome of chemotherapy of a malignant tumour depends on the number of residual cells capable of indefinite multiplication. For this reason, during recent years, inhibition of colony-forming cells has been employed to an increasing extent as an endpoint for *in vitro* chemosensitivity testing of human tumours. Although it is not proven that these cells are identical with the tumour stem cells *in situ* capable of re-growing a tumour, it is generally assumed that the clonogenic cells *in vitro* represent stem cells *in vivo* (Steel, 1977).

A substantial shortcoming of colony-forming assays based on growth in semi-solid medium is that a high percentage of tumours cannot be tested owing to insufficient growth. Furthermore, in tumours growing *in vitro*, plating efficiencies (PE) obtained are in general low, permitting only one out of every 10^4–10^6 cells in a tumour to be assayed. This raises the important question as to whether clonogenic cells really reflect the chemosensitivity of the stem cells. Attempts to develop a reliable routine method that can be used in planning chemotherapy of cancer patients have made it clear that extensive investigations of different available methods must be carried out to establish optimal conditions for particular tumour cells studied.

Courtenay has described two variants of a new soft agar method (Courtenay, 1976; Courtenay and Mills, 1978) and has shown that factors included in the assay stimulate colony growth from tumour cells. In this chapter data obtained with the Courtenay assay are presented, including colony growth, sensitivity to cancer chemotherapeutic agents, and correlations with clinical responses. As far as possible, the results will be compared with those obtained using the more widely known method described by Hamburger and Salmon (1977).

II. The Courtenay soft agar method

The method (Courtenay and Mills, 1978) is described in detail in Chapter 9, and Fig. 1 compares the procedure with the Hamburger and Salmon method. The distinguishing features of the Courtenay assay are the presence of washed rat red blood cells (RBC), the use of tubes instead of Petri dishes, a replenishable liquid medium, and hypoxic atmosphere (5% O_2, 5% CO_2, 90% N_2). The liquid medium is added after 5–7 days of incubation at 37°C; it can be removed and fresh medium added every week if necessary. Fig. 2 shows a

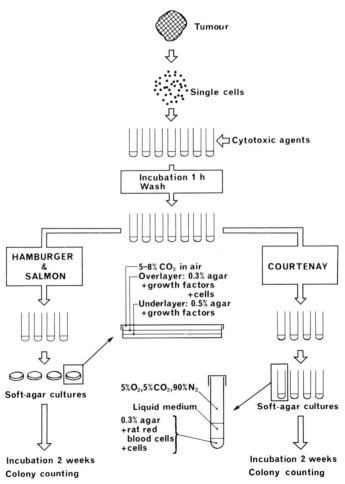

Fig. 1   Soft agar assays of Courtenay and of Hamburger and Salmon.

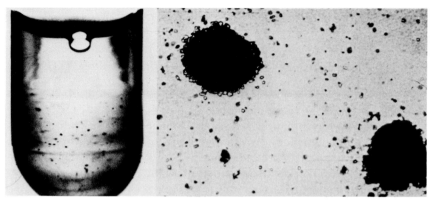

Fig. 2 A soft agar culture of melanoma colonies, macroscopically (left) and in the stereo microscope, × 50 (right). The agar is squeezed between the top and bottom of a Contact Petri dish.

culture of melanoma colonies macro- and micro-scopically after 2 weeks incubation.

III. Colony growth

A. Identification of colonies

Colony formation from non-malignant cells has not been reported in the Courtenay assay. In our studies of human melanomas (Tveit *et al.*, 1981b, 1982) light- and electron-microscopic examination, chromosome counts, and isoenzyme studies showed that the soft agar colonies were derived from human malignant cells. However, in this method as well as in other methods, there is no assurance that in each case all colonies scored are formed from malignant cells. It should be noted that colony formation in agar from macrophage progenitors has been demonstrated by Selby *et al.* (1980) when cells from human melanoma xenografts were cultivated in diffusion chambers *in vivo*.

In the colony-forming assays it is possible that cell aggregates scored as colonies are not colonies derived from single cells but are formed from pre-existing cell clumps. If such clumps are present, the dose–response curves might be expected to show a plateau and chemosensitivity data will be difficult to interpret. It is therefore important to remove clumps from the cell suspensions by sedimentation and filtration before plating in agar. When suspensions of only single cells (after disaggregation mechanically or enzymatically) were employed, in general the dose–response curves declined to zero growth (100% colony inhibition) using the Courtenay assay (Tveit *et al.*, 1981b, 1982).

B. Plating efficiency

Courtenay *et al.* (1978) observed colony formation in 22 out of 48 human tumour specimens of various histological types. Melanomas and ovarian carcinomas grew more frequently in agar than other tumour types. Rupniak *et al.* (1982) found poor colony growth in primary tumours of neuroblastomas, squamous cell carcinomas of the head and neck, and colorectal carcinomas. In contrast, their results obtained with metastatic tumour material were relatively encouraging. In our laboratory we have grown 379 human tumours in the Courtenay system primarily metastatic melanomas, breast cancers, and ovarian carcinomas. Data on colony growth are given in Table 1. Melanomas gave the highest PE (number of colonies as a percentage of number of viable cells plated) and breast cancers the lowest. If sufficient cells were available, colony formation was adequate (>30 colonies in control cultures) for chemosensitivity measurement in approximately 70% of the melanomas, in 50–60% of ovarian carcinomas, in 50% of breast cancer metastases, and in about 40% of primary breast carcinomas.

Table 1   Plating efficiency of human tumours

Tumours	Number (and percentage) of samples giving PE (%):					
	<0.01	0.01–0.09	0.1–0.9	1.0–9.9	>10.0	Total
Malignant melanoma	58 (24.9)	24 (10.3)	95 (40.8)	53 (22.7)	3 (1.3)	233 (100)
Breast carcinoma	54 (54.0)	19 (19.0)	24 (24.0)	3 (3.0)	0 (0)	100 (100)
Ovarian carcinoma	8 (27.6)	9 (31.0)	6 (20.7)	6 (20.7)	0 (0)	29 (100)
Soft-tissue sarcoma	3 (25.0)	4 (33.3)	5 (41.7)	0 (0)	0 (0)	12 (100)
Glioma	1 (20.0)	2 (40.0)	2 (40.0)	0 (0)	0 (0)	5 (100)
Total	124 (32.7)	58 (15.3)	132 (34.8)	62 (16.4)	3 (0.8)	379 (100)

To establish whether the Courtenay method or that of Hamburger and Salmon gave the most adequate growth of tumour cells from biopsy specimens in soft agar, tumour cells from the same samples were grown concurrently using the two different methods. Plating efficiencies obtained with melanomas, ovarian carcinomas, gliomas, and breast cancers are listed in Table 2. For melanomas considerably higher PE values were obtained in the Courtenay assay (Tveit *et al.*, 1981a). The reason for this was shown to be the presence of rat RBC and low oxygen (5%) concentration in the Courtenay assay (Tveit *et al.*, 1981a). In most cases of ovarian carcinomas approximately the same PE were obtained with the two methods (Tveit and Endresen, unpublished) although two tumours grew better in the Courtenay method. Gliomas showed better colony growth in the Courtenay procedure (Endresen

Table 2   Plating efficiency (%) of patients' tumours using two different soft agar methods

Tumour		Courtenay–Mills	Hamburger–Salmon
Melanoma	1.	0.01	0
	2.	0.07	0.01
	3.	0	0
	4.	7.7	0.09
	5.	10.1	0
	6.	0.6	0.002
	7.	0	0
	8.	0.9	0.07
	9.	2.4	0.3
Ovarian	1.	0	0
	2.	0.044	0
	3.	0.45	0 (clusters)
	4.	1.28	1.03
	5.	0.02	0.015
	6.	0	0
	7.	0 (clusters)	0 (clusters)
	8.	0 (clusters)	0
	9.	0.35	0.40
Glioma	1.	0.17	0.002
	2.	0.18	0.03
	3.	0.01	0 (clusters)
	4.	0.03	0
	5.	0	0
Breast	1.	0.14	0.14
	2.	0.054	0.047

et al., 1981) whereas the two breast carcinomas examined gave similar PE with both methods.

An important finding in our study was that the Courtenay method, in contrast to the Hamburger and Salmon method, gives a linear relationship between the number of cells plated and the number of colonies formed (Tveit *et al.*, 1981a, 1982). In Fig. 3 this relationship is shown for a patient's

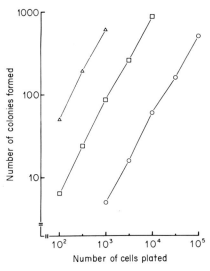

Fig. 3   Relationship between number of cells plated and number of colonies formed for a melanoma cell line (△), a xenograft (□), and a surgical specimen (○).

melanoma, a xenografted melanoma, and a melanoma cell line. When less than 10^4 cells are plated, the presence of RBC seems in most cases to be necessary for this linear relationship (Tveit *et al.*, 1981a,b).

IV. *In vitro* chemosensitivity

Dose–response curves or survival curves were determined after incubation of cells with various concentrations of different drugs *in vitro* and cultivation in soft agar. Characteristic curves are shown for five melanomas treated with DTIC and abrin in Fig. 4. Resistant tumours have dose–response curves of similar shape to those of sensitive tumours, and plateaus are not in general seen using the Courtenay assay.

Sensitivity of melanoma cells treated with CCNU, vinblastine, abrin, and in some cases also DTIC, was found to be considerably lower in the Courtenay assay than in the Hamburger and Salmon assay (Tveit *et al.*, 1981a).

Representative curves obtained with the two assays on the same samples of treated tumour cells are shown in Fig. 5. Recently we have also obtained evidence that similar differences in sensitivity are found for other tumour types and other drugs (Tveit and Endresen, unpublished). Several reasons for these observed differences in sensitivity have been discussed previously (Tveit

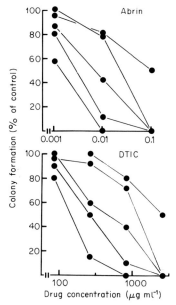

Fig. 4 Dose–response curves for five patients' melanomas treated *in vitro* with DTIC or abrin.

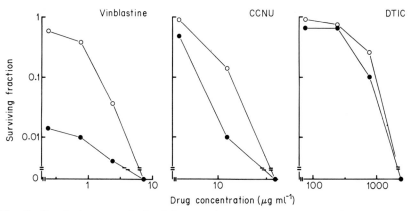

Fig. 5 Survival curves obtained for a melanoma treated *in vitro* with vinblastine, CCNU, or DTIC, and assayed with the method of Courtenay (O) and of Hamburger and Salmon (●).

et al., 1981a). It is not unexpected that different culture conditions, which may select for different populations of clonogenic cells, also may exhibit different sensitivities to antitumour agents. It is also possible that the Hamburger and Salmon method employs a substance that is cytotoxic when combined with antitumour agents. Moreover, the lack of linearity in the Hamburger and Salmon method between cell number and colony number at low cell density (Tveit *et al.*, 1981a) may contribute to the higher sensitivities observed with this method.

Because of the different sensitivities found in the two soft agar assays studied, the same evaluation procedure for *in vitro* sensitivity testing cannot be used. In both assays criteria for *in vitro* sensitivity versus resistance have to be established on empirical grounds, by careful comparisons with *in vivo* responses.

V. *In vitro/in vivo* correlations of sensitivity

A. Correlations to responses of xenografts

The use of *in vitro* clonogenic assays to predict clinical responses to chemotherapy is based on the assumption that the *in vivo* response is correlated closely with the *in vitro* sensitivity of the clonogenic cells assayed. However, this is not *a priori* certain for at least two reasons: (i) *in vivo* response may be determined not only by the intrinsic cellular chemosensitivity, but may be influenced to some degree also by other factors (e.g. drug penetration, natural defence mechanisms, and immune reactions); (ii) clonogenic cells assayed *in vitro* may not represent the cells *in situ* that are responsible for the *in vivo* response, but may be a subpopulation selected by the particular conditions used *in vitro*.

Because of these factors it is necessary to look carefully at the *in vitro/in vivo* relationship regarding drug sensitivity. This can be done by using murine tumours or human tumour xenografts in immune-deprived animals where response to chemotherapy can be assessed quantitatively. In such experiments correlations were obtained for xenografted melanomas treated with melphalan, MeCCNU, and adriamycin (Bateman *et al.*, 1980), and with DTIC, CCNU, vinblastine, procarbazine, abrin, and ricin (Tveit *et al.*, 1980). Results for DTIC, abrin, and ricin have been shown in Chapter 16. For all nine agents a positive *in vitro/in vivo* correlation was found, indicating that there is a close relationship between *in vivo* response and *in vitro* sensitivity of the cells that are clonogenic in the Courtenay assay. If such positive correlations had not been found, good correlations to clinical responses would not have been expected.

B. Correlations with clinical responses

Although the use of human xenografts provides important information regarding the usefulness of an *in vitro* assay, the clinical value of such tests can only be established on the basis of retrospective and prospective clinical trials. So far, only data from two laboratories using the Courtenay assay give correlations with clinical responses. Rupniak *et al.* (1982) found, in a small number of patients with ovarian carcinomas, good correlations between *in vitro* resistance and clinical resistance. In our laboratory we have concentrated mainly on human melanomas.

In our studies we have quantitated the *in vitro* sensitivity by determination of the ID_{50} (the concentration required to inhibit colony formation by 50%) from the dose–response curves, and by means of the calibration curves obtained on melanoma xenografts the ID_{50} values have been converted into the *in vivo* term "expected growth delay" (EGD) (Tveit *et al.*, 1982). So far, 72 correlations with clinical responses have been carried out in 58 patients (Fig. 6). All patients previously treated with the drug tested had low *in vitro* sensitivity (EGD $\leqslant 1.2$). Previously untreated patients were classified in four

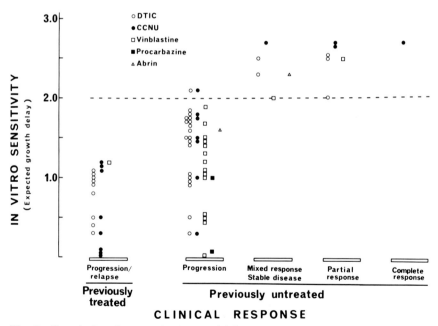

Fig. 6 Correlations between *in vitro* sensitivity (expected growth delay) and clinical response in 58 melanoma patients, either previously treated with the drug tested (14 patients) or previously untreated (44 patients).

groups with respect to response. Patients with complete response (1 patient), partial response (6 patients), and mixed response or stable disease after prior progression (5 patients) had EGD values between 2.0 and 3.0. Patients with progression had EGD values ≤2.1. Thus, in melanomas *in vitro* sensitivity and clinical response seem to be well correlated, in agreement with findings in melanoma xenografts. Patients with EGD values >2.0 have a high probability of clinical response, whereas patients with values <2.0 do not seem to respond.

A few of the patients included in Fig. 6 received chemotherapy on the basis of *in vitro* results. Two patients who responded were tested both before and after chemotherapy was given (response followed by relapse). In both cases the tumour was considerably more resistant after relapse than before treatment (Fig. 7).

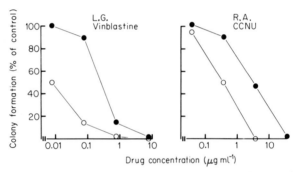

Fig. 7   Dose–response curves for two patients before (○) and after (●) chemotherapy with the drug indicated. The EGD values were: L.G., 2.5 (before) and 1.2 (after); R.A., 2.7 (before) and 1.1 (after).

VI. Conclusions and future prospects

For melanoma cells the Courtenay assay gives good culture conditions, with high enough plating efficiency for sensitivity testing in about 70% of cases. In melanomas, *in vitro* sensitivity of the clonogenic cells and *in vivo* response is well correlated for a number of different drugs tested, and positive correlations with clinical responses have been obtained. These data are promising for future use of the assay in predicting individual responses to chemotherapy. For other tumour types the Courtenay assay gives lower plating efficiency. *In vitro/in vivo* correlations have not yet been established, either in xenografts or in clinical specimens. Such investigations are under way.

Since *in vitro* chemosensitivity testing in individual patients may considerably improve clinical chemotherapy in the future, basic work concerning growth conditions and calibration of *in vitro* assays should be pursued in a systematic way. Growth factors other than those currently used may be included to optimize colony growth for different tumour types. The relationship between *in vitro* sensitivity and *in vivo* response to chemotherapy, including correlations with clinical results, has to be established for all tumour types and all drugs. Such investigations will require a concerted effort in many institutions.

Acknowledgements

This work was supported by the Norwegian Cancer Society.

References

Bateman, A. E., Selby, P. J., Steel, G. G. and Towse, G. D. W. (1980). *In vitro* chemosensitivity tests on xenografted human melanomas. *Br. J. Cancer* **41**, 189–198.

Courtenay, V. D. (1976). A soft agar colony assay for Lewis lung tumour and B16 melanoma taken directly from the mouse. *Br. J. Cancer* **34**, 39–45.

Courtenay, V. D. and Mills, J. (1978). An *in vitro* colony assay for human tumours grown in immune-suppressed mice and treated *in vivo* with cytotoxic agents. *Br. J. Cancer* **37**, 261–268.

Courtenay, V. D., Selby, P. J., Smith, I. E., Mills, J. and Peckham, M. J. (1978). Growth of human tumour cell colonies from biopsies using two soft-agar techniques. *Br. J. Cancer* **38**, 77–81.

Endresen, L., Tveit, K. M. and Rugstad, H. E. (1981). Colony forming ability in soft agar of human solid tumours. Influence of rat erythrocytes and oxygen concentration on plating efficiency (Abstract). Third NCI-EORTC Symposium on New Drugs in Cancer Therapy, Brussels.

Hamburger, A. W. and Salmon, S. E. (1977). Primary bioassay of human tumor stem cells. *Science* **197**, 461–463.

Rupniak, H. T., Marks, P., Watkins, S., Bourne, G., Slevin, M., Bancroft-Livingston, G. H., Simmons, C. A. and Hill, B. T. (1982). Drug sensitivities of human tumor cells obtained directly from biopsy material. Proc. 12th Int. Congress of Chemotherapy, pp. 1274–1276. ASM Publications, Washington.

Selby, P. J., Courtenay, V. D., McElwain, T. J., Peckham, M. J. and Steel, G. G. (1980). Colony growth and clonogenic cell survival in human melanoma xenografts treated with chemotherapy. *Br. J. Cancer* **42**, 438–447.

Steel, G. G. (1977). *Growth Kinetics of Tumours*. Clarendon Press, Oxford.

Tveit, K. M., Fodstad, Ø., Olsnes, S. and Pihl, A. (1980). *In vitro* sensitivity of human melanoma xenografts to cytotoxic drugs: correlation to *in vivo* chemosensitivity. *Int. J. Cancer* **26**, 717–722.

Tveit, K. M., Endresen, L., Rugstad, H. E., Fodstad, Ø. and Pihl, A. (1981a). Comparison of two soft agar methods for assaying chemosensitivity of human tumours *in vitro*: malignant melanomas. *Br. J. Cancer* **44**, 539–544.

Tveit, K. M., Fodstad, Ø. and Pihl, A. (1981b). Cultivation of human melanomas in soft agar: factors influencing plating efficiency and chemosensitivity. *Int. J. Cancer* **28,** 329–334.

Tveit, K. M., Fodstad, Ø., Lotsberg, J., Vaage, S. and Pihl, A. (1982). Colony growth and chemosensitivity *in vitro* of human melanoma biopsies: relationship to clinical parameters. *Int. J. Cancer* **29,** 533–538.

26. Conclusions, Problems, Recent Developments, and Future Perspectives

B. T. HILL and P. P. DENDY

The concept of developing an *in vitro* test that will accurately predict the correct chemotherapeutic treatment for an individual patient with cancer is not new. However, during the last 5 years many laboratories, throughout the world, have attempted to exploit the significant advances that have been made in successfully culturing human tumour cells to re-examine this idea. The foregoing chapters in this book have provided a comprehensive review of the current status of the majority of these endeavours and in this final chapter we will attempt to highlight the main conclusions drawn and suggest fruitful areas for further research.

The laboratory research worker confronted with a biopsy specimen faces numerous challenges which include: precise tumour cell identification and characterization; successful disaggregation of the tissue to provide "viable" and "representative" tissue explants, slices, or tumour cell suspensions; selection of the assay procedure to be adopted and the conditions for drug exposures, followed ultimately by accurate data analyses.

Chapters in Section I provide details of the current state of knowledge of the main differences that have been identified between "normal" and "tumour" cells. Although no single property or even group of properties may be considered specific for human tumour cell identification, biochemical and immunological methods of recognition, coupled with physical methods of sorting "viable" cell populations, may soon provide samples of human tumour cells of adequate purity specifically for drug sensitivity evaluation. These techniques might also prove of particular value in tackling the problem of tumour cell heterogeneity. For example, Smith et al. (1981) have detected heterogeneity in response to adriamycin amongst breast carcinoma cultures as well as heterogeneity among subpopulations within a single carcinoma, whilst Rosenblum et al. (1981) emphasize in their studies with brain tumours that clonal heterogeneity might play an important role in determining tumour response to drugs. Historically, superiority was implied or claimed by proponents of the clonogenic assay system over other methodologies since growth of cells in soft agar was considered a marker for neoplasia. However, the recent reports of colony formation in soft agar by tissue from a patient with fibrocystic disease of the breast (Von Hoff *et al.*, 1981c), from patients with parathyroid hyperplasia (Bradley *et al.*, 1980), and from benign prostatic hypertrophy tissue (Sarosdy *et al.*, 1982) sound another word of caution in this interpretation. It is therefore imperative that future studies closely examine histologic, karyologic, and other factors to ascertain the exact nature of the cells being evaluated.

Chapters in Section II provide a comprehensive survey of the major methodologies employed for investigating drug sensitivities, and Table 1 in Chapter 19 summarizes the chief advantages and disadvantages of each approach. Mechanical disaggregation of tissue has been used in most of these studies, although recent evidence tends to favour the use of enzymatic methods with the clonogenic assays as discussed in Chapter 8 and further supported by a recent publication which emphasizes that under these conditions quantity is reduced but quality improved resulting in significantly elevated cloning efficiencies (Hamburger *et al.*, 1982). The emphasis in Section II is on clonogenic assays used on either direct biopsy specimens or established cell lines. Indeed several groups suggest that, if fresh tumour material is maintained in culture for a few passages before assay, enhanced cloning efficiencies result (e.g. Smith *et al.*, 1981; Rosenblum *et al.*, 1981). However, the use of multicellular spheroids, discussed in Chapter 13, is likely to receive more attention in the future. This type of three-dimensional structure is particularly suited for addressing problems of drug accessibility and evaluating the differential responses of hypoxic versus oxic tumour cells to drugs and radiation. Organ culture remains an attractive model since such a wide range of tumour types can be studied using this technique, as reviewed in Chapter 14. The only animal *in vivo* screening system considered here employs human tumour xenografts (see Chapters 15 and 16). The Norwegian group have stated that testing of chemosensitivity of xenografts is too time-consuming to be of practical value for individual patients. Instead they consider xenografts as important tools in validating *in vitro* assays of chemosensitivity since drug responses in xenografts in nude mice can be measured quantitatively and reproducibly, as discussed in Chapter 16. The ability to grow human tumours in nude mice has also proved valuable for removing mycoplasma contamination from human tumour cell lines by one *in vivo* passage, and preliminary data suggest that for certain tumour types this *in vivo* environment is ideal for the initial establishment of tumour cell lines from biopsy material that can then subsequently be taken into culture.

Accurate assessment of cell survival requires the use of a clonogenic assay. The various types of assay and modifications are reviewed in Chapter 8, and full laboratory details of three of these procedures are provided in Chapters 9–11. A major disadvantage of these assays, when considering their role in predictive, individualized drug sensitivity testing, is the period of time that has to elapse before a result is obtained. Indeed, the short-term nature of the vital dye exclusion assays (Weisenthal et al., 1983, and Chapter 21) and the radioactive incorporation assays involving nucleic acid or protein synthesis (see Chapters 6 and 7) is certainly one of their major advantages. Recent attempts to benefit from the specific advantages of these various methodologies have included: (i) an assay based on ^{3}H-thymidine incorporation by acid-precipitable material of tumour cells grown in a soft agar system, which provides data in 5 days (Tanigawa et al., 1982); (ii) application of an autoradiographic technique applied to double layer agar culture to measure depression of labelling index, providing results in 8–10 days (Elson et al., 1982); (iii) use of a cell-containing liquid top layer and a soft-agar bottom layer, measuring ^{3}H-thymidine incorporation into acid-precipitable material by scintillation counting (Friedman and Glaubiger, 1982). In each of these examples the authors claim good correlations between results obtained using these modified methods and those from parallel colony forming assays. Indeed, Livingston et al. (1980) believe that their labelling index perturbation test and the "stem" cell assay system of Hamburger and Salmon measure effects of drug exposure on similar subpopulations of cells which are critical to continued cell renewal, namely, the fraction actively involved in DNA synthesis. So these published results are encouraging, and it is hoped that they will provide impetus for other investigators. However, the overriding factor as to whether one specific in vitro sensitivity test method is superior to another depends on which provides the best degree of clinical correlation.

Chapters in Section III provide encouraging evidence of the increasing collaboration between clinicians and scientists. Data now available from several groups, using different methodologies in retrospective studies, have shown correlations between in vitro drug sensitivities and relapse-free survival (see e.g. Chapters 20, 23, and 24). Von Hoff et al. (1981b) have also suggested that the number of colonies growing in a cloning assay may be used as a prognostic factor for survival. This finding of a correlation between agar clonogenicity and patient survival was also reported by Bertoncello et al. (1982). However, this latter group cautioned against any general optimism on the basis of these findings since problems relating to inherent tumour heterogeneity, quality of sample, and tissue disaggregation meant that only 36% of all specimens received could be evaluated. Indeed, it is salutary to remember the failed experiments and the fact, as pointed out by Von Hoff et al. (1981a), that the human tumour colony forming assay, as now constituted, and even when carried out in this major cancer centre, can provide useful sensitivity information for only about 25% of the general oncology patients. Furthermore, many of the reported results involve studies only with restricted tumour types, the most favoured being ovarian ascites and metastatic melanomas. However, evidence continues to accrue, particularly with the clonogenic assays, that many other "solid" tumours can be grown *in vitro*; see, for example, the recent reports of success with breast cancer (Sandbach *et al.*, 1982) and with urologic malignancies (Sarosdy *et al.*, 1982). Optimization of culture conditions, as discussed in Chapters 8 and 12, may enable such studies to be extended not only to other tumour types but also for enhancing the cloning efficiencies obtained which are frequently disappointingly low.

The rank order of sensitivity among patients depends strongly on the selected *in vitro* test dose; see, for example, Daniels *et al.* (1981). Thus selection of the "appropriate" test dose for each drug is critical for optimal validity. The methods currently adopted are reviewed in Chapter 17, but meanwhile the debate surrounding selection of "ideal" *in vitro* drug concentrations and exposure times continues and can only be resolved by further studies. Similarly controversy surrounds the selection of endpoints for the laboratory assays. These are frequently varied depending not only on the assay but also on the tumour type being studied, as discussed in Chapter 19. Indeed it is of interest that in a recent comparative study of two assay methods, monolayer cloning versus microtitration, good clinical correlations were obtained with both assays when ID_{50} values were used, but with ID_{90} values the cloning assays alone provided results that correlated with clinical data, suggesting that the cloning technique is superior in determining low surviving fractions (Morgan *et al.*, 1983). These data add weight to the argument that different assays may have specific values depending on the problem under investigation. Similarly certain assay methodologies may prove advantageous for particular tumour types.

In general, results of laboratory/clinical correlative studies have been encouraging. For example, the pattern of *in vitro* sensitivity for specific tumour types is similar to current clinical experience, as shown by the following examples. (i) In urological tumours the highest *in vitro* sensitivity rate was seen in testicular cancer, a disease in which patients are now effectively treated with multiple drug therapy, whilst renal cell, bladder, and prostate cancer demonstrated refractoriness to drugs currently in use clinically, as they have in the cloning system (Sarosdy *et al.*, 1982), although these authors caution that the definition of "sensitivity" *in vitro* is somewhat arbitrary. (ii) Melanoma cells have proved resistant to most agents tested, both before and after drug exposure *in vitro*, and this would correlate with the fact that clinical chemotherapy in this tumour has proved so unsuccessful (Meyskens *et al.*, 1981). (iii) In ovarian cancer, tumours from pretreated patients prove less responsive *in vitro* to most drugs than those from untreated patients, a finding confirmed by clinical data (Alberts *et al.*, 1981).

Whilst there remain several protagonists of the value of these predictive assays for individualizing therapy (see e.g. Mann *et al.*, 1982, and Chapters 20 and 25) other groups favour alternative approaches which include evaluation of new drugs or analogues in Phase II *in vitro* trials (see Chapters 19 and 24). However, all investigators realize the necessity for prospective, randomized, clinical trials involving large numbers of patients and taking into account the statistical considerations, discussed in Chapter 18. These studies will require standardization not only of the laboratory assay methods, which may require more rigid control of test reagents and conditions, but also standardized clinical protocols *and*, most important, standards for assessing response to therapy. We suggest that these latter clinical problems certainly represent the major hurdles. Indeed, improved methods for assessing clinical responses to therapy are definitely needed. Present hopes are pinned on the use of tumour specific monoclonal antibodies but recent developments in diagnostic imaging techniques, notably X-ray computerized whole-body transmission tomography, ultrasound, and nuclear magnetic resonance imaging, can be expected to play an increasingly important role.

Suggestions for future investigations have been included in several of the chapters and specifically in the overviews provided in Chapters 8, 12, and 19. Some of these proposals will involve new approaches whilst others place emphasis on consolidating existing data. These ideas can be summarized best under four main headings; a few examples are listed below.

1. *New or improved methodologies*

(i) Optimization of culture conditions, tissue disaggregation techniques, and cloning efficiencies.

(ii) Improved storage procedures and recovery of "viable" cell populations after cryopreservation.

(iii) Intercomparisons of results of drug sensitivity using different screening assay procedures.

2. *Studies of basic tumour biology*

(i) Establishment of proliferative characteristics of human tumour clonogenic cells; for example, Meyskens *et al.* (1983) have initiated such studies with melanoma.

(ii) Studies of tumour–host interactions; for example, Asano and Mandel (1981) have suggested that clonal growth of T-lymphocytes infiltrating the tumour should prove useful for investigating lymphocyte–tumour relationships *in vivo*, and Durie *et al.* (1982) have provided evidence of amyloid production in human myeloma stem cell culture and propose that further use of the clonogenic assay will permit detailed studies of the interactions between myeloma cells and macrophages in amyloid deposition.

(iii) Study of the self-renewal capacity of clonogenic human tumour cells; indeed preliminary data are already available for ovarian tumours (Buick and MacKillop, 1981) and melanomas (Thomson and Meyskens, 1982).

3. *Laboratory chemotherapeutic and pharmacological studies*

(i) Investigate the development and mechanism(s) of drug resistance; for example, Meyskens *et al.* (1981) suggested that "resistant" colonies derived from melanoma cultures provide a valuable source of material for such work, and the demonstration by Hofmann *et al.* (1981) that drug resistance in multiple myeloma is associated with high *in vitro* incorporation of ^{3}H-thymidine merits further study.

(ii) Extend the range of agents tested; for example, by using the drug bioactivation method described by Lieber *et al.* (1981), evaluating the interferons as reported by Epstein and Marcus (1981), considering radio-sensitizers and radioprotectors and drug combinations with or without hormones.

(iii) Optimization and standardization of drug exposure conditions; for example, the stability of drugs in culture should be established if continuous exposure is selected, and the influence of different serum concentrations on drug sensitivities should be investigated.

4. *Clinical studies*

(i) Evaluate the relationship between hormone receptor status and response to cytotoxic chemotherapy; for example, Sandbach *et al.* (1982) reported no correlation between oestrogen receptor status and sensitivity to a variety of antitumour agents including adriamycin, whilst in contrast Kaufmann (1982) found that response to adriamycin *in vitro* correlated negatively with oestrogen and/or progesterone receptor content.

(ii) Establish the prognostic value of these drug sensitivity assays in terms of effects on survival and perhaps as suggested by Von Hoff *et al.* (1981a) for the selection of patients for adjuvant chemotherapy, as opposed to watchful waiting.

(iii) Use assays to monitor drug treatment efficacy; this may be of particular value where repeat biopsies are possible or successive samples can be obtained from bronchial or peritoneal washing.

(iv) Determine the value of these clonogenic assays as an index of malignant or biological potential of a tumour; for example, Stanisic and Buick (1980) have reported that cluster growth in the clonogenic assay provided the first indicator of malignancy in two patients with transitional cell carcinomas of the bladder, and Von Hoff *et al.* (1981b) have used the clonogenic assay successfully to document marrow involvement by small cell lung cancer and neuroblastoma.

In conclusion, it is clear that the use of surgical biopsy material *in vitro* is providing a rich source of valuable biological experiments. When the studies are directed towards drug sensitivity testing, the clinical objective is well defined and of the utmost importance. Many groups would claim that the use of predictive tests has already improved the quality of life of some patients and, although we are still a long way from a routine test service, the recent increased interest in this type of work suggests that progress will not only be maintained but should accelerate during the next few years. The fact that most successes in drug sensitivity testing relate to the accurate prediction of drug resistance might be expected since most evaluations are carried out on tumour samples from heavily pretreated patients and/or those with advanced disease. Under these circumstances the Goldie–Coldman mathematical model (1979) would predict that such tumours would contain a high proportion of drug-resistance phenotypes. Therefore more accurate information about sensitivity might be obtained if these tests were carried out on tumours at the time of their initial diagnosis. In this way valuable information for optimal adjuvant chemotherapy may become available.

References

Alberts, D. S., Chen, H. S. G., Salmon, S. E., Surwit, E. A., Young, L., Moon, T. E. and Meyskens, F. L. (1981). Chemotherapy of ovarian cancer directed by the human tumour stem cell assay. *Cancer Chemother. Pharmacol.* **6**, 279–285.

Asano, S. and Mandel, T. (1981). Colonies formed in agar from human breast cancer and their identification as T-lymphocytes. *J. Nat. Cancer Inst.* **67**, 25–32.

Bertoncello, I., Bradley, T. R., Campbell, J. J., Day, A. J., McDonald, I. A., McLeish, G. R., Quinn, M. A., Rome, R. and Hodgson, G. S. (1982). Limitations of the clonal agar assay for the assessment of primary human ovarian tumour biopsies. *Br. J. Cancer* **45**, 803–811.

Bradley, E. C., Reichert, C. M., Brennan, M. F. and Von Hoff, D. D. (1980). Direct cloning of human parathyroid hyperplasia cells in soft-agar. *Cancer Res.* **40**, 3694–3696.

Buick, R. N. and MacKillop, W. J. (1981). Measurement of self-renewal in culture of clonogenic cells from human ovarian carcinoma. *Br. J. Cancer* **44**, 349–355.

Daniels, J. R., Daniels, A. M., Luck, E. E., Whitman, B., Casagrande, J. T. and Skinner, D. G. (1981). Chemosensitivity of human neoplasms with *in vitro* clone formation. *Cancer Chemother. Pharmacol.* **6**, 245–251.

Durie, B. G., Persky, B., Soehnlen, B. J., Grogan, T. M. and Salmon, S. E. (1982). Amyloid production in human myeloma stem-cell culture, with morphologic evidence of amyloid secretion by associated macrophages. *New Engl. J. Med.* **307**, 1689–1692.

Elson, D. L., Osborne, C. K., Livingston, R. B. and Von Hoff, D. D. (1982). Methods for determining chemosensitivity of MCF-7 cells in double layer agar culture: labelling index depression and colony count inhibition. *Stem Cells* **2**, 34–44.

Epstein, L. B. and Marcus, S. G. (1981). Review of experience with interferon and drug sensitivity testing of ovarian carcinoma in semisolid agar culture. *Cancer Chemother. Pharmacol.* **6**, 273–277.

Friedman, H. M. and Glaubiger, D. L. (1982). Assessment of *in vitro* drug sensitivity of human tumor cells using ^{3}H-thymidine incorporation in a modified human tumor stem cell assay. *Cancer Res.* **42**, 4683–4689.

Goldie, J. H. and Coldman, A. J. (1979). A mathematical model for relating the drug sensitivity of tumors to their spontaneous mutation rate. *Cancer Treat. Rep.* **63**, 1727–1731.

Hamburger, A. W., White, C. P. and Tencer, K. (1982). Effect of enzymatic disaggregation on proliferation of human tumor cells in soft agar. *J. Nat. Cancer Inst.* **68**, 945–949.

Hofmann, V., Salmon, S. E. and Durie, B. G. (1981). Drug resistance in multiple myeloma associated with high *in vitro* incorporation of ^{3}H-thymidine. *Blood* **58**, 471–476.

Kaufmann, M. (1982). Nucleic acid precursor incorporation assay for testing tumour sensitivity and clinical applications. *Drugs Exp. Clin. Res.* **7**, 345–358.

Lieber, M. M., Ames, M. M., Powis, G. and Kovach, J. S. (1981). Anticancer drug testing *in vitro*: use of an activating system with the human tumor stem cell assay. *Life Sci.* **28**, 287–293.

Livingston, R. B., Titus, G. A. and Heibrun, L. K. (1980). *In vitro* effects on DNA synthesis as a predictor of biological effect from chemotherapy. *Cancer Res.* **40**, 2209–2212.

Mann, B. D., Kern, D. H., Guilano, A. E., Burk, M. W., Campbell, M. A., Kaiser, L. R. and Morton, D. L. (1982). Clinical correlations with drug sensitivities in the clonogenic assay. *Arch. Surg.* **117**, 33–36.

Meyskens, F. L., Moon, T. E., Dana, B., Gilmartin, E., Casey, W. J., G-Chen, H. S., Franks, D. H., Young, L. and Salmon, S. E. (1981). Quantitation of drug sensitivity by human metastatic melanoma colony-forming units. *Br. J. Cancer* **44**, 787–797.

Meyskens, F. L., Thomson, S. P., Moon, T. E. and Salmon, S. E. (1983). Cellular proliferation of metastatic malignant melanoma tumor colony forming units in soft agar. (in press)

Morgan, D., Freshney, R. I., Darling, J. L., Thomas, D. G. T. and Celik, F. (1983). Assay of anticancer drugs in tissue culture: cell cultures of biopsies from human astrocytoma. *Br. J. Cancer* (in press).

Rosenblum, M. L., Dougherty, D. V., Reese, C. and Wilson, C. B. (1981). Potentials and possible pitfalls of human stem cell analysis. *Cancer Chemother. Pharmacol.* **6**, 227–235.

Sandbach, J., Von Hoff, D. D., Clark, G., Cruz, A. B., O'Brien, M. and the South Central Texas Human Tumor Cloning Group. (1982). Direct cloning of human breast cancer in soft agar culture. *Cancer* **50**, 1315–1321.

Sarosdy, M. F., Lamm, D. L., Radwin, H. M. and Von Hoff, D. D. (1982). Clonogenic assay and *in vitro* chemosensitivity testing of human urologic malignancies. *Cancer* **50**, 1332–1338.

Smith, H. S., Hackett, A. J., Lan, S. and Stampfer, M. R. (1981). Use of an efficient method for culturing human mammary epithelial cells to study adriamycin sensitivity. *Cancer Chemother. Pharmacol.* **6**, 237–244.

Stanisic, T. M. and Buick, R. N. (1980). *In vitro* clonal assay for bladder cancer: clinical correlation with states of urothelium in 33 patients. *J. Urol.* **124**, 30–33.

Tanigawa, N., Kern, D. H., Hikasa, Y. and Morton, D. L. (1982). Rapid assay for evaluating the chemosensitivity of human tumors in soft agar culture. *Cancer Res.* **42**, 2159–2164.

Thomson, S. P. and Meyskens, F. L. (1982). Method for measurement of self-renewal capacity of clonogenic cells from biopsies of metastatic human malignant melanoma. *Cancer Res.* **42**, 4606–4613.

Von Hoff, D. D., Casper, J., Bradley, E., Sandbach, J., Jones, D. and Makuch, R. (1981a). Association between human tumor colony-forming assay results and response of an individual patient's tumor to chemotherapy. *Am. J. Med.* **70**, 1027–1032.

Von Hoff, D. D., Cowan, J., Harris, G. and Reisdorf, G. (1981b). Human tumour cloning: feasibility and clinical correlations. *Cancer Chemother. Pharmacol.* **6**, 265–271.

Von Hoff, D. D., Sandbach, J., Osborne, G. K., Metelmann, C., Clark, G. M. and O'Brien, M. (1981c). Potential and problems with the growth of breast cancer in a human tumor cloning system. *Breast Cancer Res. Treat.* **1**, 141–148.

Weisenthal, L. M., Marsden, J. A., Dill, P. L. and Macaluso, C. K. (1983). A novel dye exclusion method for testing *in vitro* chemosensitivity of human tumors. *Cancer Res.* **43**, 749–757.

Index